Transplantation

Editors

AMAN MAHAJAN
CHRISTOPHER WRAY

ANESTHESIOLOGY CLINICS

www.anesthesiology.theclinics.com

Consulting Editor
LEE A. FLEISHER

September 2017 • Volume 35 • Number 3

ELSEVIER

1600 John F. Kennedy Boulevard • Suite 1800 • Philadelphia, Pennsylvania, 19103-2899

http://www.theclinics.com

ANESTHESIOLOGY CLINICS Volume 35, Number 3
September 2017 ISSN 1932-2275, ISBN-13: 978-0-323-55266-0

Editor: Katie Pfaff
Developmental Editor: Kristen Helm

Anesthesiology Clinics (ISSN 1932-2275) is published quarterly by Elsevier Inc., 360 Park Avenue South, New York, NY 10010-1710. Months of issue are March, June, September, and December. Periodicals postage paid at New York, NY and at additional mailing offices. Subscription prices are $100.00 per year (US student/resident), $333.00 per year (US individuals), $404.00 per year (Canadian individuals), $620.00 per year (US institutions), $783.00 per year (Canadian institutions), $225.00 per year (Canadian and foreign student/resident), $460.00 per year (foreign individuals), and $783.00 per year (foreign institutions). To receive student and resident rate, orders must be accompanied by name of affiliated institution, date of term, and the *signature* of program/residency coordinator on institutions letterhead. Orders will be billed at individual rate until proof of status is received. Foreign air speed delivery is included in all *Clinics'* subscription prices. All prices are subject to change without notice. POSTMASTER: Send address changes to *Anesthesiology Clinics,* Elsevier Health Sciences Division, Subscription Customer Service, 3251 Riverport Lane, Maryland Heights, MO 63043. Customer Service (orders, claims, online, change of address): Elsevier Health Sciences Division, Subscription Customer Service, 3251 Riverport Lane, Maryland Heights, MO 63043. **Tel:1-800-654-2452 (U.S. and Canada); 314-447-8871 (outside U.S. and Canada). Fax: 314-447-8029. E-mail: journalscustomerservice-usa@elsevier.com (for print support); journalsonlinesupport-usa@elsevier.com (for online support).**

Reprints. For copies of 100 or more of articles in this publication, please contact the Commercial Reprints Department, Elsevier Inc., 360 Park Avenue South, New York, NY 10010-1710. Tel.: 212-633-3874; Fax: 212-633-3820; E-mail: reprints@elsevier.com.

Anesthesiology Clinics, is also published in Spanish by McGraw-Hill Inter-americana Editores S. A., P.O. Box 5-237, 06500 Mexico D. F., Mexico.

Anesthesiology Clinics, is covered in *MEDLINE/PubMed (Index Medicus), Current Contents/Clinical Medicine, Excerpta Medica, ISI/BIOMED,* and *Chemical Abstracts.*

Contributors

CONSULTING EDITOR

LEE A. FLEISHER, MD, FACC
Robert D. Dripps Professor and Chair of Anesthesiology and Critical Care, Professor of Medicine, Perelman School of Medicine at University of Pennsylvania, Philadelphia, Pennsylvania

EDITORS

AMAN MAHAJAN, MD, PhD
Ronald L. Katz MD Professor and Chair, Department of Anesthesiology and Perioperative Medicine, Professor of Anesthesiology and Bioengineering, Executive Director, UCLA Perioperative Services, Co-Director, UCLA Cardiac Arrhythmia Center, Neurocardiology Research Center, UCLA Health, Los Angeles, California

CHRISTOPHER WRAY, MD
Associate Professor, Department of Anesthesiology, University of California Los Angeles, Los Angeles, California

AUTHORS

DIETER ADELMANN, MD
Assistant Professor, Department of Anesthesiology and Perioperative Care, University of California San Francisco, San Francisco, California

JOHN ANDERSON-DAM, MD
HS Assistant Clinical Professor, Department of Anesthesiology and Perioperative Medicine, Ronald Reagan UCLA Medical Center, David Geffen School of Medicine at UCLA, Los Angeles, California

MICHAEL BENGGON, MD
Assistant Professor, Department of Anesthesiology, Loma Linda Medical Center, Loma Linda, California

MICHELLE BRAUNFELD, MD
Professor and Vice Chair, Department of Anesthesiology and Perioperative Medicine, David Geffen School of Medicine at UCLA, Chief, Department of Anesthesiology, VA Greater Los Angeles Healthcare System, Los Angeles, California

JEREMY D. DEER, MD
Associate Fellowship Director, Director of Education, Attending Physician, Pediatric Anesthesiology, Ann & Robert H. Lurie Children's Hospital of Chicago, Assistant Professor of Anesthesiology, Northwestern University Feinberg School of Medicine, Chicago, Illinois

VIJAY S. GORANTLA, MD, PhD, FRCS
Associate Professor of Surgery, Director, Vascularized Composite Allotransplantation Program, Departments of Surgery, Ophthalmology, and Bioengineering, Military Medical Consultant in Reconstructive Transplantation, US Air Force, Wake Forest Institute for Regenerative Medicine, Wake Forest Baptist Medical Center, Winston-Salem, North Carolina

REED HARVEY, MD
Assistant Professor, Department of Anesthesiology, Ronald Reagan UCLA Medical Center, University of California Los Angeles, Los Angeles, California

JOSHUA HERBORN, MD
Assistant Professor, Department of Anesthesiology, Northwestern University Feinberg School of Medicine, Chicago, Illinois

CURTIS D. HOLT, PharmD
Director, Clinical Research Program, Clinical Professor, UCLA Department of Surgery, Dumont-UCLA Transplant Center, David Geffen School of Medicine at UCLA, Los Angeles, California

DAME W. IDOSSA, MD
Resident, Internal Medicine, Mayo Clinic, Rochester, Minnesota

KATE KRONISH, MD
Assistant Professor, Department of Anesthesiology and Perioperative Care, University of California San Francisco, San Francisco, California

JASWANTH MADISETTY, MD
Assistant Professor, Department of Anesthesiology and Pain Management, William P. Clements University Hospital, The University of Texas Southwestern Medical Center, Dallas, Texas

AARON M. MITTEL, MD
Clinical Fellow, Department of Anesthesiology, Columbia University Medical Center, College of Physicians and Surgeons, Columbia University, New York, New York

CHRISTINE NGUYEN-BUCKLEY, MD
Clinical Instructor, Department of Anesthesiology, David Geffen School of Medicine at UCLA, Los Angeles, California

ALINA NICOARA, MD, FASE
Assistant Professor of Anesthesiology, Division of Cardiothoracic Anesthesia, Department of Anesthesiology, Duke University Medical Center, Durham, North Carolina

SURAJ PARULKAR, MD
Instructor, Department of Anesthesiology, Northwestern University Feinberg School of Medicine, Chicago, Illinois

RAYMOND M. PLANINSIC, MD
Professor of Anesthesiology, Department of Anesthesiology, University of Pittsburgh Medical Center, Pittsburgh, Pennsylvania

MICHAEL A. RAMSAY, MD, FRCA
Chairman, Department of Anesthesiology, Baylor University Medical Center, Dallas, Texas

DAVINDER RAMSINGH, MD
Associate Professor, Department of Anesthesiology, Loma Linda Medical Center, Loma Linda, California

JAY S. RAVAL, MD
Assistant Professor, Division of Transfusion Medicine, Department of Pathology and Laboratory Medicine, Transfusion Medicine Service, Hematopoietic Progenitor Cell Laboratory, University of North Carolina at Chapel Hill, Chapel Hill, North Carolina

ALEC RUNYON, MD
PGY-4, Department of Anesthesiology, Loma Linda Medical Center, Loma Linda, California

DOUGLAS ALANO SIMONETTO, MD
Assistant Professor of Medicine, Department of Gastroenterology and Hepatology, Mayo Clinic, Rochester, Minnesota

SANTHANAM SURESH, MD
Chair, Department of Pediatric Anesthesiology, Ann & Robert H. Lurie Children's Hospital of Chicago, Professor of Anesthesiology and Pediatrics, Northwestern University Feinberg School of Medicine, Chicago, Illinois

GEBHARD WAGENER, MD
Professor, Department of Anesthesiology, Columbia University Medical Center, College of Physicians and Surgeons, Columbia University, New York, New York

CYNTHIA WANG, MD
Assistant Professor, Department of Anesthesiology and Pain Management, William P. Clements University Hospital, The University of Texas Southwestern Medical Center, Dallas, Texas

NICHOLAS R. WASSON, MD
Director, Pediatric Transplant Anesthesia, Attending Physician, Pediatric Anesthesiology, Ann & Robert H. Lurie Children's Hospital of Chicago, Assistant Professor of Anesthesiology, Northwestern University Feinberg School of Medicine, Chicago, Illinois

MELISSA WONG, MD
Clinical Instructor, Division of Liver and Pancreas Transplantation, Department of Surgery, David Geffen School of Medicine at UCLA, Los Angeles, California

VICTOR W. XIA, MD
Clinical Professor, Department of Anesthesiology and Perioperative Medicine, Ronald Reagan UCLA Medical Center, David Geffen School of Medicine at UCLA, Los Angeles, California

Contents

Mechanisms of rejection, new pharmacologic approaches, and genomic medicine are major foci for current research in transplantation. It is hoped that these new agents and personalized immunosuppression will provide for less toxic regimens that are effective in preventing both acute and chronic allograft rejection. Until new agents are available, practitioners must use various combinations of currently approved agents to find the best regimens for improved long-term outcomes.

Since the first liver transplant was performed in 1963, great advancements have been made in hepatic transplantation. Surgical techniques have been revised and improved, diagnostic methods for identifying and preventing infections have been developed, and a more conservative use of immunosuppressive agents has resulted in better long-term posttransplant outcomes. A total of 7841 liver transplantations were performed in the United States in 2016, resulting in greater than 85% survival at 1 year posttransplant. However, technical surgical complications, infections, rejections, and chronic medical conditions persist. This article discusses the infectious complications and malignancies that may arise after liver transplantation.

The shortage of suitable organs is the biggest obstacle for transplants. At present, most organs for transplant in the United States are from donation after neurologic determination of death (brain death). Potential organs for transplant need to maintain their viability during a series of insults, including the original disease, physiologic derangements during the dying process, ischemia, and reperfusion. Proper donor management before, during, and after procurement has potential to increase the number and quality of organs from donors. Anesthesiologists need to understand the physiologic derangements associated with brain death and the updated donor management during the periprocurement period.

as they pertain to heart transplantation. The preanesthesia and intraoperative considerations are also discussed. Finally, management after transplantation is also reviewed.

Anesthesia for Lung Transplantation

Alina Nicoara and John Anderson-Dam

Perioperative management of patients undergoing lung transplantation is challenging and requires constant communication among the surgical, anesthesia, perfusion, and nursing teams. Although all aspects of anesthetic management are important, certain intraoperative strategies (mechanical ventilation, fluid management, extracorporeal mechanical support deployment) have tremendous impact on the subsequent evolution of the lung transplant recipient, especially with respect to allograft function, and should be carefully considered. This review highlights some of the intraoperative anesthetic challenges and opportunities during lung transplantation.

Anesthesia for Liver Transplantation

Dieter Adelmann, Kate Kronish, and Michael A. Ramsay

The provision of anesthesia for a liver transplant program requires a dedicated team of anesthesiologists. Liver transplant anesthesiologists must have an understanding of liver physiology and anatomy; the spectrum of clinical disease associated with liver dysfunction; the impact of warm and cold ischemia times, surgical techniques in liver transplantation, and the impact of ischemia-reperfusion syndrome; and optimal practices to protect the liver. The team must provide a 24-hour service, be actively involved in the selection committee process, and stay current with advances in the subspecialty.

Anesthesia for Intestinal Transplantation

Christine Nguyen-Buckley and Melissa Wong

The diagnosis of irreversible intestinal failure confers significant morbidity, mortality, and decreased quality of life. Patients with irreversible intestinal failure may be treated with intestinal transplantation. Intestinal transplantation may include intestine only, liver-intestine, or other visceral elements. Intestinal transplantation candidates present with systemic manifestations of intestinal failure requiring multidisciplinary evaluation at an intestinal transplantation center. Central access may be difficult in intestinal transplantation candidates. Intestinal transplantation is a complex operation with potential for hemodynamic and metabolic instability. Patient and graft survival are improving, but graft failure remains the most common postoperative complication.

Anesthesia and Perioperative Care in Reconstructive Transplantation

Raymond M. Planinsic, Jay S. Raval, and Vijay S. Gorantla

Reconstructive transplantation of vascularized composite allografts (VCAs), such as upper extremity, craniofacial, abdominal, lower extremity, or genitourinary transplants, has emerged as a cutting-edge specialty, with more than 50 programs in the United States and 30 programs across the world performing these procedures. Most VCAs involve complicated technical planning and preparation, protracted surgery, and complex immunosuppressive or immunomodulatory protocols, each associated with unique anesthesiology challenges. This article outlines key procedural, patient, and protocol-related aspects of VCA relevant to anesthesiology management with the goal of ensuring patient safety and optimizing surgical, immunologic, and functional outcomes.

Joshua Herborn and Suraj Parulkar

As solid organ transplantation increases and patient survival improves, it will become more common for these patients to present for nontransplant surgery. Recipients may present with medical problems unique to the transplant, and important considerations are necessary to keep the transplanted organ functioning. A comprehensive preoperative examination with specific focus on graft functioning is required, and the anesthesiologist needs pay close attention to considerations of immunosuppressive regimens, blood product administration, and the risk benefits of invasive monitoring in these immunosuppressed patients. This article reviews the posttransplant physiology and anesthetic considerations for patients after solid organ transplantation.

ANESTHESIOLOGY CLINICS

THE CLINICS ARE AVAILABLE ONLINE!
Access your subscription at:
www.theclinics.com

Foreword

Transplantation Anesthesia: The Role of the Anesthesiologist

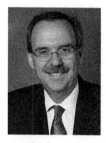

Lee A. Fleisher, MD, FACC
Consulting Editor

Anesthesiologists have been engaged in perioperative management of the transplant patient since transplantation surgery began in the 1960s. Cardiac and liver transplant anesthesia teams were common when I was training, while lung transplantation can involve either cardiac or thoracic anesthesia teams. Kidney transplant anesthesia was usually part of the routine noncardiac team, but optimal management protocols clearly impact organ survival. Today, it is becoming more common to see other organ transplants and management strategies being better defined to optimize both patient and organ survival.

In identifying a center with a large and diverse practice, the University of California in Los Angeles (UCLA) has always been a leader. In fact, the quality of their outcomes led them to propose the first "bundles" in transplant care. To edit this issue, I have asked Drs Mahajan and Wray from UCLA. Aman Mahajan, MD, PhD is Professor of Anesthesiology and Bioengineering. He is the Chair of the Department of Anesthesiology at the David Geffen School of Medicine at UCLA with expertise in Cardiothoracic Anesthesiology, Cardiac Electrophysiology, and Echocardiography. Christopher Wray, MD is Associate Clinical Professor for Liver Transplant and Cardiothoracic Anesthesiology and Co-Director for Liver Transplant Anesthesiology. Together, they have brought together a phenomenal group of authors to educate us on best current practices.

Lee A. Fleisher, MD, FACC
Perelman School of Medicine at
University of Pennsylvania
3400 Spruce Street, Dulles 680
Philadelphia, PA 19104, USA

E-mail address:
Lee.Fleisher@uphs.upenn.edu

Anesthesiology Clin 35 (2017) xiii
http://dx.doi.org/10.1016/j.anclin.2017.06.002
1932-2275/17/© 2017 Published by Elsevier Inc.

anesthesiology.theclinics.com

Preface

Organ Transplantation: A Systematic Review

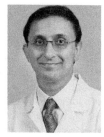 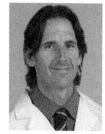

Aman Mahajan, MD, PhD   Christopher Wray, MD
Editors

Organ transplantation has evolved significantly since its initial inception in the 1960s. Advances in surgical techniques, immunosuppression, and perioperative management strategies have resulted in continued improvements in graft viability and posttransplant patient survival. Organ transplantation is now widespread and growing on an international level. In concordance with these developments, the field of transplant anesthesiology has evolved as well. Today, highly specialized anesthesia teams are crucial to the success of transplant programs. Transplant anesthesiologists are involved in all aspects of the perioperative care of transplant patients, including the preoperative selection of transplant candidates, the intraoperative management of complex transplant surgeries, and the postoperative critical care of transplant recipients. Anesthesiologists in these teams have driven crucial research and patient care strategies that are central to the progress of organ transplantation. Heart and lung transplant teams rely on specially trained cardiac anesthesia teams. Pediatric anesthesiologists are routinely involved in all phases of pediatric transplantation. Most centers now employ liver transplant anesthesia groups that are dedicated to the specialized perioperative care of the liver transplant patient. Recent development of transplant anesthesia fellowships has contributed to the growth of transplant anesthesia.

This issue of *Anesthesiology Clinics* provides an updated survey of topics central to the anesthetic care of transplant patients. Experts in their respective fields have contributed state-of-the-art reviews of all categories of transplant anesthesia by organ system. Current research and updated clinical strategies for the anesthetic management of cardiac, lung, liver, kidney/pancreas, and intestinal transplants as well as the management of the organ donor are reviewed in individual articles. Specialized topics central to the care of transplant patients are discussed as well. These include an overview of transplant immunosuppression, a review of posttransplant infection and malignancies, and an update on coagulation management and transfusion in

Anesthesiology Clin 35 (2017) xv–xvi
http://dx.doi.org/10.1016/j.anclin.2017.06.001
1932-2275/17/© 2017 Published by Elsevier Inc.

transplant patients. Pediatric experts provide a review of the anesthetic management of pediatric liver and kidney transplant. Reconstructive transplantation is an emerging field and includes hand, face, and tissue composite transplants. Experts in the anesthetic management of reconstructive transplantation provide a review of this novel surgical specialty. As organ transplantation has become widespread, recipients are frequently undergoing nontransplant surgical procedures after successful transplant. An article reviews the anesthetic considerations in transplant recipients for nontransplant surgery with attention to each transplant organ system.

Organ transplantation is a dynamic sphere; future changes and challenges are expected. Age limits for transplant candidates are increasing in conjunction with an aging population. Chronic illnesses in older candidates may affect postoperative survival and impact transplant candidacy. End-stage organ disease patterns are also changing; therapies for specific diseases such as hepatitis C virus infection and diabetes may alter future indications for transplantation. Increasingly complex surgical and medical treatment paradigms have been employed in the management of transplant patients. The transplant anesthesiologist is a crucial member of the transplant team and has an important role in future advances. Updated knowledge of the anesthetic considerations for organ transplantation is necessary for both the transplant anesthesiologist and the anesthesiologist involved in the care of patients prior to and after transplant.

Aman Mahajan, MD, PhD
Department of Anesthesiology &
Perioperative Medicine
UCLA Perioperative Services
UCLA Cardiac Arrhythmia Center &
UCLA Neurocardiology Research Center
UCLA Health System
757 Westwood Plaza, Suite 2331-L
Los Angeles, CA 90095-7403, USA

Christopher Wray, MD
Department of Anesthesiology
University of California Los Angeles
757 Westwood Plaza
Suite 3325
Los Angeles, CA 90095, USA

E-mail addresses:
AMahajan@mednet.ucla.edu (A. Mahajan)
CWray@mednet.ucla.edu (C. Wray)

Overview of Immunosuppressive Therapy in Solid Organ Transplantation

Curtis D. Holt, PharmD

KEYWORDS

- Solid organ transplantation • Immunosuppression • Immunosuppressive strategies

KEY POINTS

- Solid organ transplantation is a life-saving treatment option for patients with end-stage organ failure.
- Lifelong immunosuppressive agents are administered to modulate a transplant recipient's immune system response to the donor organ by using induction, maintenance, and rescue therapy.
- Clinicians must comprehend the implications of using immunosuppressive agents; these include their mechanisms of action, pharmacokinetics, dosing and monitoring strategies, clinical efficacy, adverse effects and drug interactions, and clinical indications.

INTRODUCTION

Improvements in surgical techniques and availability of immunosuppressive options have led to current successes in the arena of solid organ transplantation. Historically, transplantation was limited by acute rejection, leading to graft loss and poor patient survival. These results have dramatically improved over recent years, with 1-year patient and allograft survival approaching or exceeding 90% for many solid organ transplant recipients. This has allowed transplantation to become the treatment of choice for many patients who would otherwise expire or require lifelong dialysis. Long-term allograft survival has not, however, kept pace with short-term success. Chronic rejection remains an unsolved and poorly understood complication in transplantation medicine. Although its occurrence is rare in liver transplants, it is a leading cause of late allograft loss in kidney transplants. Although transplant clinicians are successfully maintaining most patients with functional grafts for 5 or more years, they have created

Clinical Research Program, UCLA Department of Surgery, Dumont-UCLA Transplant Center, David Geffen School of Medicine at UCLA, 650 CE Young Drive South, Room 77-123CHS, Los Angeles, CA 90095-7054, USA
E-mail address: cholt@mednet.ucla.edu

Anesthesiology Clin 35 (2017) 365–380
http://dx.doi.org/10.1016/j.anclin.2017.04.001

a large population at risk for chronic rejection and other complications, such as infection, lymphoproliferative diseases, and organ dysfunction related to chronic exposure to immunosuppressants. In this review, the immunology of transplant rejection and the immunosuppressive agents currently in use in adult solid organ transplantation are described.

TRANSPLANT IMMUNOLOGY

The immune system is the major barrier to long-term graft survival in solid organ transplant recipients. Donor organs are detected as foreign material by the recipient immune system and may be attacked and rejected. The ultimate goal of transplant recipients is graft acceptance, also known as tolerance, ideally without the use of long-term immunosuppressant medication. The major known pathways involved in acute rejection are outlined.

RECOGNITION

Identification of self or nonself occurs on chromosome 6 of the human genome. Within this chromosome is the major histocompatibility complex, also referred to as HLA complex. It contains the coding sequences of several different genes that code for HLA molecules. The purpose of HLA molecules is to display peptides on the surface of immune system cells so they can be identified as self or foreign. In transplant rejection, these peptides are usually components of a donor's HLA molecules that have been captured and broken down for display on a recipient's own HLA molecule. Antigen-presenting cells (APCs) are cells that display HLA molecules with their respective peptides. In transplant rejection, APCs can be of donor or recipient origin and may include passenger cells transplanted with the organ and/or the organ's own cell lines.[1] Recipient interaction occurs when passenger cells migrate to secondary lymphoid tissues or when recipient cells encounter graft vasculature.

PROCESSING

Immune system activation occurs when APCs display their foreign peptides to an immunologic target cell. In the cell-mediated response of transplantation, this target is the T lymphocyte. Each T cell displays thousands of individual T-cell receptors and each can bind thousands of HLA-peptide complexes.[1–5] The T-cell receptor is coupled with a cluster of differentiation (CD) molecule, specifically the CD3 molecule, and forms a complex responsible for T-cell activation.[6] A wide array of CD molecules exists among various immune cells. In addition, secondary signals via other pathways are required for full cellular activation.[5,7] On the surface of T cells, various molecules interact with APCs, providing secondary signals and increasing cytokine production, resulting in full stimulation of the immune response.[8–10]

MECHANISMS OF TARGET CELL DESTRUCTION

T cells possess 2 mechanisms for target cell destruction. One mechanism is used by cytotoxic CD8$^+$ cells; a second mechanism is used by cytotoxic CD4$^+$ cells. Both mechanisms result in activation of pathways that lead to destruction and cellular death of foreign cells.[11] In addition to T cells, other immunologic components contribute to graft rejection. Encounters between B cells and donor HLA molecules lead to the display of donor HLA–derived peptides on B-cell receptors. Subsequent interactions with T cells lead to immune globulin production against the donor HLA.[4] These antibodies bind to target donor HLA molecules and trigger foreign cell destruction via the complement cascade and natural killer (NK) cell binding to antibody-coated cells.[11]

PREEXISTING SENSITIZATION

Transplant recipients may encounter immune stimulatory substances prior to transplant through pregnancy, blood transfusions, implantable devices, or previous transplant. Development of reactivity may result from responses to passenger cells in transfusions, from antibodies to paternal HLA in pregnancy, or to biomaterial in medical devices. These pretransplant exposures may sensitize recipients and contribute to rejection or decreased graft survival.[12–17] Presence of these antibodies is generally determined by histocompatibility testing performed prior to transplant. Recipient serum is tested against a pool of lymphocytes from donors with known HLA markers. The amount of reactivity between the recipient and the lymphocyte pool is graded as a percentage and correlates with a recipient's risk of positive reactivity with donors from the normal population. The resulting percentage is termed, panel reactive antibody. Various measures have been used to decrease the amount of panel reactive antibodies, including plasmapheresis, intravenous immunoglobulin, and pretransplant immunosuppression.[18–21]

CHRONIC REJECTION

One of the major barriers to long-term graft survival is chronic rejection. The hallmark of chronic rejection is progressive loss of organ function due to fibrosis or sclerosis. The exact cause of chronic rejection is unknown; however, acute rejection is often considered a risk factor.[18–25] An acute rejection episode may contribute to an initial allograft insult that provides the spark to trigger the progressive mechanisms that lead to functional deterioration of the allograft. A detailed description of chronic rejection is beyond the scope of this review; however, successful immunosuppression in the early post-transplant phase may block mechanisms that contribute to chronic rejection.[15]

IMMUNOSUPPRESSIVE STRATEGIES

Patient survival and allograft survival ultimately rely on appropriate host immune system modulation. A lifelong immunosuppressive regimen is required in solid organ transplant recipients to suppress the recipient immune response to the transplanted organ. Immunosuppressive agents are administered during the perioperative period to prevent organ rejection. It is important for transplant anesthesiologists to understand the basic pharmacology of common immunosuppressive agents.

Initial immunosuppressive induction therapy provides intense, short-term immunosuppression during the perioperative and immediate postoperative periods.[26] A select group of agents is used for induction therapy (**Table 1**). In general, induction agents

Table 1	
Induction immunosuppressive agents	
Agent	**Classification**
Alemtuzumab (Campath)	T-cell–depleting monoclonal antibody
Equine antithymocyte globulin (Thymoglobulin)	T-cell–depleting polyclonal antibody
Basiliximab (Simulect)	IL-2 receptor antagonist
Belatacept (Nulojix)	Second messenger signal inhibitor

act by depleting T cells, resulting in reduced acute rejection rates and enhanced graft survival. Induction agents may also be used in patients who are at high risk for early rejection to reduce the dosage of calcineurin blockers or to eliminate the use of corticosteroids.[27,28] An anesthesiologist is often responsible for administration of induction agents during the intraoperative period.

Maintenance immunosuppression consisting of multiple medications that target different areas of the immune response occurs in the postoperative period (**Table 2**). Historically, maintenance regimens included azathioprine and corticosteroids. This drug regimen was inadequate, however, in preventing rejection. Introduction of cyclosporine in the early 1980s led to enhanced patient and allograft survival and reduced rejection rates. Currently, most transplant centers use a triple-drug regimen that includes the second-generation calcineurin inhibitor (CNI) tacrolimus, the antiproliferative agent mycophenolic acid, and a corticosteroid. These agents are carefully selected based on organ type, and dosages are individually titrated to prevent rejection while avoiding adverse effects. In general, higher dosages of maintenance immunosuppressive agents are used in the early post-transplant phase. Dosages are gradually reduced over the first year to minimize toxicity. Maintenance regimens are lifelong; however, triple-drug regimens may be reduced to double-drug or single-drug regimens depending on an individual patient's clinical course. Recent studies suggest a benefit to converting from calcineurin-based regimens to rapamycin-based therapy to preserve long-term renal function.[28–30] Individual immunosuppressive agents are reviewed.

COMMONLY USED IMMUNOSUPPRESSIVE AGENTS
Corticosteroids

Corticosteroid therapy has been a cornerstone of immunosuppression in transplant patients for several decades. Corticosteroids have many immunosuppressive mechanisms. They seem to inhibit interleukin (IL) synthesis in macrophages and monocytes.[31,32] They also inhibit expression of many cytokine genes and induce programmed cell death in murine T cells in immature thymocytes. These potent, nonspecific immunosuppressant effects contribute to their effectiveness in many areas of transplantation.

Prednisolone, prednisone, and methylprednisolone are the most commonly used corticosteroid preparations in transplantation. They are all converted to active prednisolone in the body. The pharmacologic half-lives of these agents persist for 24 hours,

Table 2 Maintenance immunosuppressive agents	
Agent	**Classification**
Methylprednisolone	Corticosteroid
Prednisone	Corticosteroid
Prednisolone	Corticosteroid
Cyclosporine (Gengraf, Neoral, and Sandimmune)	CNI
Tacrolimus (Prograf, Astagraf XR, and Envarsus XL)	CNI
Mycophenolic acid (CellCept and Myfortic)	Antimetabolite
Azathioprine (Imuran)	Antimetabolite
Everolimus (Zortress)	mTOR receptor
Sirolimus (Rapamune)	mTOR receptor

so that once-daily administration is adequate. Corticosteroids are metabolized by hepatic microsomal enzyme systems. Drugs that induce or inhibit these enzymes may affect plasma prednisolone levels. Dose adjustments may be indicated when interacting drugs are administered, although adjustments are usually not required in patients with renal or hepatic dysfunction. Dosages vary according to protocols established at each transplant center. Typically, the highest dose of steroid is prescribed at the time of transplantation. Standard steroid regimens may include methylprednisolone initial doses ranging from 250 mg to 1000 mg followed by a taper over the next 3 days to 10 days.[32,33] Use of other immunosuppressive induction agents may allow for lower corticosteroid dosing or even steroid-free maintenance therapy regimens. Administration of preoperative steroids 1 hour prior to administration of antithymocyte globulin may minimize the cytokine release syndrome associated with antithymocyte globulin.[34] In general, intraoperative corticosteroid administration regimens are individualized by center and organ transplant type. Steroids also remain first-line therapy for suspected allograft rejection, with dosing regimens recommended for 3 days to 10 days.[32,33]

Although the immunosuppressive utility of corticosteroid administration is well established, the side effects and morbidity associated with chronic administration of corticosteroids are significant. The magnitude of acute and chronic side effects associated with steroid use stems from the presence of steroid receptors on nearly every cell in the body. Chronic corticosteroid use induces glucose intolerance, weight gain, osteoporosis, hypertension, hyperlipidemia, growth inhibition, and other systemic complications that have negative impacts on graft survival.[35] In addition, patient quality of life may be adversely affected due to the development of acne, hirsutism, and cushingoid features. The introduction of nonsteroidal immunosuppressive agents has prompted interest in steroid-sparing immunosuppressive regimens.[36,37] Abrupt withdrawal of corticosteroids, however, often precipitates an exaggerated immune response that can trigger accelerated graft rejection. Prolonged steroid taper regimens over a 3-month to 6-month period along with intensive organ function monitoring is standard in renal transplant recipients.

INHIBITORS OF T-CELL PROLIFERATION
Mycophenolic Acids (Mycophenolate Mofetil and Myfortic)

The mechanism of action of the mycophenolic acids (MPAs) is based on interference with purine synthesis.[38] In normal cells, guanine and adenine nucleotides are synthesized in a pathway that relies on the purine enzyme, inosine monophosphate dehydrogenase (IMPDH). IMPDH is inhibited by MPAs, resulting in depletion of guanosine nucleotide and nucleosides.[38–40] This results in selective inhibition of T-lymphocyte and B-lymphocyte proliferation with minimal effects on other organ systems, because proliferating T cells and B cells are dependent on the de novo pathway for purine synthesis.[38–40] MPAs produce many immunosuppressant effects, including inhibition of B-lymphocyte and T-lymphocyte proliferative responses and reduction of proliferative responses to alloantigenic stimulation in human lymphocytes.[38–40]

After gastrointestinal (GI) absorption, mycophenolate mofetil (MMF) is rapidly hydrolyzed by the liver to its biologically active form, MPA.[38–41] MPA undergoes glucuronidation in the liver and kidney to form the inactive metabolite, mycophenolic acid glucuronide (MPAG).[40,41] MPAG is eliminated in the urine and excreted in bile. MPAG may be reconverted to MPA, however, by undergoing hydrolysis. In patients with renal dysfunction, MPAG may accumulate and reconvert to the active acid form of the drug, possibly leading to excessive immunosuppression or toxicity.

Plasma concentrations peak within 1 hour to 3 hours after a single oral dose, with secondary peaks occurring within 6 hours to 12 hours as a result of enterohepatic circulation.[40,41] The elimination half-life of MPA is approximately 17 hours after administration.[40,41] Dosage adjustments are recommended in patients with renal dysfunction.[40–42] No dosage adjustments are recommended in patients with hepatic dysfunction. MPA is extensively bound to albumin; however, the pharmacologic effects are due to unbound MPA.[40,41,43]

Pharmacokinetic drug interaction studies with MMF have been conducted with a variety of drugs common in transplant patients.[40,41,44,45] The most commonly reported adverse effects due to MMF in renal allograft recipients were GI, hematologic, and infectious.[46,47] Nephrotoxicity, neurotoxicity, and hepatotoxicity are uncommon with the MPAs. The usual initial dose of MMF is 1g orally twice daily. In patients with severe chronic renal failure, lower dosages are indicated.

Mycophenolic acid sodium

Mycophenolate acid sodium (Myfortic) is an enteric-coated formulation of the sodium salt of mycophenolic acid.[48] The mechanism of action is the same as MMF. Enteric coating allows the delayed release of mycophenolic acid into the small intestine, ameliorating some of the GI side effects.

CALCINEURIN INHIBITORS
Cyclosporine

The clinical availability of cyclosporine in the early 1980s not only dramatically improved kidney graft survival rates but also accounted for the widespread acceptance of extrarenal transplants. Cyclosporine suppresses the synthesis of IL-2 and other cytokines by inhibiting intracellular calcineurin and subsequent cytokine transcription[49] (**Table 3**). Patients treated with cyclosporine experience an approximate 50% reduction in calcineurin activity, thereby maintaining a degree of immune responsiveness that is sufficient to maintain host defenses.

Cyclosporine is widely distributed into both blood cells and plasma.[50] Although cyclosporine does not readily penetrate the blood-brain barrier, liver transplant patients with low serum cholesterol levels seem to have an increased risk of serious central nervous system effects. Cyclosporine is extensively metabolized by gut and hepatic cytochrome P450IIIA isoenzymes.[50,51] Many metabolites have been isolated; however, metabolite AM1 is the predominant metabolite and has 10% of the immunosuppressant activity of the parent compound. Cyclosporine is prone to significant drug interactions in patients with hepatic dysfunction and advanced age. Cyclosporine is excreted in the bile and does not need to be modified in the presence of renal dysfunction.

Measurement of cyclosporine levels is critical due to the complex pharmacokinetic profile, described previously. Therapeutic ranges are based on many factors,

Table 3
Comparison of selected immunosuppressive agents' mechanisms of action

	Everolimus/Sirolimus	Cyclosporine	Tacrolimus
Binding protein	FKBP-12	Cyclophylin	FKBP-12
Enzyme	mTOR	Calcineurin	Calcineurin
Effect on IL-2	Inhibit cellular response	Inhibits production	Inhibits production
Cell cycle	Inhibit G_1-S Phase	Inhibits G_0-G_1	Inhibits G_0-G_1

including the type of organ transplant. Drug interactions not only increase or decrease cyclosporine levels but also may augment nephrotoxicity (**Table 4**). Gut metabolism via cytochrome enzymes plays a major role in cyclosporine bioavailability and potential drug interactions. Inducers or inhibitors of cytochrome P450IIIA enzymes may interfere with the biotransformation and/or oral bioavailability of cyclosporine, resulting in clinically significant decreases or increases in cyclosporine levels respectively. Due to the complex medical conditions of most transplant patients, use of interacting drugs is sometimes unavoidable. Close monitoring of cyclosporine concentrations is mandatory along with the understanding of the significance of each drug interaction.

The most common side effect of cyclosporine is nephrotoxicity, occurring in approximately 25% of patients.[50,52] Cyclosporine produces dose-related, reversible renal vasoconstriction that particularly affects the afferent arterioles. Cyclosporine-induced renal vasoconstriction may manifest as delayed recovery of early malfunctioning renal allografts or as a transient elevation in serum creatinine that is difficult to differentiate from other causes of renal allograft dysfunction.[52] Chronic interstitial fibrosis frequently occurs in kidneys of patients receiving chronic cyclosporine therapy as well. Thrombotic microangiopathy is a less common form of cyclosporine toxicity that is similar to hemolytic uremic syndrome and is associated with poor graft prognosis unless aggressive medical interventions are undertaken.[52,53] Other cyclosporine renal effects that require monitoring, such as impaired sodium excretion, hyperkalemia, hyperchloremic acidosis, and hypomagnesemia, add to the complex management of these patients. Many clinical approaches have been undertaken to modify the renal effects of cyclosporine nephrotoxicity. Some centers augment immunosuppression with other non-nephrotoxic agents, such as MMF or basiliximab.[54–56]

Table 4
Drug interactions with calcineurin blockers

Cytochrome Inhibitors (Immediate Onset): Increase Calcineurin Inhibitor Concentrations

Antibiotic	Antifungal	Protease Inhibitors	Calcium Channel Blockers	Selective Serotonin Reuptake Inhibitors	Others
Erythromycin	Fluconazole	Ritonavir	Diltiazem	Fluoxetine	Amiodarone
Clarithromycin	Itraconazole	Saquinavir	Verapamil	Paroxetine	Cannabinoids
Norfloxacin	Ketoconazole	Indinavir	Nicardipine	Sertraline	Cimetidine
Metronidazole	Voriconazole	Nelfinavir			Valproic acid
	Posaconazole				Grapefruit juice
	Isavuconazole				Red wine

Cytochrome Inducers (Slow, Time-dependent Process): Decrease Calcineurin Inhibitor Concentrations

Antileptic Drugs	Antituberculars	Others
Carbamazepine	Rifampin	Dexamethasone
Phenytoin	Isoniazid	Griseofulvin
Ethosuximide		St John's wort
Phenobarb/primidone		

Pharmacodynamic Drug Interactions: Enhanced Risk of Renal Toxicity

Aminoglycosides, amphotericin B, acyclovir, ciprofloxacin, trimethoprim/sulfamethoxazole, vancomycin
Cyclooxygenase 2 inhibitors, NSAIDs, angiotensin-converting enzyme inhibitors, loop diuretics

Cyclosporine also exhibits other nonrenal toxicities, including elevations of serum aminotransferase and bilirubin levels, cholelithiasis, hirsutism, and gingival hyperplasia.[50,52,53] Hyperlipidemia and glucose intolerance associated with cyclosporine administration are compounded by the administration of steroids. Severe neurologic complications, such as posterior reversible encephalopathy syndrome and central pontine myelinolysis, have also been reported.[57,58]

Typical initial oral doses of cyclosporine are 5 mg/kg/d to 15 mg/kg/d given in 2 divided doses. Drug concentration monitoring should direct dosage adjustments to achieve target levels. The initial dosing of cyclosporine is dependent on many factors. Some centers administer the first dose prior to surgery whereas others omit preoperative cyclosporine altogether. Delayed cyclosporine administration necessitates the administration of another potent immunosuppressant to prevent rejection in the early postoperative period. Once cyclosporine therapy has been initiated, dosage adjustments are empiric based on cyclosporine levels, organ function, and toxicity.

Tacrolimus

Tacrolimus (Prograf) is a macrolide agent that was derived from *Streptomyces tsukubaensis* in 1985. Since its approval by the Food and Drug Administration for preventing rejection in liver and kidney allograft recipients, the drug has been evaluated in many types of organ transplantation. On a cellular level, tacrolimus and cyclosporine have similar effects; however, tacrolimus seems 10 times to 100 times more potent in its ability to inhibit IL-2 and T-cell activation[59] (see **Table 3**). Clinically, a reduction in IL-2 concentration is thought to minimize the immune response associated with allograft rejection, although other cytokines are also inhibited by tacrolimus.[59] Several multicenter, randomized controlled trials using tacrolimus for maintenance immunosuppression in solid organ transplant recipients have been conducted, which demonstrated that the drug is effective or more effective compared with cyclosporine-based immunosuppressive regimens.[60–63] Most transplant centers use tacrolimus-based immunosuppression as first-line therapy to prevent rejection.

After oral administration, tacrolimus is poorly absorbed, resulting in low plasma peak concentrations.[59,64] The time to peak absorption after an oral dose varies from 0.5 hours to 4 hours and is impacted by factors that affect GI absorption. Tacrolimus is highly lipophilic and undergoes extensive tissue distribution. Tacrolimus is primarily bound by albumin and alpha-1-acid glycoprotein.[59,64] The drug undergoes complete hepatic metabolism prior to elimination from the body.[64] The mechanism of tacrolimus elimination seems to be via hepatic and gut cytochrome P450 mechanisms with inactive metabolites excretion in bile. Mean elimination half-life in liver allograft recipients is approximately 8 hours; clearance is reduced in patients with significant hepatic impairment.[59,64] Because tacrolimus is metabolized by the cytochrome P450 isoenzyme CYP3A, several potential drug interactions are possible (see **Table 4**). Additional monitoring to reduce the risk of either toxicity or rejection is necessary.

Adverse effects associated with tacrolimus are often dose and concentration dependent. Similar to other immunosuppressive agents, tacrolimus can cause nephrotoxicity, neurotoxicity, and an increased risk of infection.[59–63] Tacrolimus seems less likely than cyclosporine to cause hypertension or hypercholesterolemia and more likely to cause insulin-dependent diabetes mellitus. Other tacrolimus-induced adverse effects include hyperkalemia, hypomagnesemia, and GI symptoms.

Oral dosing of tacrolimus is the preferred route of administration and is initiated in the early post-transplant phase. Oral dosages are usually started at 0.1 mg/kg/d to 0.3 mg/kg/d in divided doses. Elderly recipients and patients with hepatic or renal dysfunction should be started on the lowest recommended dosages to avoid the risk of toxicity. New modified-release formulations of tacrolimus (Astagraf XL and Envarsus XR) offer the benefit of once-daily dosing.

INHIBITORS OF LATE T-CELL FUNCTION
Mammalian Target of Rapamycin Inhibitors

The inhibitors of mammalian target of rapamycin (mTOR) include 2 drugs: sirolimus (Rapamune) and everolimus (Zortress).[65–68] In contrast to the CNIs, the mTOR inhibitors do not affect the early phase of T-cell activation. The mTOR inhibitors act late in the cell cycle, preventing IL-2–mediated T-cell proliferation (see **Table 3**). These agents have demonstrated immunosuppressive synergy with cyclosporine and tacrolimus and are not considered nephrotoxic or neurotoxic when used alone.

Sirolimus

Sirolimus is a macrolide antibiotic structurally related to tacrolimus. The immunosuppression mechanism occurs by interaction between sirolimus and the rapamycin and FK-binding protein 12 (FKBP-12) target, resulting in failure of T cells to enter the division cycle[65,69] (see **Table 3**). Sirolimus is metabolized via the cytochrome P450IIIA isozyme system. It has a drug interaction profile similar to that of cyclosporine and tacrolimus. Sirolimus is initiated at least 30 days after transplant with a loading dose of 3 mg to 6 mg, followed by once daily maintenance doses of 1 mg to 3 mg.

Everolimus

Everolimus, a structural analog of sirolimus, has a mechanism of action identical to that of sirolimus but has increased bioavailability and a shorter half-life.[67,68] Once inside the cell, it binds to FKBP-12. This complex then binds mTOR, resulting in blockade of IL-2 and IL-5 driven proliferation of T lymphocytes and B lymphocytes. The drug has been approved for use in both liver and kidney transplant recipients. Everolimus should not be administered in liver transplant recipients until at least 30 days post-transplant to reduce the potential risk of hepatic artery thrombosis.[68]

Drug interactions must be considered with the mTOR inhibitors. Because they are considered synergistic with cyclosporine, use of an mTOR inhibitor in combination with a lower-dose calcineurin CNI may reduce long-term nephrotoxicity. Changes in cyclosporine dosing require titration of the everolimus dose.[70] Several studies have reported improved renal function after a switch from CNI-based immune suppression to mTOR-based regimens.[71–73] Major adverse effects associated with the mTOR inhibitors include hypertriglyceridemia, hypercholesterolemia, leukopenia, mucositis, edema, proteinuria, poor wound healing, and thrombocytopenia.

INTERLEUKIN 2 RECEPTOR ANTAGONISTS
Basiliximab

Basiliximab is a chimeric monoclonal antibody containing both murine and human antibody sequences.[74] This agent competitively inhibits the alpha subunit of the IL-2 receptor (IL-2α [CD25]). The IL-2α target receptor is selectively expressed on activated T lymphocytes that are critical in the cellular immune response associated with allograft rejection.

The terminal half-life of basiliximab is approximately 7 days.[74,75] No significant drug interactions have been reported for basiliximab. This agent has been used in combination with most of the drugs commonly used in solid organ transplant recipients with no increase in adverse effects.[74,75] The incidence of adverse reactions reported with basiliximab was essentially equal to that in placebo-treated patients in clinical trials.[74,75] A cytokine release syndrome that historically was common with muromonab CD3 (OKT3) has not been noted with basiliximab. In addition, infections and malignancies were similar in basiliximab and placebo groups in clinical trials.[76,77]

Basiliximab decreases the incidence of acute rejection when used as induction therapy in combination with maintenance immunosuppression. Basiliximab requires two 20-mg intravenous doses at the time of transplant and another 20 mg 4 days later.[78] At many centers, an anesthesiologist is responsible for administration of a preoperative dose of basiliximab for kidney transplant.

POLYCLONAL ANTIBODIES
Antithymocyte Globulin

Antithymocyte globulin (Thymoglobulin) is a polyclonal antibody obtained by immunization of rabbits with human thymocytes. The solution is pasteurized to increase viral safety, then concentrated and provided in a lyophilized form.[79] This product is Food and Drug Administration approved for treatment of allograft rejection.[79] The agent has also been used in several transplant recipients off-label as induction immunosuppressant therapy.[80–82] Thymoglobulin consists of antibodies specific for T-cell epitopes. The mechanism of action may be linked to the lysis of peripheral lymphocytes, uptake of lymphocytes by the reticuloendothelial system, and masking of lymphocyte receptors. The plasma half-life is 44 hours with a terminal half-life of 13 days.[79–82] As with other polyclonal preparations, there are large variations in half-life between individuals. Adverse effects include leukopenia, fever, chills, infection, and malignancies.[79–82] The recommended dose is 1.5 mg/kg/d diluted in 250-mL normal saline and infused through a central line with a 0.2-μm filter.[79–82] The first dose should be infused over 6 hours with subsequent doses infused over 4 hours. Premedications, including methylprednisolone 1 hour prior to administration along with acetaminophen and diphenhydramine, are standard at most centers.[79–82] The current recommended length of therapy for the treatment of rejection is 7 days to 10 days. Daily monitoring for toxicity should include white blood cell and platelet counts. As with any antilymphocyte preparation, administration of antiviral, antifungal, and antibacterial prophylaxis for 1 month to 3 months post-therapy is warranted to protect patients during the most intense time of immunosuppression.

MONOCLONAL ANTIBODIES

New biologic agents, including monoclonal antibodies and receptor-fusion proteins, are promising alternatives due to their lack of immunogenicity and prolonged biologic effects. Because these agents are typically more specific and more selective, they are considered less toxic although less efficacious. These agents interfere with various targets involved in allograft recognition and rejection. Target molecules include those involved with immune cell interactions, signaling mechanisms, and T-cell proliferation.

Alemtuzumab

Alemtuzumab (Campath) is a recombinant DNA–derived humanized anti-CD52 monoclonal antibody currently approved for treatment of B-cell chronic lymphocytic leukemia.[83–85] It targets T lymphocytes and B lymphocytes, NK cells, macrophages, and monocytes. After intravenous administration, alemtuzumab completely depletes lymphocytes from the circulation and the periphery. The average half-life of the drug is approximately 12 days. Recent studies have reported that the drug can be used for desensitization prior to transplant, for induction therapy, and for treatment of antibody-mediated rejection (AMR).[86–88] Many induction protocols recommend a single 30-mg perioperative dose followed by 30 mg 24 hours later.[84,85] The most significant adverse events are prolonged lymphopenia, infusion reactions (hypotension, rigors, fever, bronchospasm, chills, and rash), and the subsequent risk of opportunistic infections. This risk is manageable with appropriate use of antimicrobial prophylaxis. Premedication with antihistamines and acetaminophen is recommended to ameliorate first-dose symptoms associated with cytokine release. Clinical experience with alemtuzumab in transplantation is limited but promising.

Rituximab

Rituximab (Rituxan) is a murine/human chimeric monoclonal antibody approved for use in treating non-Hodgkin lymphomas. Within the field of transplantation, it has been used primarily for desensitization, for cases of post-transplant lymphoproliferative disorder, and for AMR.[89–91] Its role as an immunosuppressant is new, with only case reports supporting its use. Rituximab is specific for the CD20 surface marker on B cells. Close monitoring during infusion is necessary given the risk of severe infusion-related events, including tumor lysis syndrome, mucocutaneous reactions, and even death.[89]

OTHER AGENTS
Bortezomib

Bortezomib (Velcade) is one of the newest agents used in desensitization protocols and for AMR. This agent is a reversible 26s proteasome inhibitor that suppresses mature plasma cell antibody production resulting in profound immunosuppressive effects.[92,93] Studies are limited, but based on data in renal transplant recipients this agent may be considered an alternative strategy against refractory AMR.

Eculizumab

Eculizumab (Soliris) is a monoclonal anti-C5 inhibitor that halts the complement cascade by inhibiting the formation of the terminal membrane attack complex. This drug has also been used in desensitization protocols and for treatment of AMR.[94,95] Case reports in solid organ transplant recipients describe limited efficacy, high cost, and enhanced risk for gram-negative bacterial infection.[94,95]

Costimulation Blockade

A costimulation blockade agent represents one of the newest classes of immunosuppressive agents available for solid organ transplant recipients. Belatacept (Nulojix), an agent that mimics soluble CTLA-4, interferes with the costimulatory system in T cells, resulting in immune dampening responses.[96–98] Belatacept is only approved for prevention of kidney transplant rejection in combination with basiliximab induction, MMF, and corticosteroids. The initial dose is 10 mg/kg intravenously on the day of transplant and continued until 12 weeks after transplantation.[96–98] Adverse effects occur in more than 20% of patients and include anemia, leukopenia, diarrhea, urinary tract infections, edema, hypertension, dyslipidemia, hyperglycemia, proteinuria, and electrolyte disorders.[96–98] There are no dosage adjustments needed in patients with renal or hepatic impairment and no drug-drug interactions.

SUMMARY

Mechanisms of rejection, new pharmacologic approaches, and genomic medicine are major foci for current research in transplantation. It is hoped that these new agents and personalized immunosuppression will provide less toxic regimens that are effective in preventing both acute and chronic allograft rejection. Until new agents are available, practitioners must use various combinations of currently approved agents in an effort to find the best regimens for improved long-term outcomes.

REFERENCES

1. Rogers NJ, Lechler RI. Allorecognition. Am J Transplant 2001;1:97–102.
2. Da silva MB, da Cunha FF, Terres FF, et al. Old game, new players: linking classical theories to new trends in transplant immunology. World J Transplant 2017;7: 1–25.
3. Klein J, Sato A. The HLA system. First of two parts. N Engl J Med 2000;343: 702–9.
4. Delves PJ, Roitt IM. The immune system. Second of two parts. N Engl J Med 2000;343:108–17.
5. Van Der Merwe PA, Davis SJ. Molecular interactions mediating T cell antigen recognition. Annu Rev Immunol 2003;21:659–84.
6. Alarcon B, Gil D, Delgado P, et al. Initiation of TCR signaling: regulation within CD3 dimers. Immunol Rev 2003;191:38–46.
7. Davis SJ, Ikemizu S, Evans EJ, et al. The nature of molecular recognition by T cells. Nat Immunol 2003;4:217–24.
8. Sayegh MH, Turka LA. The role of T-cell costimulatory activation pathways in transplant rejection. N Engl J Med 1998;338:1813–21.
9. Chambers CA, Allison JP. Costimulatory regulation of T cell function. Curr Opin Cell Biol 1999;11:203–10.
10. Agnello D, Lankford CS, Bream J, et al. Cytokines and transcription factors that regulate T helper cell differentiation: new players and new insights. J Clin Immunol 2003;23:147–61.
11. Le Moine A, Goldman M, Abramowicz D. Multiple pathways to allograft rejection. Transplantation 2002;73:1373–81.
12. Julius M, Maroun CR, Haughn L. Distinct roles for CD4 and CD8 as co-receptors in antigen receptor signalling. Immunol Today 1993;14:177–83.
13. Frasca L, Amendola A, Hornick P, et al. Role of donor and recipient antigen-presenting cells in priming and maintaining T cells with indirect allospecificity. Transplantation 1998;66:1238–43.
14. Minami Y, Kono T, Miyazaki T, et al. The IL-2 receptor complex: its structure, function, and target genes. Annu Rev Immunol 1993;11:245–68.
15. Waldmann TA, Dubois S, Tagaya Y. Contrasting roles of IL-2 and IL-15 in the life and death of lymphocytes: implications for immunotherapy. Immunity 2001;14: 105–10.
16. van Kampen CA, Versteeg-van der Voort Maarschalk MF, Langerak-Langerak J, et al. Pregnancy can induce long-persisting primed CTLs specific for inherited paternal HLA antigens. Hum Immunol 2001;62:201–7.
17. Katznelson STS, Cecka JM. Handbook of kidney transplantation. In: Danovitch GM, editor. Lippincott Williams and Wilkins handbook. Philadephia: Lippincott Williams & Wilkins; 2001. p. xiii, 443, [3] of plates.
18. Tyan DB, Li VA, Czer L, et al. Intravenous immunoglobulin suppression of HLA alloantibody in highly sensitized transplant candidates and transplantation with a histoincompatible organ. Transplantation 1994;57:553–62.
19. Itescu S, Burke E, Lietz K, et al. Intravenous pulse administration of cyclophosphamide is an effective and safe treatment for sensitized cardiac allograft recipients. Circulation 2002;105:1214–9.

20. Schmid C, Garritsen HS, Kelsch R, et al. Suppression of panel-reactive anti-bodies by treatment with mycophenolate mofetil. Thorac Cardiovasc Surg 1998;46:161–2.
21. Schweitzer EJ, Wilson JS, Fernandez-Vina M, et al. A high panel-reactive anti-body rescue protocol for cross-match-positive live donor kidney transplants. Transplantation 2000;70:1531–6.
22. Pisani BA, Mullen GM, Malinowska K, et al. Plasmapheresis with intravenous immunoglobulin G is effective in patients with elevated panel reactive antibody prior to cardiac transplantation. J Heart Lung Transplant 1999;18:701–6.
23. Taylor DO, Edwards LB, Mohacsi PJ, et al. The registry of the International Society for Heart and Lung Transplantation: twentieth official adult heart transplant report–2003. J Heart Lung Transplant 2003;22:616–24.
24. McLaren AJ, Fuggle SV, Welsh KI, et al. Chronic allograft failure in human renal transplantation: a multivariate risk factor analysis. Ann Surg 2000;232:98–103.
25. Behrendt D, Ganz P, Fang JC. Cardiac allograft vasculopathy. Curr Opin Cardiol 2000;15:422–9.
26. Hill P, Cross NB, Barnett AN, et al. Polyclonal and monoclonal antibodies for in-duction therapy in kidney transplant recipients. Cochrane Database Syst Rev 2017;11:1.
27. Ekberg H. Calcineurin inhibitor sparing in renal transplantation. Transplantation 2008;86:761–7.
28. Giessing M, Fuller TF, Tuelimann M, et al. Steroid and calcineurin inhibitor free immunosuppression in kidney transplantation: state of the art and future develop-ments. World J Urol 2007;25:325–32.
29. Husing A, Schmidt M, Beckebaum S, et al. Long term renal function in liver trans-plant recipients after conversion from calcineurin inhibitors to mTOR inhibiotrs. Ann Transplant 2015;26:707–13.
30. Gude E, Gullestad L, Arora S, et al. Benefit of early conversion from CNI based to everolimus based immunosuppression in heart transplantation. J Heart Lung Transplant 2010;29:641–7.
31. Vacca A, Martinotti S, Screpanti I, et al. Transcriptional regulation of the inter-leukin 2 gene by glucocorticoid hormones. J Biol Chem 1990;265:8075–80.
32. Vacca A, Felli P, Farina AR, et al. Glucocorticoid receptor mediated suppression of the interleukin 2 gene expression through impairment of the *cooperativity be-tween nuclear factor of activated t cells and AP1 enhancer* elements. J Exp Med 1992;175:637–46.
33. Moini M, Schilsky ML, Tichy EM. Review on immunosuppression in liver trans-plantation. World J Hepatol 2015;7:1355–68.
34. Karam S, Wall RK. Current state of immunosuppression: past, present, and future. Crit Rev Eukaryot Gene Expr 2015;25:113–34.
35. Dhanasekaran R. Management of immunosuppression in liver transplantation. Clin Liver Dis 2017;21:337–53.
36. Oplez G, Dohler B, Laux G, et al. Long term prospective study of steroid withdra-walm in kidney and heart transplant recipients. Am J Transplant 2005;5(4 pt 1):720–8.
37. Kasiske BL, Chakkera HA, Louis TA, et al. A meta analysis of immunosuppression withdrawal trials in renal transplantation. J Am Soc Nephrol 2000;11:1910–7.
38. Sollinger HW, Eugui EM, Allison AC. RS-61443: mechanism of action, experi-mental and early clinical results. Clin Transplant 1991;5:523–6.
39. Sievers T, Rossi SJ, Ghobrial R, et al. Mycophenolate mofetil: a new immunosup-pressive in transplantation. Pharmacotherapy 1997;17:1178–97.

40. Fulton B, Markham A. Mycophenolate mofetil. A review of its pharmacodynamic and pharmacokinetic properties and clinical efficacy in renal transplantation. Drugs 1996;51:278–98.

41. Shaw LM. Mycophenolate mofetil: pharmacokinetic strategies for optimizing immunosuppression. Drug Metabol Drug Interact 1997;14:33–40.

42. Cellcept " (mycophenolate mofetil) capsule. Syntex, Roche Pharmaceuticals [Package Insert]. Nutley, NJ: 1995.

43. Hood KA, Zarembski DG. Mycophenolate mofetil: a unique immunosuppressive agent. Am J Health Syst Pharm 1997;54:285–94.

44. Mignat C. Clinically significant drug interactions with new immunosuppressive agents. Drug Saf 1997;16:267.

45. Trotter JF. Drugs that interact with immunosuppressive agents. Semin Gastrointest Dis 1998;9:147.

46. Neff RT, Hurst FP, Falta EM, et al. Progressive multifocal leukoencephalopathy and use of mycophemolate mofetil after kidney transplantation. Transplantation 2008;27:1474–8.

47. Manfro RC, Vedolin L, Cantarelli M, et al. Progressive multifocal leukoencephalopathy in a kidney transplant recipient after conversion to mycophenolic acid therapy. Transpl Infect Dis 2009;11:189–90.

48. Sanford M, Keating GM. Enteric coated mycophenolate sodium: a review of its use in the prevention of renal transplant rejection. Drugs 2008;68:2505–33.

49. Schreiber SL. The mechanism of action of cyclosporine A and FK506. Immunol Today 1992;13:136–42.

50. Kahan BD. Cyclosporine. N Engl J Med 1989;321:1725–38.

51. Ptachcinski RJ. Clinical pharmacokinetics of cyclosporine. Clin Pharmacokinet 1986;11:107–32.

52. Shah MB, Martin JE, Schroeder TJ, et al. The evaluation of the safety and tolerability of two formulations of cyclosporine: neoral and sandimmune. A meta-analysis. Transplantation 1999;67(11):1411–7.

53. Flechner SM, Kobashigawa J, Klintmalm G. Calcineurin inhibitor sparing regimens in solid organ transplantation: focus on improving renal function and nephrotoxicity. Clin Transplant 2008;22:1–15.

54. Mathis AS, Eqloff G, Ghin HL. Calcineurin inhibitor sparing strategies in renal transplantation. World J Transplant 2014;24:57–80.

55. Farkas SA, Schnitzbauer AA, Kirchner G, et al. Calcineurin minimization protocols in liver transplantation. Transpl Int 2009;22:49–60.

56. Thibault G, Paintuad G, Legendre C, et al. CD25 blockade in kidney transplant patients randomized to standard dose or high dose basiliximab with cyclosporine or high dose basilimab in a calcineurin free regimen. Transpl Int 2016;29:184–95.

57. Yu J, Zheng SS, Liang TB, et al. Possible causes of central pontine myelinolysis after liver transplantation. World J Gastroenterol 2004;10:2540–3.

58. Harirchian MH, Ghaffarpour M, Tabaeizadeh M, et al. Immunosuppressive drugs, an emerging cause of posterior reversible encephalopathy syndrome: case series. J Stroke Cerebrovasc Dis 2015;24:191–5.

59. Plosker GL. Tacrolimus: a further update of its pharmacology and therapeutic use in the management of organ transplantation. Drugs 2000;59:324.

60. The U.S. Multicenter FK 506 Liver Study Group. A comparison of tacrolimus (FK 506) and cyclosporine for immunosuppression in liver transplantation. N Engl J Med 1994;331:1110–5.

61. European FK 506 Multicentre Liver Study Group. Randomized trial comparing tacrolimus (FK 506) and cyclosporin in prevention of liver allograft rejection. Lancet 1994;344:423–8.

62. Shapiro R, Jordan ML, Scantlebury VP, et al. A prospective randomized trial of FK 506 based immunosuppression after renal transplantation. Transplantation 1995; 27:485–90.

63. Wu Q, Marescaux C, Wolff V, et al. Tacrolimus associated posterior reversible encephalopathy syndrome after solid organ transplantation. Eur Neurol 2010;64: 169177.

64. Venkataramanan R. Clinical pharmacokinetics of tacrolimus. Clin Pharmacokinet 1995;29:404–30.

65. Ingle G, Sievers TM, Holt CD. Sirolimus: The Newest Immunosuppressive for Solid Organ Transplantation. Ann Pharmacother 2000;34:1044.

66. Fine NM, Kushwaha SS. Recent advances in mammalian traget of rapamycin inhibitor use in heart and lung transplantation. Transplantation 2016;100:2558–68.

67. Pascual J. Everolimus in clinical practice-renal transplanattion. Nephrol Dial Transplant 2006;21(suppl 3):18–23.

68. Gabardi S, Baroletti SA. Everolimus: a proliferation signal inhibitor with clinical applications in organ transplantation, oncology, and cardiology. Pharmacotherapy 2010;30:1044–56.

69. Moris R. Modes of action of FK506, cyclosporin A and rapamycin. Transplant Proc 1994;26:3272–5.

70. Van Gelder T, Fischer L, Shihab F, et al. Optimizing everolimus exposure when combined with calcineurin inhibitors in solid organ transplantation. Transplant Rev 2017. [Epub ahead of print].

71. Schena FP, Pascoe MD, Alberu J, et al. Conversion from calcineurin inhibitors to sirolimus maintenance therapy in renal allograft recipients: 24 month efficacy and safety results from the CONVERT trial. Transplantation 2009;87:233–42.

72. Witzke O, Sommerer C, Arns W. Everolimus immunosuppression in kidney transplantation: what is the optimal strategy. Transplant Rev 2016;30:3–12.

73. Langer RM, Hene R, Vitko S, et al. Everolimus plus early tacrolimus minimization: a phase II, randomized, open label, multicenter trial in renal transplantation. Transpl Int 2012;25:592–602.

74. Berard JL, Velez RL, Freeman RB, et al. A review of interleukin 2 receptor antagonists in solid organ transplantation. Pharmacotherapy 1999;19:1127–37.

75. Van Gelder T, Warle M, TerMeulen RG. Anti-interleukin 2 receptoe antibodies: what is the basis for choice? Drugs 2004;64:1737–41.

76. Chapman TM, Keating GM. Basiliximab: a review of its use as induction therapy in renal transplantation. Drugs 2003;24:2801–35.

77. McKeage K, McCormack PL. Basiliximab: a review of its use as induction therapy in renal transplantation. BioDrugs 2010;24:55–76.

78. Henry ML, Rajab A. The use of basiliximab in solid organ transplantation. Expert Opin Pharmacother 2002;11:1657–63.

79. Mohty M, Bacigalupo A, Saliba F, et al. New directions for rabbit antithymocyte globulin (Thymoglobulin) in solid organ tranplants, stem cell transplants and autoimmunity. Drugs 2014;74:1605–34.

80. Deeks ED, Keating GM. Rabbit antithymocyte globulin (thymoglobulin): a review of its use in the prevention and treatment of acute renal allograft rejection. Drugs 2009;69:1483.

81. Gaber AO, Monaco AP, Russell JA, et al. Rabbit antithymocyte globulin (thymoglobulin): 25 years and new frontiers in solid organ transplantation and haematology. Drugs 2010;70:691–732.
82. Hardinger KL. Rabbit antithymocyte globulin induction therapy in adult renal transplantation. Pharmacotherapy 2006;26:1771–83.
83. Morris PJ, Russell NK. Alemtuzumab (campath 1H): a systematic review in organ transplantation. Transplantation 2006;81:1361–7.
84. Hale G. The CD 52 antigen and the development of campath antibodies. Cytotherapy 2001;3:137–43.
85. Ferrajoli A, O'Brien S, Keating MJ. Alemtuzumab: a novel monoclonal antibody. Expert Opin Biol Ther 2001;1:1059–65.
86. Kim M, Martin ST, Townsend KR, et al. Antibody-mediated rejection in kidney transplantation: a review of pathophysiology, diagnosis, and treatment options. Pharmacotherapy 2014;34:733–44.
87. LaMattina JC, Mezrich JD, Hofmann RM, et al. Alemtuzumab as compared to alternative contemporary induction regimens. Transpl Int 2012;25:518–26.
88. Willcombe M, Roufosse C, Brookes P, et al. Antibody-mediated rejection after alemtuzumab induction: incidence, risk factors, and predictors of poor outcome. Transplantation 2011;92:176–82.
89. Sadaka B, Alloway RR, Woodle ES. Management of antibody-mediated rejection in transplantation. Surg Clin North Am 2013;93:1451–66.
90. Ravichandran AK, Schilling JD, Novak E, et al. Rituximab is associated with improved survival in cardiac allograft patients with antibody-mediated rejection: a single center review. Clin Transplant 2013;27:961–7.
91. Macklin PS, Morris PJ, Knight SR. A systematic review of the use of rituximab for desensitization in renal transplantation. Transplantation 2014;98:794–805.
92. Lee J, Kim BS, Park Y, et al. The effect of bortezomib on antibody-mediated rejection after kidney transplantation. Yonsei Med J 2015;56:1638–42.
93. Paterno F, Shiller M, Tillery G, et al. Bortezomib for acute antibody-mediated rejection in liver transplantation. Am J Transplant 2012;12:2526–31.
94. Tran D, Boucher A, Collette S, et al. Eculizumab for the treatment of severe antibody-mediated rejection: a case report and review of the literature. Case Rep Transpl 2016;2016:9874261.
95. Yelken B, Arpalı E, Görcin S, et al. Eculizumab for treatment of refractory antibody-mediated rejection in kidney transplant patients: a single-center experience. Transplant Proc 2015;47:1754–9.
96. Herr F, Brunel M, Roders N, et al. Co-stimulation blockade plus T-cell depletion in transplant patients: towards a steroid- and calcineurin inhibitor-free future? Drugs 2016;76:1589–600.
97. Satyananda V, Shapiro R. Belatacept in kidney transplantation. Curr Opin Organ Transpl 2014;19:573–7.
98. Martin ST, Tichy EM, Gabardi S. Belatacept: a novel biologic for maintenance immunosuppression after renal transplantation. Pharmacotherapy 2011;31:394–407.

Infectious Complications and Malignancies Arising After Liver Transplantation

Dame W. Idossa, MD[a], Douglas Alano Simonetto, MD[b],*

KEYWORDS

- Liver transplantation • Immunosuppression • Infection • Malignancy • Mortality

KEY POINTS

- Infection is the most frequent cause of death immediately after liver transplantation.
- Bacterial pathogens are the leading cause of infection after liver transplantation, most often occurring within the first month after surgery.
- Viral infections cause the majority of febrile episodes between 1 and 6 months after liver transplant.
- Invasive fungal infections are common in posttransplant patients.
- The risk of malignancy is 2 to 4 times higher in transplant recipients compared with their nontransplanted counterparts.

INTRODUCTION

Since the first liver transplant was performed in 1963, great advancements have been made in the field of hepatic transplantation. Surgical techniques have been revised and improved; diagnostic methods for identifying and preventing infections have been developed, and more conservative use of immunosuppressive agents have resulted in better long-term posttransplant outcomes. Despite the myriad advancements made since the initial liver transplants of the 1960s, technical surgical complications, infections, rejections, and chronic medical conditions such as renal failure, diabetes, dyslipidemia, osteopenia, coronary artery disease, and malignancy persist.[1] In this review, we discuss the infectious complications and malignancies that may arise after liver transplantation as a result of the procedure itself, and from posttransplant immunosuppression.

Disclosure Statement: The authors have nothing to disclose.
[a] Internal Medicine, Mayo Clinic, 200 First Street Southwest, Rochester, MN 55905, USA;
[b] Department of Gastroenterology and Hepatology, Mayo Clinic, 200 First Street Southwest, Rochester, MN 55905, USA
* Corresponding author.
E-mail address: Simonetto.douglas@mayo.edu

Anesthesiology Clin 35 (2017) 381–393
http://dx.doi.org/10.1016/j.anclin.2017.04.002
1932-2275/17/© 2017 Elsevier Inc. All rights reserved.

anesthesiology.theclinics.com

INFECTIOUS COMPLICATIONS

In many centers, infection is the most frequent cause of death immediately after liver transplantation. Unfortunately, the diagnosis is often delayed owing to the effects of immunosuppressive agents, inhibiting the usual inflammatory responses and clinical signs of an infectious state.[2] Such a delay in diagnosis leads to increased morbidity and mortality in these posttransplant patients. Infectious complications can be categorized into those occurring within the first month (early), between 1 to 6 months (intermediate), and after 6 months (late) after transplantation. Understanding these complications may help to optimize management strategies, support patient quality of life, and improve long-term outcomes after liver transplantation.[3]

EARLY BACTERIAL INFECTIONS

Bacterial pathogens are the leading cause of infection after liver transplantation, most often occurring within the first month after transplant. These infections usually involve the surgical site, peritoneal space, bloodstream, and respiratory tract.[4–7] The most common bacterial pathogens include *Enterococcus* species, *Streptococcus viridans*, *Staphylococcus aureus*, and members of the *Enterobacteriaceae* family.[3] The rate of infection with multidrug-resistant organisms is steadily increasing in patients with previous antibiotic exposure, recurrent hospitalizations, and invasive interventions such as mechanical ventilation and indwelling devices. In some centers, the prevalence rate of methicillin-resistant *S aureus* colonization may exceed 80%,[8,9] whereas vancomycin-resistant enterococcus colonization may reach up to 55%.[10]

Surgical wound infections are commonly seen within the first month of transplantation.[11] These infections are commonly caused by gram-positive cocci such as *S aureus* and *Enterococcus*, and less commonly by gram-negative organisms such as *Escherichia coli*, *Acinetobacter*, and *Pseudomonas*.[12] Intraabdominal infections including cholangitis, peritonitis, bile leak, and intraabdominal abscesses are also common early in the postoperative period.[13] **Tables 1** and **2** present the most common causative pathogens and the risk factors associated with these infections.

Bloodstream infections are also a serious and common occurrence postoperatively, with associated mortality rates of 24% to 36% in liver transplant recipients.[14,15] Specific organisms responsible for bacteremia vary between transplant centers. Gram-positive cocci were considered to be the most common causative agents of early

Table 1			
Common pathogens early in the postoperative phase			
Surgical Wound	**Intraabdominal**	**Bloodstream**	**Respiratory Tract**
Staphylococcus aureus	*Staphylococcus aureus*	Specific organisms vary between transplant centers	*Staphylococcus aureus*
Enterococci spp	*Enterococci* spp		*Pseudomonas aeruginosa*
Escherichia coli[a]	*Acinetobacter*		*Klebsiella*
Acinetobacter spp[a]	*Pseudomonas aeruginosa*		*Enterobacter*
Pseudomonas aeruginosa[a]	*Klebsiella*		*Haemophilus influenza*
	Clostridium difficile		*Stenotrophomonas maltophilia*
			Serratia marcescens

[a] Less commonly associated.

Table 2
Risk factors associated with early postoperative infections

Surgical Wound	Intraabdominal	Bloodstream	Respiratory Tract
HLA mismatching	Pretransplant ascites	Old age	Prolonged mechanical
Preoperative antibiotic	Renal replacement	Prolonged central	ventilation
use	therapy	venous access	Massive transfusions
Previous liver/kidney	Surgical wound	UNOS class I or IIA	Malnutrition
transplant	infection	Diabetes	
Surgeon inexperience	Reoperation	Renal dysfunction	
Biliary leaks	Hepatic artery	Hypoalbuminemia	
Prolonged surgical time	thrombosis		
Reoperation			
Choledochojejunal/			
hepaticojejunal			
reconstruction			
>4 U of blood			
transfused			
intraoperatively			
Intraoperative			
vasopressor use			
Combined liver–kidney			
transplantation			
Preoperative			
mechanical			
ventilation			
Perioperative			
hyperglycemia			

Abbreviation: UNOS, United Network for Organ Sharing.

posttransplant bacteremia. However, recent studies have demonstrated a possible shift toward gram-negative organisms.[15–17] For example, the proportion of gram-negative bacteremia at 1 transplant center increased from 25% during the period 1989 to 1993 to 51.8% during the period of 1998 to 2003, whereas gram-positive bacteremia decreased from 75% to 48.2% during the same period.[15] **Table 2** presents the risk factors most commonly associated with blood stream infections.

Respiratory tract infections are among the leading causes of sepsis and mortality after liver transplantation.[13] The long duration and technical complexity of liver transplantation often lead to prolonged mechanical ventilation and massive transfusions. These interventions increase the risk for respiratory tract infections early in the postoperative period. In addition, immunosuppression, underlying edematous state, and malnutrition increase the likelihood of hospital-acquired pneumonia. **Table 1** reports common causative agents of respiratory tract infections in liver transplant recipients.

INTERMEDIATE AND LATE BACTERIAL INFECTIONS

During the intermediate posttransplant period (2–6 months), opportunistic infections may occur owing to the higher levels of immunosuppression.[18] Infections with *Listeria monocytogenes* and *Nocardia* species may develop in this period. In addition, reactivation of latent infections, including those caused by *Mycobacterium* species, may also be seen.[14,18]

The rate of bacterial infections significantly decreases in the late period (>6 months) after transplantation. This is partly owing to the tapering of immunosuppressive agents in those with satisfactory allograft function.[18] These patients more often develop community-acquired infections, similar to those seen in the general population, although at an increased rate.[18]

VIRAL INFECTIONS

Aside from allograft rejection, viral infections are responsible for causing the majority of febrile episodes occurring between 1 to 6 months after liver transplantation. The most common viral pathogens include herpesviruses such as cytomegalovirus (CMV), Epstein-Barr virus (EBV), varicella zoster virus, as well as polyomavirus BK, adenovirus, and recurrent hepatitis.[18]

HERPES VIRUSES

CMV is the most common viral infection that influences outcome after liver transplantation.[19,20] CMV infection occurs through the reactivation of the latent virus in response to immunosuppression or through de novo transmission of CMV from a seropositive donor to a seronegative recipient.[21] Without prophylaxis, CMV infections develop in 36% to 100% of solid organ transplant recipients, and symptomatic disease occurs in 11% to 72%, most often during the first 100 days after transplantation.[18,22] Clinical manifestations of CMV infections can be owing to the direct effects of viral replication, including fever, malaise, and cytopenias, but may also arise from the indirect effects of the virus on the host's immune response. These indirect effects can lead to increased risk of other opportunistic infections and tissue-invasive disease with end-organ damage.[23,24] CMV infection can also lead to increased risk of bacteremia, invasive fungal infections, and an almost 4-fold increase in risk of death during the first year after liver transplant.[25] The risk for CMV infection is greatest in cases of mismatch, where the donor is CMV seropositive and recipient is CMV seronegative. CMV infections can be greatly reduced by prophylaxis with ganciclovir or valganciclovir for high-risk groups or by close surveillance, early diagnosis, and treatment of all transplant recipients.[26]

Primary EBV infection is uncommon in the general adult population in the United States, given that approximately 90% to 95% of adults are seropositive. Thus, many patients undergoing liver transplantation have already been exposed at the time of the procedure.[20] Those who have not been infected before transplantation may be exposed to EBV from seropositive donors or transfusions with non–leukoreduced blood products.[20] EBV infection is commonly associated with posttransplant lymphoproliferative disorder (PTLD).[20]

HSV infection is rare, but it can be seen very early in the posttransplant period, likely from reactivation of the virus in the setting of immunosuppression. The clinical presentation is often nonspecific with fevers, leukopenia, abnormal liver function tests without jaundice, and right upper quadrant abdominal pain. Some patients can also present with mucocutaneous lesions. For patients not on prophylaxis for CMV, acyclovir is recommended for the first 1 to 3 months after transplantation.[20]

Varicella zoster virus infection is also rare and it can present as chickenpox or herpes zoster. Patients that develop either of these diseases may be treated with valaciclovir or famciclovir in the outpatient setting.[20]

HEPATITIDES RELEVANT TO LIVER TRANSPLANTATION
Hepatitis B

Recurrence of hepatitis B virus (HBV) after liver transplantation is a major cause of allograft dysfunction, cirrhosis, and graft failure. Thus, prevention of recurrence is extremely important. Before the advent of HBV treatments, recurrence of HBV after transplant in hepatitis B surface antigen–positive patients was almost universal.[27] This was especially true for patients undergoing liver transplantation for HBV-related cirrhosis. Fortunately, now more than 90% of recurrent HBV infections can be clinically controlled by antiviral treatment (nucleos[t]ide analogues) in combination with hepatitis B immunoglobulins (HBIg).[27,28]

There is substantial risk of acquiring de novo HBV infection in recipients who receive liver transplant from donors who are anti-hepatitis B core positive. The risk seems to be decreased, but not eliminated, in recipients who have protective surface antibody from vaccination. Therefore, the risk of acquiring HBV infection cannot be prevented solely by matching anti-hepatitis B core positive livers to recipients with anti-HB surface antibody. Administration of prophylactic antiviral therapy is essential in such settings. Prophylaxis with HBIg monotherapy has been shown to be inferior to antiviral therapy owing to the inability of the HBIg to inhibit HBV replication.[29] In patients receiving lamivudine monotherapy, the incidence of de novo infections was found to be 2.7% as compared with 3.6% in patients receiving combination therapy with lamivudine and HBIg.[30] Thus, antiviral monotherapy can be used in the effort to prevent de novo hepatitis B infections in posttransplant patients.[31]

Hepatitis C

Recurrence of hepatitis C virus (HCV) infection after liver transplantation is one of the leading causes of graft failure. Recurrence rates of HCV are almost universal, occurring in more than 95% of transplanted patients with a prior diagnosis of HCV.[32] There is also an accelerated disease progression after graft infection, which results in a higher morbidity and rates in posttransplant patients compared with their nontransplanted counterparts. In the past, treatment options involved combination of interferon-based regimens and ribavirin, which have not been shown to improve patient or graft outcomes. Sustained virologic response in liver transplant patients with HCV reoccurrence treated with interferon/ribavirin-based regimens were shown to be roughly 30%.[33,34] However, studies with sofosbuvir-based therapies have demonstrated promising results in treatment of HCV infections. Sofosbuvir is a direct-acting antiviral agent that inhibits HCV RNA replication. Multiple studies have demonstrated superiority of sofosbuvir-based therapy when compared with the previous standard of care across all HCV genotypes.[35–38] Sofosbuvir-based antiviral therapy for recurrent HCV after liver transplantation has also been shown to have 85% to 91% sustained virologic response.[39,40]

COMMON FUNGAL INFECTIONS IN LIVER TRANSPLANTATION

Invasive fungal infections are frequently seen in liver transplant patients, with incidence ranging from 5% to 42% of transplant recipients. The most common fungal infections are attributed to *Candida* species, followed by *Aspergillus*, with associated mortality rates of 30% to 50% and 65% to 90%, respectively.[3] Endemic mycoses owing to *Histoplasma capsulatum*, *Coccidiodes immitis*, and *Blastomyces dermatitidis* may also occur in liver recipients from endemic regions. Last, prolonged immunosuppression after liver transplants can also lead to opportunistic infections, including *Pneumocystis jirovecii*-associated pneumonitis. However, the use of prophylactic antibiotics, such as trimethoprim-sulfamethoxazole, within the first year after transplantation has significantly reduced the incidence of *Pneumocystis* infections in this population.[3,41]

Candida Species

Infections owing to *Candida* species—*Candida albicans, C glabrata*, and *C tropicalis*—are the most common invasive fungal infections among liver transplant recipients, accounting for 30% to 50% of all invasive fungal infections in this population.[3] Candida infections are associated with complicated surgical procedures, including reexploration, retransplantation, and large blood product transfusion requirements.[42] Early in the postoperative period, *Candida* species may cause surgical wound infections, leading to candidemia, peritonitis, hepatic and abdominal abscesses, endophthalmitis, esophagitis, and urinary tract infections.[43] The overall mortality associated with invasive fungal infections can be as high as 77%.[44] As mentioned, CMV infections have also been shown to increase the risk of invasive fungal infections. Thus, effective CMV prophylaxis among high-risk patients significantly decreases the incidence of invasive *Candida* infection.[20]

Current recommendations support antifungal prophylaxis against *Candida* in high-risk liver recipients.[43,45] Duration of prophylaxis is not well-defined, but should be given for at least 7 to 14 days.[20] Fluconazole, echinocandins, and amphotericin are all possible therapies used for targeted prophylaxis. However, echinocandins are becoming the leading choice given the increase rates of fluconazole-resistant *Candida* species, as well as their lack of interaction with calcineurin inhibitors.[20,44] Antifungal prophylaxis in high-risk patients has reduced the incidence of fungal infections; however, a metaanalysis has not shown any improvement in overall mortality.[46] Treatment of invasive candidiasis after liver transplantation requires combination of antifungal therapy, elimination of the source of infection, and reduction of immunosuppression whenever possible. The reduction of immunosuppression should be balanced against the risk of graft rejection.

Aspergillus Species

Aspergillus is the second most common fungal infection observed after liver transplantation. It is often seen within the first month after transplant and can be life threatening. The most common Aspergillus species include *Aspergillus fumigatus* (73%), *A flavus* (14%), and *A terreus* (8%).[47] Infection with these organisms is the result of the inhalation of airborne spores, which initially result in pulmonary infection, with subsequent extrapulmonary dissemination to virtually any other organ.[3] Risk factors for *Aspergillus* infections include prolonged surgery, excessive blood loss, retransplantation, steroid-resistant rejection, renal failure (particularly the need for dialysis), CMV infection, diabetes, and prolonged use of broad-spectrum antibiotics.[47] The overall 1-year survival in patients with invasive aspergillus infections is 35%. Survival is higher in patients with a single organ involvement, those diagnosed more than 30 days after transplantation, those without renal failure, and patients treated with antifungal agents such as voriconazole.[47]

Given the high mortality risk associated with *Aspergillus* infection, antifungal prophylaxis should be given for high-risk liver transplant recipients.[48] Currently, targeted prophylaxis is used most frequently during the initial hospital stay or for the first month after transplantation.[49,50] Similar to infections associated with *Candida* species, prophylaxis can decrease the incidence of superficial and invasive fungal infections, however it does not reduced the overall mortality.[46,50]

The current guidelines recommend voriconazole as first-line choice for the treatment of invasive aspergillosis owing to associated higher response rates, improved survival, and fewer severe side effects when compared with amphotericin B.[47,48] Lipid formulations of amphotericin B can be used as second-line therapy.[48] Echinocandins are also effective for treatment, but they have been used mainly as salvage therapy for invasive aspergillosis.[3,20,48] The Infectious Disease Society of America recommends combination antifungal regimens as salvage therapy for nonresponsive cases of invasive aspergillosis, but the efficacy of this approach remains controversial.[43,48] Surgical excision or debridement remains an integral part of the management of invasive aspergillosis.

MALIGNANCIES ASSOCIATED WITH LIVER TRANSPLANTATION

The risk of malignancy is 2 to 4 times higher in transplant recipients compared with their nontransplanted counterparts. Cancer is expected to surpass cardiovascular complications as the primary cause of death in transplant recipients within the next 2 decades.[51,52] Recurrence of pretransplant cancers, including hepatocellular carcinoma (HCC) and cholangiocarcinoma, as well as de novo neoplasms can occur. At 10 years after transplantation, neoplasms account for almost 30% of deaths in this population.[51,53] This is in part owing to the long-term exposure to immunosuppressive agents, which increase the risk of malignancy.

Dermatologic Cancers

Skin cancer is the most common malignancy after transplantation, representing roughly 30% of all de novo malignancies. The most common type of skin cancer in this population is squamous cell carcinoma, followed by basal cell carcinoma and melanoma.[51] The most important risk factors include increased intensity and longer duration of immunosuppressive therapy, human papillomavirus infection, and a history of increased ultraviolet exposure.[54] Immunosuppression can lead to reduced immune surveillance and thereby facilitate the survival and proliferation of atypical cells. In addition, some agents such as azathioprine and cyclosporine have been shown to have direct carcinogenic effects.[55] Infections with human papilloma virus, Merkel cell polyomavirus, and human herpes viruses have also been shown to contribute to the development of squamous cell carcinoma, Merkel cell carcinoma, and Kaposi sarcoma, respectively.[56,57] Prevention strategies include routine dermatologic examination, protection from sunlight exposure with sunscreen and protective clothing, and modulation of immunosuppressive therapy. Interestingly, regimens that include mammalian target of rapamycin inhibitors, such as sirolimus and everolimus, rather than calcineurin inhibitors have been shown to reduce the risk for skin cancer and prolong the time to onset in kidney transplant recipients.[58]

Hematologic Cancers

PTLD encompasses a heterogeneous group of diseases characterized by excessive proliferation of lymphoid cells. Liver transplant recipients have an intermediate risk of PTLD. The pathogenesis of PTLD is multifactorial. Primarily, it is associated with infection or reactivation of EBV, especially in seronegative recipients from seropositive donors.[59] Other viruses, such as HCV, have been observed more frequently in liver transplant recipients who develop PTLD as compared with those who are not infected.[60] HCV is thought to induce clonal expansion of B lymphocytes and it has been associated with extrahepatic lymphoproliferative disorders. Other risk factors for the development of PTLD include increased intensity of immunosuppression and the use of certain immunosuppressive agents, including muromonab-CD3 (OKT3) and cyclosporine. Surveillance for PTLD via measurement of EBV DNA has been proposed. Progressively increasing EBV DNA should prompt investigation for PTLD by physical examination, imaging, and excisional biopsy of any suspicious lymph nodes.

Treatment options for established PTLD include reduction of immunosuppression, targeting of B cells with monoclonal antibodies, and chemotherapy.[61] Preemptive therapy with antiviral therapy including ganciclovir and valganciclovir has been shown to reduce the incidence of PTLD in pediatric EBV-seronegative solid organ transplant recipients.[62]

Hepatocellular Carcinoma Recurrence

Liver transplantation is the most effective treatment option for the treatment of HCC. The 5-year disease-free survival rate after liver transplantation is estimated to be 60% to 80%.[63] Recurrence of HCC after liver transplantation is associated with a worse prognosis.[64] Risk factors for HCC recurrence after transplant include increased preoperative serum alpha-fetoprotein levels, advanced tumor stage, and evidence of angiolymphatic invasion. The immunosuppressive agent of choice can also affect HCC recurrence rates. The calcineurin inhibitors cyclosporine and tacrolimus have shown to have a dose-dependent increase in the risk of HCC recurrence.[65] Other studies have suggested a reduction in the risk of HCC recurrence with the use of mammalian target of rapamycin inhibitors.[66,67] However, mammalian target of rapamycin inhibitors are associated with an increased risk of rejection, hepatic artery thrombosis, and impaired wound healing, as compared with calcineurin inhibitors.[68]

DIFFERENCES IN POSTTRANSPLANT INFECTIONS AND MALIGNANCIES BETWEEN LIVER AND KIDNEY TRANSPLANT RECIPIENTS

Similar to liver transplantation, postoperative infections cause the majority of morbidity and mortality associated with renal transplantation. Most of the life-threatening infections occur in the first 6 months after transplantation, owing to postoperative complications as well as high levels of immunosuppression early in the postoperative period.[69,70] The most common infections after renal transplantation include urinary tract infection (50%–75%), lower respiratory tract infection (9%), and diarrheal illnesses.[71,72] **Table 3** lists common causative agents responsible for urinary, respiratory, and gastrointestinal infection after renal transplantation.

Table 3
Common infections and causative agents in renal transplants

Urinary Tract Infection	Respiratory Tract Infections	Gastrointestinal Infection
Enterobacteriaceae spp (including ESBL)	*Staphylococcus aureus* (MRSA)	*Escherichia coli*
Pseudomonas aeruginosa	*Streptococcal* spp	*Clostridium difficile*
CMV	VRE	Shigella
Type 1 human polyomavirus (BKV)	*Legionella* spp	Salmonella
	Chlamydophila pneumonia	*Yersinia* species
	CMV	CMV
	RSV	Cryptosporidia
	Influenza and parainfluenza viruses	Microsporidia
	Pneumocystis jirovecii	
	Candida albicans	
	Aspergillus fumigatus	
	Histoplasmosis	

Abbreviations: CMV, cytomegalovirus; ESBL, extended spectrum beta-lactamase; MRSA, methicillin-resistant *Staphylococcus aureus*; RSV, respiratory syncytial virus; VRE, vancomycin-resistant enterococcus.

Malignancy is the third most common cause of death in renal transplant recipients. This is partly owing to chronic immunosuppression, which can impair immune surveillance. Similar to liver transplantation, nonmelanoma skin cancers account for the majority of malignancies after renal transplantation (40%–53%). Kaposi sarcoma, thought to be caused by reactivation of human herpesvirus 8, can also be commonly seen after renal transplantation.[73] In addition, the incidence of Kaposi sarcoma in transplant recipients may be as high as 500 times that in healthy individuals.[74] Renal transplant recipients also have a 20-fold greater risk of developing PTLD, squamous cell carcinoma of the eye, and cancers involving the anogenital region as compared with the general population.

SUMMARY

Infectious complications and the development of malignancies remain important causes of morbidity and mortality among liver transplant recipients. Infectious complications can be reduced dramatically with early detection and use of perioperative prophylactic antimicrobials. Mortality associated with malignancies can be reduced with vigilant surveillance, early detection, and modulation of immunosuppressive agents as appropriate.

REFERENCES

1. Moreno R, Berenguer M. Post-liver transplantation medical complications. Ann Hepatol 2006;5(2):77–85.
2. Moon DB, Lee SG. Liver transplantation. Gut Liver 2009;3(3):145–65.
3. Romero FA, Razonable RR. Infections in liver transplant recipients. World J Hepatol 2011;3(4):83–92.
4. Moreno A, Cervera C, Gavalda J, et al. Bloodstream infections among transplant recipients: results of a nationwide surveillance in Spain. Am J Transplant 2007; 7(11):2579–86.
5. Bert F, Larroque B, Paugam-Burtz C, et al. Microbial epidemiology and outcome of bloodstream infections in liver transplant recipients: an analysis of 259 episodes. Liver Transpl 2010;16(3):393–401.
6. del Pozo JL. Update and actual trends on bacterial infections following liver transplantation. World J Gastroenterol 2008;14(32):4977–83.
7. Kawecki D, Chmura A, Pacholczyk M, et al. Bacterial infections in the early period after liver transplantation: etiological agents and their susceptibility. Med Sci Monit 2009;15(12):Cr628–37.
8. Garzoni C. Multiply resistant gram-positive bacteria methicillin-resistant, vancomycin-intermediate and vancomycin-resistant Staphylococcus aureus (MRSA, VISA, VRSA) in solid organ transplant recipients. Am J Transplant 2009;9(Suppl 4):S41–9.
9. van Delden C, Blumberg EA. Multidrug resistant gram-negative bacteria in solid organ transplant recipients. Am J Transplant 2009;9(Suppl 4):S27–34.
10. Munoz P. Multiply resistant gram-positive bacteria: vancomycin-resistant enterococcus in solid organ transplant recipients. Am J Transplant 2009;9(Suppl 4): S50–6.
11. Hellinger WC, Crook JE, Heckman MG, et al. Surgical site infection after liver transplantation: risk factors and association with graft loss or death. Transplantation 2009;87(9):1387–93.

12. Freire MP, Soares Oshiro IC, Bonazzi PR, et al. Surgical site infections in liver transplant recipients in the model for end-stage liver disease era: an analysis of the epidemiology, risk factors, and outcomes. Liver Transpl 2013;19(9):1011–9.

13. Chelala L, Kovacs CS, Taege AJ, et al. Common infectious complications of liver transplant. Cleve Clin J Med 2015;82(11):773–84.

14. Kim SI. Bacterial infection after liver transplantation. World J Gastroenterol 2014; 20(20):6211–20.

15. Singh N, Wagener MM, Obman A, et al. Bacteremias in liver transplant recipients: shift toward gram-negative bacteria as predominant pathogens. Liver Transpl 2004;10(7):844–9.

16. Al-Hasan MN, Razonable RR, Eckel-Passow JE, et al. Incidence rate and outcome of Gram-negative bloodstream infection in solid organ transplant recipients. Am J Transplant 2009;9(4):835–43.

17. Shi SH, Kong HS, Xu J, et al. Multidrug resistant gram-negative bacilli as predominant bacteremic pathogens in liver transplant recipients. Transpl Infect Dis 2009; 11(5):405–12.

18. Fishman JA. Infection in solid-organ transplant recipients. N Engl J Med 2007; 357(25):2601–14.

19. Razonable RR, Emery VC. Management of CMV infection and disease in transplant patients. 27-29 February 2004. Herpes 2004;11(3):77–86.

20. Hernandez Mdel P, Martin P, Simkins J. Infectious complications after liver transplantation. Gastroenterol Hepatol 2015;11(11):741–53.

21. Bodro M, Sabe N, Llado L, et al. Prophylaxis versus preemptive therapy for cytomegalovirus disease in high-risk liver transplant recipients. Liver Transpl 2012; 18(9):1093–9.

22. Hodson EM, Jones CA, Webster AC, et al. Antiviral medications to prevent cytomegalovirus disease and early death in recipients of solid-organ transplants: a systematic review of randomised controlled trials. Lancet 2005;365(9477): 2105–15.

23. Ljungman P, Griffiths P, Paya C. Definitions of cytomegalovirus infection and disease in transplant recipients. Clin Infect Dis 2002;34(8):1094–7.

24. Beam E, Razonable RR. Cytomegalovirus in solid organ transplantation: epidemiology, prevention, and treatment. Curr Infect Dis Rep 2012;14(6):633–41.

25. George MJ, Snydman DR, Werner BG, et al. The independent role of cytomegalovirus as a risk factor for invasive fungal disease in orthotopic liver transplant recipients. Boston Center for Liver Transplantation CMVIG-Study Group. Cytogam, MedImmune, Inc. Gaithersburg, Maryland. Am J Med 1997;103(2):106–13.

26. Azevedo LS, Pierrotti LC, Abdala E, et al. Cytomegalovirus infection in transplant recipients. Clinics (Sao Paulo) 2015;70(7):515–23.

27. Maiwall R, Kumar M. Prevention and treatment of recurrent hepatitis B after liver transplantation. J Clin Transl Hepatol 2016;4(1):54–65.

28. Chien RN, Liaw YF. Nucleos(t)ide analogues for hepatitis B virus: strategies for long-term success. Best Pract Res Clin Gastroenterol 2008;22(6):1081–92.

29. Roche B, Roque-Afonso AM, Sebagh M, et al. Escape hepatitis B virus mutations in recipients of antibody to hepatitis B core antigen-positive liver grafts receiving hepatitis B immunoglobulins. Liver Transpl 2010;16(7):885–94.

30. Saab S, Waterman B, Chi AC, et al. Comparison of different immunoprophylaxis regimens after liver transplantation with hepatitis B core antibody-positive donors: a systematic review. Liver Transpl 2010;16(3):300–7.

31. John S, Andersson KL, Kotton CN, et al. Prophylaxis of hepatitis B infection in solid organ transplant recipients. Therap Adv Gastroenterol 2013;6(4):309–19.

32. Dhanasekaran R, Firpi RJ. Challenges of recurrent hepatitis C in the liver transplant patient. World J Gastroenterol 2014;20(13):3391–400.
33. Berenguer M. Systematic review of the treatment of established recurrent hepatitis C with pegylated interferon in combination with ribavirin. J Hepatol 2008; 49(2):274–87.
34. Xirouchakis E, Triantos C, Manousou P, et al. Pegylated-interferon and ribavirin in liver transplant candidates and recipients with HCV cirrhosis: systematic review and meta-analysis of prospective controlled studies. J Viral Hepat 2008;15(10): 699–709.
35. Gane EJ, Stedman CA, Hyland RH, et al. Nucleotide polymerase inhibitor sofosbuvir plus ribavirin for hepatitis C. N Engl J Med 2013;368(1):34–44.
36. Kowdley KV, Lawitz E, Crespo I, et al. Sofosbuvir with pegylated interferon alfa-2a and ribavirin for treatment-naive patients with hepatitis C genotype-1 infection (ATOMIC): an open-label, randomised, multicentre phase 2 trial. Lancet 2013; 381(9883):2100–7.
37. Lawitz E, Lalezari JP, Hassanein T, et al. Sofosbuvir in combination with peginterferon alfa-2a and ribavirin for non-cirrhotic, treatment-naive patients with genotypes 1, 2, and 3 hepatitis C infection: a randomised, double-blind, phase 2 trial. Lancet Infect Dis 2013;13(5):401–8.
38. Jacobson IM, Gordon SC, Kowdley KV, et al. Sofosbuvir for hepatitis C genotype 2 or 3 in patients without treatment options. N Engl J Med 2013;368(20):1867–77.
39. Ajlan A, Al-Jedai A, Elsiesy H, et al. Sofosbuvir-based therapy for genotype 4 HCV recurrence post-liver transplant treatment-experienced patients. Can J Gastroenterol Hepatol 2016;2016:2872371.
40. Faisal N, Bilodeau M, Aljudaibi B, et al. Sofosbuvir-based antiviral therapy is highly effective in recurrent hepatitis c in liver transplant recipients: Canadian multicenter "real-life" experience. Transplantation 2016;100(5):1059–65.
41. Martin SI, Fishman JA. Pneumocystis pneumonia in solid organ transplant recipients. Am J Transplant 2009;9(Suppl 4):S227–33.
42. Silveira FP, Kusne S. Candida infections in solid organ transplantation. Am J Transplant 2013;13(Suppl 4):220–7.
43. Pappas PG, Kauffman CA, Andes DR, et al. Clinical practice guideline for the management of candidiasis: 2016 update by the Infectious Diseases Society of America. Clin Infect Dis 2016;62(4):e1–50.
44. Singh N. Fungal infections in the recipients of solid organ transplantation. Infect Dis Clin North Am 2003;17(1):113–34, viii.
45. Pappas PG, Silveira FP. Candida in solid organ transplant recipients. Am J Transplant 2009;9(Suppl 4):S173–9.
46. Cruciani M, Mengoli C, Malena M, et al. Antifungal prophylaxis in liver transplant patients: a systematic review and meta-analysis. Liver Transpl 2006;12(5):850–8.
47. Barchiesi F, Mazzocato S, Mazzanti S, et al. Invasive aspergillosis in liver transplant recipients: epidemiology, clinical characteristics, treatment, and outcomes in 116 cases. Liver Transpl 2015;21(2):204–12.
48. Singh N, Husain S. Aspergillosis in solid organ transplantation. Am J Transplant 2013;13(Suppl 4):228–41.
49. Singh N, Wagener MM, Cacciarelli TV, et al. Antifungal management practices in liver transplant recipients. Am J Transplant 2008;8(2):426–31.
50. Singh N, Husain S. Invasive aspergillosis in solid organ transplant recipients. Am J Transplant 2009;9(Suppl 4):S180–91.
51. Burra P, Rodriguez-Castro KI. Neoplastic disease after liver transplantation: Focus on de novo neoplasms. World J Gastroenterol 2015;21(29):8753–68.

52. Zhou J, Hu Z, Zhang Q, et al. Spectrum of de novo cancers and predictors in liver transplantation: analysis of the scientific registry of transplant recipients database. PLoS One 2016;11(5):e0155179.

53. Schrem H, Kurok M, Kaltenborn A, et al. Incidence and long-term risk of de novo malignancies after liver transplantation with implications for prevention and detection. Liver Transpl 2013;19(11):1252–61.

54. Berg D, Otley CC. Skin cancer in organ transplant recipients: epidemiology, pathogenesis, and management. J Am Acad Dermatol 2002;47(1):1–17 [quiz: 18–20].

55. Einollahi B, Nemati E, Lessan-Pezeshki M, et al. Skin cancer after renal transplantation: Results of a multicenter study in Iran. Ann Transplant 2010;15(3):44–50.

56. Arron ST, Jennings L, Nindl I, et al. Viral oncogenesis and its role in nonmelanoma skin cancer. Br J Dermatol 2011;164(6):1201–13.

57. Rangwala S, Tsai K. Roles of the immune system in skin cancer. Br J Dermatol 2011;165(5):953–65.

58. Euvrard S, Morelon E, Rostaing L, et al. Sirolimus and secondary skin-cancer prevention in kidney transplantation. N Engl J Med 2012;367(4):329–39.

59. Dierickx D, Tousseyn T, De Wolf-Peeters C, et al. Management of posttransplant lymphoproliferative disorders following solid organ transplant: an update. Leuk Lymphoma 2011;52(6):950–61.

60. Burra P, Buda A, Livi U, et al. Occurrence of post-transplant lymphoproliferative disorders among over thousand adult recipients: any role for hepatitis C infection? Eur J Gastroenterol Hepatol 2006;18(10):1065–70.

61. Kamdar KY, Rooney CM, Heslop HE. Post-transplant lymphoproliferative disease following liver transplantation. Curr Opin Organ Transplant 2011;16(3):274–80.

62. Hierro L, Diez-Dorado R, Diaz C, et al. Efficacy and safety of valganciclovir in liver-transplanted children infected with Epstein-Barr virus. Liver Transpl 2008; 14(8):1185–93.

63. Castroagudin JF, Molina E, Bustamante M, et al. Orthotopic liver transplantation for hepatocellular carcinoma: a thirteen-year single-center experience. Transplant Proc 2008;40(9):2975–7.

64. Welker MW, Bechstein WO, Zeuzem S, et al. Recurrent hepatocellular carcinoma after liver transplantation - an emerging clinical challenge. Transpl Int 2013;26(2): 109–18.

65. Rodriguez-Peralvarez M, Tsochatzis E, Naveas MC, et al. Reduced exposure to calcineurin inhibitors early after liver transplantation prevents recurrence of hepatocellular carcinoma. J Hepatol 2013;59(6):1193–9.

66. Vivarelli M, Dazzi A, Zanello M, et al. Effect of different immunosuppressive schedules on recurrence-free survival after liver transplantation for hepatocellular carcinoma. Transplantation 2010;89(2):227–31.

67. Schnitzbauer AA, Zuelke C, Graeb C, et al. A prospective randomised, open-labeled, trial comparing sirolimus-containing versus mTOR-inhibitor-free immunosuppression in patients undergoing liver transplantation for hepatocellular carcinoma. BMC Cancer 2010;10:190.

68. Abdelmalek MF, Humar A, Stickel F, et al. Sirolimus conversion regimen versus continued calcineurin inhibitors in liver allograft recipients: a randomized trial. Am J Transplant 2012;12(3):694–705.

69. Yalci A, Celebi ZK, Ozbas B, et al. Evaluation of infectious complications in the first year after kidney transplantation. Transplant Proc 2015;47(5):1429–32.

70. Anastasopoulos NA, Duni A, Peschos D, et al. The spectrum of infectious diseases in kidney transplantation: a review of the classification, pathogens and clinical manifestations. In Vivo 2015;29(4):415–22.

71. Becerra BJ, Becerra MB, Safdar N. A nationwide assessment of the burden of urinary tract infection among renal transplant recipients. J Transplant 2015;2015: 854640.
72. Hoyo I, Linares L, Cervera C, et al. Epidemiology of pneumonia in kidney transplantation. Transplant Proc 2010;42(8):2938–40.
73. Rama I, Grinyo JM. Malignancy after renal transplantation: the role of immunosuppression. Nat Rev Nephrol 2010;6(9):511–9.
74. Campistol JM, Schena FP. Kaposi's sarcoma in renal transplant recipients–the impact of proliferation signal inhibitors. Nephrol Dial Transplant 2007;22(Suppl 1):i17–22.

Anesthesia Management of Organ Donors

Victor W. Xia, MD[a],*, Michelle Braunfeld, MD[b,c]

KEYWORDS

- Organ transplant • Organ donor • Brain death • Ischemia and reperfusion injury
- Standardized donor management

KEY POINTS

- Most organs in the United States are procured from donation after neurologic determination of death (brain death), but organs from donation after circulatory death (cardiac death) and living organ donors are increasing.
- Physiologic derangements are common in potential donors: in order to maintain the viability of the organs for transplant, management should be started early.
- Expansion of the donor pool through the inclusion of extended criteria and high-risk donors addresses organ shortage but presents new challenges in donor management and organ transplantation.
- Ischemia/reperfusion injury in organ transplants is unavoidable; however, proper management can lessen the likelihood of postoperative graft failure and improve outcome.
- Standardized donor management has been shown to improve the number of organs transplanted per donor and the quality of the grafts.

INTRODUCTION

Worldwide, the shortage of suitable organs is the biggest obstacle for organ transplants. The discrepancy between need and supply of the suitable organs is wide and increasing. At present, organs for transplant in the United State are predominantly from donation after neurologic determination of death (brain death). To address this growing problem, the donor pool has been expanded to include organs from donation after circulatory determination of death (cardiac death) and extended criteria donors.[1] These organs theoretically have a higher risk of developing perioperative dysfunction, presenting unique challenges for donor management and organ transplantation. In

Disclosure: The authors have no commercial or financial conflicts of interest to disclose.
a Department of Anesthesiology and Perioperative Medicine, Ronald Reagan UCLA Medical Center, David Geffen School of Medicine at UCLA, 757 Westwood Plaza, Suite 3325, Los Angeles, CA 90095, USA; b Department of Anesthesiology and Perioperative Medicine, David Geffen School of Medicine at UCLA, Los Angeles, CA, USA; c Department of Anesthesiology, Greater Los Angeles VA Hospital, Los Angeles, CA, USA
* Corresponding author.
E-mail address: vxia@mednet.ucla.edu

addition, a large percentage of donated organs are not used for transplant.[2] Most unused organs are refused because of poor quality. Proper donor management has a potential to increase the number and quality of organs procured from donors.[3]

Because anesthesiologists play a key role in maintaining hemodynamic and physiologic stability of donors and preserving function in donated organs, it is important for anesthesiologists to understand the physiologic changes associated with organ donation and to provide proper care to the donors. This article discusses physiologic derangements of various organ systems associated with organ donation and the latest developments in management for organ donors before, during, and after procurement.

MANAGEMENT OF ORGAN DONORS BEFORE PROCUREMENT

Physiologic response to death is a complex process during which multisystem derangements are commonly seen. First, preexisting comorbidities or trauma may have caused severe damage to vital organs. In addition, the process of brain death results in physiologic derangements of various organ systems. If not managed properly, these derangements lead to severe injury to the organs, making them unsuitable for transplant. The proper management of organ donors should start in the intensive care unit (ICU) even before donation is being considered and should continue during the entire donation process until transplant. The goal of management before the declaration of brain death is to optimize the chance of survival. Once brain death is declared, the goal of donor management is shifted to preserve the viability of potential transplant organs. Physiologic responses in individual systems to death and recommended clinical management are discussed later (**Fig. 1**).

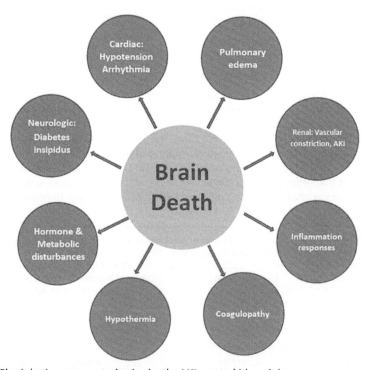

Fig. 1. Physiologic response to brain death. AKI, acute kidney injury.

Cardiovascular

The initial cardiovascular response to brain death is hypertensive crisis, which results from catecholamine release. This response is followed by persistent hypotension. The cause of persistent hypotension is multifactorial and includes loss of central sympathetic outflow, decreased cardiac output, blunted hemostatic responses, severe peripheral vasodilatation (vasoplegia), and hypovolemia caused by diabetes insipidus.[4] The initial hypertension can be treated with adrenergic antagonists such as esmolol, although this must be considered in concert with measures to decrease intracranial pressure to preserve cerebral perfusion.[2] Subsequent hypotension is usually first managed by fluid resuscitation with either normal saline or a balanced salt solution. Because starch-based colloids are associated with delayed graft function, they should not be routinely used.[5] When hemodynamic instability remains after adequate fluid resuscitation, vasoactive and/or inotropic drugs should be considered. Dopamine is usually the drug of choice in this setting. Vasopressin is increasingly used as a first-line or second-line agent in hemodynamic management, because it has been shown to have additional advantages, including improvement in vasodilatory shock, reduced requirement for catecholamines, and treatment of diabetes insipidus.[2,6,7] Norepinephrine is another commonly used vasoactive agent. However, norepinephrine in high doses is associated with posttransplant complications, including cardiac graft dysfunction and recipient mortality.[8]

Respiratory

Pulmonary injury is commonly seen in deceased donors. The increase in hydrostatic pressure in the pulmonary circulation as a result of increased systemic vascular resistance in donors can lead to pulmonary capillary leakage and pulmonary edema. Sympathetic activity triggers a systemic inflammatory response, initiating infiltration of neutrophils and lung injury. Hormonal instability reduces alveolar fluid clearance, resulting in significant accumulation of extravascular lung water and further lung injury.[9,10]

Current pulmonary management for potential lung donors favors lung protective management, which includes a small tidal volume (6–8 mL/kg), low fraction of inspired oxygen (Fio_2), high positive end-expiratory pressure (PEEP; 8–10 cm H_2O), and pulmonary recruitment maneuvers.[11] Management of acute respiratory distress syndrome in potential donors is the same as for other patients. Aerosolized terbutaline has been shown to increase alveolar fluid clearance via β-adrenergic stimulation.[12] A large amount of resuscitation fluid and/or high doses of vasopressors are associated with impaired graft function in potential lung donors and should be avoided.[9] Reversible processes, such as secretions, pulmonary edema, and atelectasis, should not be used as grounds for exclusion. Fluid restriction has been shown to increase the numbers of lung grafts available for transplant.[9]

Renal

Renal vasoconstriction is common in the setting of hypotension. Prolonged renal vasoconstriction can lead to acute kidney injury and renal failure. Diabetes insipidus, which is common and may occur in up to 80% of donors, leads to polyuria and can contribute hypotension. Vasopressin is often used in donors who require vasoconstriction. When vasoconstriction is not needed, desmopressin is the drug of the choice. Although liberal fluid administration may benefit renal grafts, recent guidelines support the goal of euvolemia in multiorgan donors.

Endocrine and Hormone

Brain death is frequently associated with disturbances of synthesis, release, and use of cortisol, thyroid hormones, antidiuretic hormone, and insulin. The development of central diabetes insipidus can result in severe fluid and electrolyte abnormalities.[9] Involvement of anterior pituitary function in brain death can lead to deficiencies in T3, T4, adrenocorticotropic hormone, thyroid-stimulating hormone, and human growth hormone. Hyperglycemia is commonly encountered in brain-dead donors caused by decreased insulin concentrations and increased insulin resistance. Hyperglycemia in donors is common and is exacerbated by steroid therapy. Poor glucose control adversely affects donor renal function.[13]

Early studies suggest that thyroid hormone replacement may increase the number of organs transplanted per donor.[4,14] However, the benefits of thyroid hormone supplement cannot be confirmed by recent studies.[2] Exogenous replacement of antidiuretic hormone in brain-dead donors has been shown to improve graft function in kidney, liver, and cardiac recipients.[9] Glycemic management should target a glucose level between 120 and 180 mg/dL by administration of insulin. Recently, a hormonal resuscitation package (steroid, vasopressin, insulin) was shown to improve not only organ retrieval rates but posttransplant patient and graft survival.[15]

Temperature

Hypothalamic function and regulation of body temperature are usually lost in brain-dead donors, with initial hyperpyrexia followed by hypothermia. Reduced metabolic rate and muscle activity in combination with peripheral vasodilatation contribute to persistent hypothermia. Normothermia (temperature >35°C) has traditionally been recommended before and during procurement. A recent trial suggests that mild donor hypothermia (34°C–35°C) in the ICU reduces delayed kidney graft function.[16]

Metabolic and Others

Polyuria and homeostatic changes can cause rapid changes to K^+, Mg^{++}, and Ca^{++}, leading to cardiac arrhythmias.[4] Hypernatremia is common in potential donors and may be associated with poor quality of donor organs. Donor hypernatremia is associated with poor transplant outcomes in liver (>155 mmol/L) and heart (>170 mmol/L).[17,18] Hypernatremia should be treated by therapy for the underlying cause (DI) and the administration of hypotonic solutions.[9] Correction of severe hypernatremia before procurement seems to attenuate posttransplant liver dysfunction.[9] One-third of brain-dead donors present with coagulopathy, which is thought to be caused by the release of tissue thromboplastin from brain tissue.[10]

A systemic inflammatory response, characterized by vasodilatation and tachycardia, together with cytokine elaboration and leukocyte migration from the intravascular space into solid organ parenchyma, occur often in donors. It is associated with graft failure and recipient mortality. Methylprednisolone can reduce the inflammatory response, modulate immune function, and improve organ quality and organ yield.[2] However, some studies fail to show benefits of steroid replacement therapy.[3,4]

Donors with Extended Criteria

Extended criteria donors have been increasingly used. Although the precise definition of an extended criteria donor has not been specified, it is generally thought that donors with advanced age, long ischemia time, preexisting comorbidities, steatosis (for liver donors), and donation after cardiac death are high risks for adverse outcomes. In addition to the increased postoperative risks (delayed graft function, higher incidence of immune-mediated rejection), extended criteria donors are associated with intraoperative complications and have implications for perioperative management.[19] In liver transplants, extended criteria donors may be associated with a higher incidence of intraoperative hyperkalemia, postreperfusion syndrome, intraoperative bleeding, and postoperative reoperation.[20,21]

Organs from Donation After Cardiac Death

Warm ischemia occurring during withdrawal of life support in donors after cardiac death can cause severe ischemia injury and microthrombosis in the donated organs. Administration of heparin before life support withdrawal reduces risk of thrombosis. Invasive premortem cannulation of the femoral artery and vein allows rapid infusion of cold preservation solution and possible extracorporeal membrane oxygenation after death. However, both techniques generate vigorous ethical debate.[9]

Standardized Donor Management

Standardized donor management with specific preset goals has been recommended by several international organizations.[3] Evidence has shown that standardized donor management can increase the number of organs transplanted per donor and the quality of donated organs.[22,23] The goals of donor management are to maintain normal hemodynamics, volume status, cardiac output, oxygenation, ventilation, electrolyte balance, acid-based status, coagulation parameters, and normothermia in potential donors (**Table 1**).[2]

Among preset goals, 4 (central venous pressure [CVP], left ventricle ejection fraction, Pao_2/Fio_2, and serum sodium level) have been associated with organ yield. Other variables (age, serum creatinine concentration, and thyroid hormone therapy) were important predictors of the number of organ recovered.[14] Early achievement of these goals is important. Donors with 4 or more organs transplanted per donor have significantly more individual goals met at the time of consent. Efforts should focus on early management in patients with catastrophic brain injury until the intent to donate is

Table 1
Donor management goals

Clinical Points	Target Range
Mean arterial pressure	>60 mm Hg
Central venous pressure	4–10 mm Hg
Ejection fraction of left ventricle	>45%
Serum sodium level	<155 mmol/L
Vasopressors	≤1 (eg, dopamine ≤10 μg/kg/min)
Pao_2/Fio_2 ratio on PEEP = 5 cm H_2O	Pao_2/Fio_2 >300
Hemoglobin level	>7 g/dL
pH value from arterial blood gas	7.3–7.45
Glucose level	<150 mg/dL
Urine output over 4 h	>1 mL/kg/h

Data from Kotloff RM, Blosser S, Fulda GJ, et al. Management of the potential organ donor in the ICU: Society of Critical Care Medicine/American College of Chest Physicians/Association of Organ Procurement Organizations consensus statement. Crit Care Med 2015;43(6):1291–325; and Malinoski DJ, Patel MS, Daly MC, et al. The impact of meeting donor management goals on the number of organs transplanted per donor: results from the United Network for Organ Sharing Region 5 prospective donor management goals study. Crit Care Med 2012;40(10):2773–80.

known,[23] because achieving these goals is also associated with a higher organ yield.[22,23]

MANAGEMENT OF ORGAN DONORS DURING PROCUREMENT SURGERY

Anesthesia for organ procurement is required for brain-dead or living donors but not for donors after cardiac death. The goal of the anesthesia management for organ procurement in brain-dead donors is to preserve viability of donated organs. An additional goal of anesthesia management for living donors is the safety of the living donor.

MANAGEMENT OF BRAIN-DEAD ORGAN DONORS

Brain-dead donors arrive in the operating room already intubated and supported by vasoactive agents. The surgical field is established via a midline laparotomy with or without extended sternotomy. A cannula placed in the aorta is used to flush the organs with cold preservation solution. Ice is applied to the surgical field to cool the organs quickly. The organs are removed with their vascular structures following isolation in an order dictated by their susceptibility to ischemia, with the heart first and the kidney last. Spinal reflexes remain intact in brain-dead donors and can cause movements on surgical stimulation, therefore administration of neuromuscular blockers is desirable. Similarly, hypertension can occur because of intact spinal reflex and surgical stimulation, and can be managed by vasodilators, opiates, and anesthetics.

Maintaining hemodynamic stability during procurement can prevent further damage to the organs. Fluids and vasoactive agents can treat blood loss and hypotension. Vasodilators such as phentolamine or alprostadil (lung recovery) may be administered during cross-clamping with the goal of decreasing systemic vascular resistance and allowing an even distribution of the preservation solution. Bradycardia in brain-dead donors does not respond to atropine, so a direct-acting chronotrope such as isoproterenol should be readily available. Heparin is usually administered before aortic cross-clamping to prevent clot formation in procured organs. Pulmonary artery catheters and CVP catheters should be withdrawn before the heart or lung is procured. Communication between the surgical team and the anesthesiologist is crucial to ensuring optimal organ quality. As soon as the organs are perfused with the cold solution, mechanical ventilation and anesthesia care may be suspended.

MANAGEMENT OF LIVING ORGAN DONORS

Living donor organ transplant has several advantages. The transplant can be scheduled as elective surgery with minimal cold ischemia time. Furthermore, the graft is not exposed to the physiologic derangements of brain death before procurement. Many studies show that living donor organ transplant is associated with a better outcome compared with deceased donor transplant.[24–26] Potential disadvantages of living organ transplant include exposing healthy donors to medical risks, decreased quality of life, and adverse financial impact.[27,28] In the past, living donors were related to the prospective recipients. Over time, the numbers of living unrelated (mostly kidney) donors have increased significantly.[24,29] Paired or chain donation, which allows 2 or more recipients with incompatible living donors to exchange organs has been widely accepted. Similar to the expansion of deceased donor criteria, living donor criteria have evolved to include donors of advanced age and those with obesity.[30]

LIVING KIDNEY DONOR

Living donor nephrectomy is routinely performed via laparoscopy.[31] The left kidney is preferred because of easier surgical exposure and longer vascular supply. The patient is placed in a lateral position. The surgical procedure begins with mobilization of the kidney, with subsequent identification and dissection of the ureter, renal vein, and artery, and separation of the adrenal vein. After clamping of the vascular structures, the kidney is retrieved through a small incision. Donor nephrectomy is performed increasingly via a retroperitoneal approach. The advantage of a retroperitoneal approach is less manipulation of intra-abdominal viscera. Other techniques, including single-incision and robotic laparoscopy, have been reported.[31,32]

Anesthetic management using general anesthesia for laparoscopic donor nephrectomy is similar to that for other patients. Standard noninvasive monitors are usually sufficient. One or 2 large-bore peripheral intravenous lines are usually placed. Blood transfusion is rare. High intra-abdominal pressure reduces venous return and has been associated with postoperative renal dysfunction.[33] Avoidance of unnecessarily high intra-abdominal pressure and adequate fluid administration seem to be good strategies to preserve kidney function. Some clinicians advocate liberal fluid administration (10–20 mL/kg/h).[33] The surgeon may request administration of furosemide or/and mannitol during the operation. Intravenous heparin (3000–5000 IU) is often administered immediately before the renal vessels are clamped.

Postoperative pain can be managed with intravenous opioids in the early postoperative period, and later with oral opioids and acetaminophen. Nonsteroidal antiinflammatory drugs should be used with caution because of concern about their potential prostaglandin-mediated adverse renal effects. Postoperative epidural analgesia should be considered for open donor nephrectomy.

Donor nephrectomy does not seem to increase long-term mortality or end-stage renal disease in the general donor population. However, the likelihood of postdonation chronic kidney disease, hypertension, and diabetes is higher among certain subgroups, such as African American and obese donors.[34] It is thought that existing studies may underestimate long-term risks of the kidney donors because of their methodology.[35] A recently developed risk projection may provide better prognostic information for the potential kidney donors.[36]

LIVING LIVER DONOR

Accurate estimation of the donor liver volume and anticipated graft size before transplant is important because it helps to avoid small-for-size syndrome in the recipient and to preserve adequate remnant liver volume in the donor.[37,38] The left lateral segment or a total left hepatic lobectomy is generally enough to provide sufficient liver mass for pediatric or small adult recipients. Right hepatic lobectomy is usually required for adult-to-adult living donor liver transplant. Left hepatic lobectomy is surgically less complex compared with right hepatic lobectomy.[39] If 1 donor cannot provide sufficient liver mass, 2 donors can be used for 1 recipient.[40]

General anesthesia is required for living liver donation surgery. Two large-bore intravenous catheters are usually placed. Standard noninvasive monitors and arterial blood pressure monitoring are typically used. Placement of a central venous catheter depends on patient condition and anesthesiologist preference. Intraoperative hemodynamic changes usually result from blood loss and manipulation of the liver. As in hepatectomy for other indications, most blood loss occurs during transection of the liver parenchyma. With improved surgical techniques and equipment, blood loss during hepatectomy has been significantly reduced. However, intraoperative massive blood loss still occurs and is a major concern for anesthesiologists. Strategies to reduce blood loss and blood transfusion include the use of low-CVP (<5 cm H_2O) technique, cell salvage, and intraoperative isovolemic hemodilution.[41,42] There are potential drawbacks of the low-CVP technique, which include the risk of CVP catheter placement and difficulty reversing hemodynamic disturbances in the event of massive bleeding. At the authors' institution, CVP placement is rarely used for monitoring in donor hepatectomy. Because peripheral venous pressure may be used as a proxy for CVP, some clinicians use it to guide fluid management.

Most patients can be extubated at the end of donor hepatectomy and cared for in a non-ICU setting. Caution is needed in the use of intravenous analgesics and opioids because the remnant liver has sustained some degree of injury.[33] After the graft is removed, fluid overload should be avoided because it may impede venous return and result in congestion of the remnant liver.[33] Nonetheless, adequate perfusion of the remnant liver should be maintained.[33]

Postoperative pain control can be achieved by patient-controlled analgesia via an intravenous or epidural catheter. The use of epidural anesthesia in living donor surgery remains controversial. Similar to other upper abdominal surgeries, postoperative epidural analgesia provides better pain control, less sedation, and decreased incidence of respiratory infection and ileus compared with intravenous patient-controlled analgesia.[43] Despite these advantages, preoperative placement of a thoracic epidural catheter is completely avoided in some centers. The development of postoperative coagulopathy (decreased platelet counts and increased prothrombin time) in patients following donor hepatectomy is a main concern.[44–46] A recent study using thromboelastometry suggests that patients may have a prothrombotic state despite increased prothrombin time in the early postoperative period after liver resection.[47]

Although living liver donor hepatectomy is safe, a wide range of donor complications, including mortality, have been reported.[48,49] A multicenter observational study of 760 adult-to-adult donor hepatectomies reported that 40% of donors had complications and 19% had more than 1 complication.[50] Infection is the most common complication. Biliary complications such as bile leak or stricture can be difficult to treat, leading to prolonged hospital stays and the possibility of further surgery.[48] Right hepatic lobectomy is associated with a higher postoperative complication rate than left hepatic lobectomy because of the increase in surgical complexity and the larger resected volume.[33,49]

MANAGEMENT OF DONATED GRAFTS AFTER PROCUREMENT

Organs after procurement are traditionally preserved in a cold (4°C) solution. University of Wisconsin (UW) solution containing adenosine and a high concentration of potassium is most widely used. Histidine-tryptophan-ketoglutarate (HTK) solution, originally developed for cardioplegia and subsequently applied to organ preservation in Europe, has gained popularity in the United States.[51] The UW solution is associated with a greater potential for hyperkalemia during organ reperfusion (particularly with the liver). However, the graft is typically flushed with colloid before reperfusion; this decreases the likelihood of severe hyperkalemia. The HTK solution is reported to be associated with poor graft function in abdominal organ transplants.[52,53] There are organ-specific solutions, such as Perfadex (Vitrolife, Goteborg, Sweden) solution for the lung and Celsior (Genzyme, Cambridge, MA) solution for the heart. Although cold ischemia time should be minimized, accepted time limits vary for different organs. Generally accepted cold ischemia times are 24 hours for the kidney, 12 hours for the liver, 6 hours for the heart, and 4 hours for the lung. Although shorter storage time is preferred, a longer storage time allows transportation of the graft to the highest acuity patient over a longer range.

In addition to static cold preservation, hypothermic continuous perfusion has recently attracted clinical interest. Potential advantages of a continuous perfusion technique include a reduction in proinflammatory cytokine expression, decreased activation of adhesion molecules and migration of leukocytes, and decreased endothelial damage and swelling. Continuous perfusion is also thought to promote increased levels of ATP.[54] Recent data suggest that organs maintained with machine perfusion may have a lower incidence of delayed graft function, particularly in high-risk donors.[19] Another advantage of the continuous perfusion technique is that the function of procured organs can be assessed during storage and may potentially be modified with pharmacologic agents.[55–57]

REFERENCES

1. Klein AS, Messersmith EE, Ratner LE, et al. Organ donation and utilization in the United States, 1999-2008. Am J Transplant 2010;10(4 Pt 2):973–86.

2. Kotloff RM, Blosser S, Fulda GJ, et al. Management of the Potential Organ Donor in the ICU: Society of Critical Care Medicine/American College of Chest Physicians/Association of Organ Procurement Organizations consensus statement. Crit Care Med 2015;43(6):1291–325.

3. Mundt HM, Yard BA, Kramer BK, et al. Optimized donor management and organ preservation before kidney transplantation. Transpl Int 2016;29(9):974–84.

4. Westphal GA. A simple bedside approach to therapeutic goals achievement during the management of deceased organ donors–An adapted version of the "VIP" approach. Clin Transplant 2016;30(2):138–44.

5. Cittanova ML, Leblanc I, Legendre C, et al. Effect of hydroxyethylstarch in brain-dead kidney donors on renal function in kidney-transplant recipients. Lancet 1996;348(9042):1620–2.

6. Chen JM, Cullinane S, Spanier TB, et al. Vasopressin deficiency and pressor hypersensitivity in hemodynamically unstable organ donors. Circulation 1999; 100(19 Suppl):II244–6.

7. Plurad DS, Bricker S, Neville A, et al. Arginine vasopressin significantly increases the rate of successful organ procurement in potential donors. Am J Surg 2012; 204(6):856–60 [discussion: 860–1].

8. Mukadam ME, Harrington DK, Wilson IC, et al. Does donor catecholamine administration affect early lung function after transplantation? J Thorac Cardiovasc Surg 2005;130(3):926–7.

9. Dare AJ, Bartlett AS, Fraser JF. Critical care of the potential organ donor. Curr Neurol Neurosci Rep 2012;12(4):456–65.

10. McKeown DW, Bonser RS, Kellum JA. Management of the heartbeating brain-dead organ donor. Br J Anaesth 2012;108(Suppl 1):i96–107.

11. Mascia L, Pasero D, Slutsky AS, et al. Effect of a lung protective strategy for organ donors on eligibility and availability of lungs for transplantation: a randomized controlled trial. JAMA 2010;304(23):2620–7.

12. Ware LB, Fang X, Wang Y, et al. Selected contribution: mechanisms that may stimulate the resolution of alveolar edema in the transplanted human lung. J Appl Physiol (1985) 2002;93(5):1869–74.

13. Blasi-Ibanez A, Hirose R, Feiner J, et al. Predictors associated with terminal renal function in deceased organ donors in the intensive care unit. Anesthesiology 2009;110(2):333–41.

14. Malinoski DJ, Daly MC, Patel MS, et al. Achieving donor management goals before deceased donor procurement is associated with more organs transplanted per donor. J Trauma 2011;71(4):990–5 [discussion: 996].

15. Rech TH, Moraes RB, Crispim D, et al. Management of the brain-dead organ donor: a systematic review and meta-analysis. Transplantation 2013;95(7):966–74.

16. Niemann CU, Feiner J, Swain S, et al. Therapeutic hypothermia in deceased organ donors and kidney-graft function. N Engl J Med 2015;373(5):405–14.

17. Totsuka E, Dodson F, Urakami A, et al. Influence of high donor serum sodium levels on early postoperative graft function in human liver transplantation: effect of correction of donor hypernatremia. Liver Transpl Surg 1999;5(5):421–8.

18. Hoefer D, Ruttmann-Ulmer E, Smits JM, et al. Donor hypo- and hypernatremia are predictors for increased 1-year mortality after cardiac transplantation. Transpl Int 2010;23(6):589–93.

19. Tso PL, Dar WA, Henry ML. With respect to elderly patients: finding kidneys in the context of new allocation concepts. Am J Transplant 2012;12(5):1091–8.

20. Xia VW, Ghobrial RM, Du B, et al. Predictors of hyperkalemia in the prereperfusion, early postreperfusion, and late postreperfusion periods during adult liver transplantation. Anesth Analg 2007;105(3):780–5.

21. Park C, Huh M, Steadman RH, et al. Extended criteria donor and severe intraoperative glucose variability: association with reoperation for hemorrhage in liver transplantation. Transplant Proc 2010;42(5):1738–43.

22. Malinoski DJ, Patel MS, Ahmed O, et al. The impact of meeting donor management goals on the development of delayed graft function in kidney transplant recipients. Am J Transplant 2013;13(4):993–1000.

23. Malinoski DJ, Patel MS, Daly MC, et al, UNOS Region 5 DMG Workgroup. The impact of meeting donor management goals on the number of organs transplanted per donor: results from the United Network for Organ Sharing Region 5 prospective donor management goals study. Crit Care Med 2012;40(10):2773–80.

24. Mandelbrot DA, Pavlakis M. Living donor practices in the United States. Adv Chronic Kidney Dis 2012;19(4):212–9.

25. Wolfe RA, Ashby VB, Milford EL, et al. Comparison of mortality in all patients on dialysis, patients on dialysis awaiting transplantation, and recipients of a first cadaveric transplant. N Engl J Med 1999;341(23):1725–30.

26. Olthoff KM, Smith AR, Abecassis M, et al. Defining long-term outcomes with living donor liver transplantation in North America. Ann Surg 2015;262(3):465–75 [discussion: 473–5].

27. Bachir NM, Larson AM. Adult liver transplantation in the United States. Am J Med Sci 2012;343(6):462–9.

28. Quintini C, Hashimoto K, Uso TD, et al. Is there an advantage of living over deceased donation in liver transplantation? Transpl Int 2012;26:11–9.

29. Freitas MC. Kidney transplantation in the US: an analysis of the OPTN/UNOS registry. Clin Transplant 2011;1–16.

30. O'Brien B, Mastoridis S, Sabharwal A, et al. Expanding the donor pool: living donor nephrectomy in the elderly and the overweight. Transplant 2012;93(11):1158–65.

31. Rocca JP, Davis E, Edye M. Live-donor nephrectomy. Mt Sinai J Med 2012;79(3): 330–41.
32. Pietrabissa A, Abelli M, Spinillo A, et al. Robotic-assisted laparoscopic donor nephrectomy with transvaginal extraction of the kidney. Am J Transplant 2010; 10(12):2708–11.
33. Feltracco P, Ori C. Anesthetic management of living transplantation. Minerva Anestesiol 2010;76(7):525–33.
34. Lentine KL, Patel A. Risks and outcomes of living donation. Adv Chronic Kidney Dis 2012;19(4):220–8.
35. Steiner RW. The risks of living kidney donation. N Engl J Med 2016;374(5): 479–80.
36. Grams ME, Sang Y, Levey AS, et al. Kidney-failure risk projection for the living kidney-donor candidate. N Engl J Med 2016;374(5):411–21.
37. Lee SG. Living-donor liver transplantation in adults. Br Med Bull 2010;94:33–48.
38. Tongyoo A, Pomfret EA, Pomposelli JJ. Accurate estimation of living donor right hemi-liver volume from portal vein diameter measurement and standard liver volume calculation. Am J Transplant 2012;12(5):1229–39.
39. Cherqui D, Soubrane O, Husson E, et al. Laparoscopic living donor hepatectomy for liver transplantation in children. Lancet 2002;359(9304):392–6.
40. Lee S, Hwang S, Park K, et al. An adult-to-adult living donor liver transplant using dual left lobe grafts. Surgery 2001;129(5):647–50.
41. Ryu HG, Nahm FS, Sohn HM, et al. Low central venous pressure with milrinone during living donor hepatectomy. Am J Transplant 2010;10(4):877–82.
42. Kim YK, Chin JH, Kang SJ, et al. Association between central venous pressure and blood loss during hepatic resection in 984 living donors. Acta Anaesthesiol Scand 2009;53(5):601–6.
43. Clarke H, Chandy T, Srinivas C, et al. Epidural analgesia provides better pain management after live liver donation: a retrospective study. Liver Transpl 2011; 17(3):315–23.
44. Choi SJ, Gwak MS, Ko JS, et al. The changes in coagulation profile and epidural catheter safety for living liver donors: a report on 6 years of our experience. Liver Transpl 2007;13(1):62–70.
45. Adachi T. Anesthetic principles in living-donor liver transplantation at Kyoto University Hospital: experiences of 760 cases. J Anesth 2003;17(2):116–24.
46. Cerutti E, Stratta C, Romagnoli R, et al. Thromboelastogram monitoring in the perioperative period of hepatectomy for adult living liver donation. Liver Transpl 2004;10(2):289–94.
47. Mallett SV, Sugavanam A, Krzanicki DA, et al. Alterations in coagulation following major liver resection. Anaesthesia 2016;71(6):657–68.
48. Abecassis MM, Fisher RA, Olthoff KM, et al. Complications of living donor hepatic lobectomy–a comprehensive report. Am J Transplant 2012;12(5):1208–17.
49. Iida T, Ogura Y, Oike F, et al. Surgery-related morbidity in living donors for liver transplantation. Transplant 2010;89(10):1276–82.
50. Middleton PF, Duffield M, Lynch SV, et al. Living donor liver transplantation–adult donor outcomes: a systematic review. Liver Transpl 2006;12(1):24–30.
51. Fridell JA, Mangus RS, Tector AJ. Clinical experience with histidine-tryptophan-ketoglutarate solution in abdominal organ preservation: a review of recent literature. Clin Transplant 2009;23(3):305–12.
52. Stewart ZA, Cameron AM, Singer AL, et al. Histidine-tryptophan-ketoglutarate (HTK) is associated with reduced graft survival in deceased donor livers, especially those donated after cardiac death. Am J Transplant 2009;9(2):286–93.

53. Stewart ZA, Lonze BE, Warren DS, et al. Histidine-tryptophan-ketoglutarate (HTK) is associated with reduced graft survival of deceased donor kidney transplants. Am J Transplant 2009;9(5):1048–54.
54. Henry SD, Nachber E, Tulipan J, et al. Hypothermic machine preservation reduces molecular markers of ischemia/reperfusion injury in human liver transplantation. Am J Transplant 2012;12:2477–86.
55. Jeevanandam V. Improving donor organ function–cold to warm preservation. World J Surg 2010;34(4):628–31.
56. Eltzschig HK, Eckle T. Ischemia and reperfusion–from mechanism to translation. Nat Med 2011;17(11):1391–401.
57. Zhai Y, Busuttil RW, Kupiec-Weglinski JW. Liver ischemia and reperfusion injury: new insights into mechanisms of innate-adaptive immune-mediated tissue inflammation. Am J Transplant 2011;11(8):1563–9.

Transfusion Medicine and Coagulation Management in Organ Transplantation

Jaswanth Madisetty, MD*, Cynthia Wang, MD

KEYWORDS

- ROTEM • Thromboelastography • Transfusion • Blood conservation
- Organ transplantation • Coagulopathy

KEY POINTS

- Blood product conservation has become increasingly important in organ transplantation.
- Improved outcomes are seen with less blood transfusion.
- New methods of assessing and managing coagulopathy have yielded significant reductions in transfused products.
- Rotational thromboelastometry is increasingly used to aid in management of coagulopathy.

INTRODUCTION

The discussion of blood product use and transfusion medicine, particularly for surgical patients, is one that is constantly evolving. High-acuity patients requiring transfusion in and out of the operating room continue to present significant challenges to clinicians. As anesthesiologists, we make decisions and initiate transfusion therapy in dynamic clinical scenarios. The need to conserve available blood products and also avoid significant transfusion-related comorbidities must be taken into consideration when caring for these patients. Anesthesiologists routinely see increasingly older patients presenting for more and more complex surgical procedures. In high-income countries such as the United States and Western Europe, patients over the age of 65 receive more than 75% of blood transfusions.[1] Increased blood product administration is associated with a variety of potential complications, from increased durations of stay and increased infection risk, to even increased mortality in a variety of surgical patients, especially liver transplant and cardiac/pulmonary cases.[2–9] These risks are

Disclosure Statement: None.
Department of Anesthesiology and Pain Management, William P. Clements University Hospital, University of Texas Southwestern Medical Center, 5323 Harry Hines Boulevard, MC 9202, Dallas, TX 75390, USA
* Corresponding author.
E-mail address: Jaswanth.madisetty@utsouthwestern.edu

Anesthesiology Clin 35 (2017) 407–420
http://dx.doi.org/10.1016/j.anclin.2017.04.004   anesthesiology.theclinics.com

in addition to the usual concerns associated with transfusion including mismatch, transfusion-associated graft-versus-host disease, transfusion-related acute lung injury, transfusion-associated circulatory overload, transmission of infectious disease, and immunomodulation. Given the impact of end-stage organ failure, these complications can have a particularly pronounced effect in the transplant population. The need to reassess transfusion strategies is, therefore, very real, and, as anesthesiologists, our intraoperative decision making plays a key role. Efforts to curtail blood product use in the surgical patient have been met with success.[10,11] In the United States, a steady decrease in the number of transfused red cell units as well as the number of donated units has been seen for several years. Although we are to be lauded for reducing the overall number of transfused units, the decrease in donated units raises concerns about the ability of blood supply to withstand critical need in mass casualty situations.[12] Nevertheless, the decrease in supply makes judicious use of products ever more important. Overall trends in blood product use have shifted toward more conservative use of products as well as targeted, factor-specific replacement, especially in the management of more complex coagulopathies. Developments in point-of-care testing have helped in this effort.[13-15] Blood product supplies are finite, and the increasing numbers of patients among the organ transplant population with extensive transfusion histories can present challenges in finding suitable blood products for cases with significant anticipated blood loss. This, along with many of the aforementioned concerns, renders making efficient use ever more important in current and future practice.[16]

HEMORRHAGE

Identifying patients at high perioperative risk for significant hemorrhage is key to successful management. In liver transplantation, several factors have been identified as increasing the likelihood of transfusion. Contrary to what is often presumed, studies have yielded equivocal findings with respect to use of coagulation tests preoperatively to determine patients at risk for surgical bleeding.[17] Often, coagulopathy as reflected in conventional laboratory testing is not a predictor for severe intraoperative bleeding in the liver transplant population. This has much to do with the complex balance between procoagulants and anticoagulants in patients with end-stage liver disease. Severity of disease (as defined by the United Network for Organ Sharing status as well as Model for End-stage Liver Disease scores), preoperative hemoglobin level, operative time, surgical approach, level of surgical expertise, and degree of portal hypertension can all portend severe hemorrhage during the intraoperative course. In cardiac surgery, advanced age, higher complexity procedures, and low preoperative hemoglobin have been identified as higher risk for bleeding and transfusion.[18] For any type of transplant procedure, extensive history of prior surgeries leading to distorted anatomy and adhesions may, in itself, increase the risk for bleeding.

Historically, protocol-based management of severe hemorrhage has been the most widely practiced; most of these protocols are derived from management of trauma patients. Massive transfusion has often been defined as greater than 6 units of packed red blood cells (PRBC). In complicated thoracic organ and abdominal organ transplantation (particularly the liver), it is not unheard of to encounter hemorrhage that requires transfusion that is orders of magnitude greater than this. This can lead to what is known as the "lethal triad" that results from massive hemorrhage and transfusion: the progressive development of coagulopathy, metabolic acidosis, and core hypothermia.[19] Despite the assumption that whole blood may be the most sensible choice for transfusion in the setting of massive hemorrhage, component therapy remains the preferred methodology. Component therapy minimizes the potential for unnecessary exposure to transfusion risk and remains the most economical way to parse out blood bank resources.

Dilutional coagulopathy is commonly seen with high volumes of blood product transfusion. Physiologically, approximately 20% to 30% of clotting factor activity is necessary for appropriate coagulation to occur. Replacement of one blood volume with only RPBC can reduce the concentration of clotting factors to one-third of the original levels. Other sources of coagulopathy also prevail in the setting of massive hemorrhage and in the transplant population. These include hyperfibrinolysis, which is commonly seen in the liver transplant and cardiac transplant recipient, and consumptive coagulopathy, which is less frequently encountered, but is more often seen when massive hemorrhage and transfusion occur. This has led to the development of commonly accepted ratios of replacement of clotting factors, fibrinogen, and platelets. In the past, transfusion protocols with fresh frozen plasma (FFP) to red blood cell ratios of 1:2 and up to 1:4 or 1:6 have been followed, but data and trends have shifted in massive transfusion protocols toward more equivalent replacement of blood and plasma in severe hemorrhage.[14] This has led many centers to develop protocols that replace blood loss with the equivalent of 1:1 FFP:PRBC ratios in the setting of massive hemorrhage. In fact, in 2005, a symposium of surgeons, anesthesiologists, hematologists, transfusion medicine specialists, and epidemiologists at the United States Army Institute of Surgical Research resulted in a consensus to create guidelines for massive transfusion in severely injured patients to include 1:1:1 ratios of PRBC:FFP:platelets.[20–22]

Appropriate monitoring and management of hypothermia and acidosis can also temper the development of worsened outcomes in massive hemorrhage. Conventional laboratory tests including prothrombin time and partial thromboplastin time can be prolonged abnormally in the setting of hypothermia. Hypothermia impairs platelet function and platelet plug formation and can, in and of itself, precipitate hyperfibrinolysis. Acidosis, when it occurs in conjunction with hypothermia, portends poor outcomes. By one estimate, when the two coexist, mortality rates can be as high as 90%.[20,23]

For centers that have access to factor concentrates, the trend has been toward using targeted replacement therapy with prothrombin complex concentrate (PCC) or fibrinogen concentrate in lieu of FFP and cryoprecipitate to correct deficiencies in coagulation. Although PCC has been used conventionally to reverse the effects of warfarin in the setting of life-threatening bleeding or perioperatively, it has found a place in transplant surgery as an effective way to treat coagulopathy while minimizing or eliminating most of the adverse effects associated with blood transfusion. PCC is a 3-factor (factors II, IX, and X) or 4-factor (II, VII, IX, X) concentrate that contains clotting factors at 25 times the levels of normal plasma. In the United States, 4-factor PCC is available predominantly. In addition to clotting factors, PCC also contains the thromboinhibitors proteins C and S, rendering the mix of PCC a balanced mix of procoagulants and anticoagulants.[24] The use of PCC was first studied in cardiac and trauma patients with favorable results.[25,26] Many have validated the role of PCC in transplantation, particularly cardiac and liver procedures. Multiple studies have shown a positive effect in reducing blood product transfusion when the administration of PCC is guided by viscoelastic testing.[11,27,28] In cardiac transplant patients who receive PCC for warfarin reversal before surgery, studies have shown an overall reduction in blood product use.[29,30]

Fibrinogen concentrate, like PCC, is available as a lyophilized powder that can be reconstituted rapidly to deliver a precise dose. It allows for more targeted repletion of fibrinogen, because it is pure and, unlike cryoprecipitate, does not contain factor VIII, XIII, or von Willebrand factor. Many have demonstrated that it, too, helps to decrease overall blood product use in liver transplantation.[27,31,32] Evidence for fibrinogen concentrate in other transplant populations, including cardiac, remains sparse. When used under the guidance of viscoelastic testing results, the incidence of thromboembolic complications is not increased with factor concentrates.

MONITORING AND DECISION MAKING

Organ transplantation presents unique challenges to intraoperative management. Perfusion and preservation of organ functionality is of utmost importance, and transfusion decisions are targeted toward that goal. Careful management of transfusion is vital to the survival of the patient and of the graft. New technologies in coagulation monitoring have helped to streamline component use and avoid unnecessary transfusion.[14,33] Conventional coagulation studies require laboratory analysis that can require a significant amount of time, potentially delaying crucial intraoperative decision making. The time lag in receiving results can be upwards of 30 minutes, during which the clinical status may have changed significantly. Also, these tests are performed on plasma samples rather than whole blood and at standard temperatures rather than actual in vivo patient temperature. As a result, only a small component of the complex hemostatic mechanism is revealed, giving an incomplete picture of overall coagulation. Given that these tests are quantitative in nature, there is no insight to the qualitative aspect of clotting; platelet counts are a prime example: thrombocytopenia does not equate to thrombocytopathia, and vice versa. The consistency of conventional testing is also questionable, because each laboratory calibrates its controls differently. An International Normalized Ratio of 2.0 from one institution, for instance, may not be precisely reproducible at another hospital. Furthermore, tests like the International Normalized Ratio are calibrated on normal, healthy volunteers, not patients with end-stage organ failure requiring transplantation. Thus, the accuracy of some of these tests in a severely ill patient population may at times be called into question.[34,35] Given these shortcomings, the trend has been toward the use of tests that take into consideration the interaction of all factors in a whole blood environment, such as viscoelastic testing.

For thoracic organ and liver transplantation patients, point-of-care viscoelastic testing of whole blood is commonly used to assess complex coagulopathies. Thromboelastography (TEG) or rotational thromboelastometry (ROTEM; Pentapharm, Germany) have emerged as the preferred methods of coagulation analysis at many centers. Viscoelastic testing has been shown to have a high negative predictive value, allowing clinical focus to be directed toward surgical or mechanical sources of bleeding in the setting of normal values. The findings gleaned from viscoelastic tests can reflect specific deficiencies in the coagulation pathway, indicating whether factor repletion is necessary, platelet transfusion is needed, or fibrinogen levels are inadequate. This avoids the so-called shotgun approach, allowing practitioners to target transfusion therapy and minimize the risks and morbidities associated with massive transfusion. Evidence over years of using viscoelastic testing in guiding transfusion therapy has shown positive results, minimizing overtransfusion and volume overload in cases of massive hemorrhage.[36]

TEG has been available for many years. Its use was first described in the setting of trauma, then in cardiothoracic surgery. Significant application to major bleeding in liver transplantation population began in the 1980s.[33] In all populations in which viscoelastic testing was used, a significant decrease in blood product use was observed.

In more recent years, ROTEM has emerged as a popular method of viscoelastic testing. Both are similar in that they measure clot formation, strength, and dissolution through a continuously applied rotational force as it is transmitted to an electrome-chanical transduction system. As it gains popularity in the United States, it has long been the preferred device in Europe. ROTEM provides a specific assay to assess for fibrinogen deficiency (FIBTEM) that TEG does not show. It may be the reason that ROTEM-based transfusion algorithms more frequently lead to fibrinogen repletion whereas TEG-based transfusion algorithms are more likely to recommend plasma transfusion or factor repletion. Nevertheless, the two modalities are grossly similar in application and efficacy, differing largely only in the type of activator/agent used in each device. Neither takes into account the effect of vascular endothelium on coagulation.[37,38]

Using ROTEM results to guide therapy relies on the ability to interpret results accurately and rapidly. Results of initial testing can be available often within 20 minutes or less. The main parameters of ROTEM that are used for interpretation are clotting time (CT, in seconds), amplitude in millimeters 10 minutes after CT (A10), maximum clot firmness (in millimeters), and percentage decrease in clot firmness.[39] These values are derived from the tracing produced when whole blood specimen is oscillated on a pin in the cup apparatus. As the clot stabilizes, the shaft rotation is altered, which results in deflection of light shined on the mirror in the apparatus. The tracing produced is interpreted by the aforementioned values[40] (**Fig. 1**).

Rotational Thromboelastometry Values

- CT—time from when sample is placed in cup until clot formation (minimal amplitude of 2 mm).
- A10 (amplitude at 10 minutes).

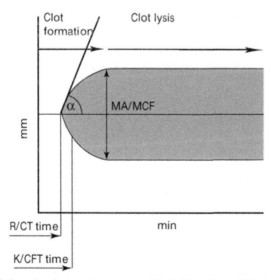

Fig. 1. Rotational thromboelastometry tracing. CT, clotting time; CFT, clot formation time; MCF, maximum clot firmness; α, alpha angle; MA, maximum amplitude; R, reaction time. (*From* Coakley M, Reddy K, Mackie I, et al. Transfusion triggers in Orthotopic liver transplantation: a comparison of the thromboelastometry analyzer, the thromboelastogram, and conventional coagulation tests. J Cardiothorac Vasc Anesth 2006;20(4):549; with permission.)

- Clot formation time—time for clot strengthening (amplitude from 2 to 20 mm).
- Maximum clot firmness (maximum clot formation)—greatest clot strength.
- Percentage decrease in clot firmness—percent clot lysis (over fixed time, often 30 minutes).

Several tracings are produced in standard ROTEM that correspond with different elements of the coagulation cascade. EXTEM, INTEM, and FIBTEM are generally the most useful tracings in making real-time intraoperative decisions in managing bleeding. EXTEM is a reflection of tissue factor–activated clot formation and corresponds with the extrinsic pathway. It has high sensitivity for detecting deficiencies in vitamin K–dependent factors. INTEM is contact activated and corresponds with the intrinsic pathway. FIBTEM incorporates tissue factor and a platelet inhibitor to assess fibrinogen levels and function. The introduction of FIBTEM has helped to identify hypofibrinogenemia more rapidly, allowing for earlier intervention. Tissue factor activation in EXTEM and FIBTEM tracings allows for more rapid results when compared with TEG.[39,40] **Fig. 2** demonstrates the correlation of ROTEM phases with various components of coagulation.

In terms of rapidly assessing ROTEM and making decisions on administration of products, some guidelines on ROTEM values can be useful. ROTEM requires precise calibration and quality assurance techniques to produce valid results and make reference ranges useful.

Generally speaking, increased CT correlates with vitamin K–specific factors and requires plasma. Formation of clot and maximum clot firmness correlate with platelet/fibrinogen levels and function. Fibrinolytic therapy is indicated when clot lysis is seen.[41]

In the setting of a low maximum amplitude (MA), indicating a lack of clot strength, both platelets and fibrinogen can play a role. Simultaneous evaluation of both INTEM and FIBTEM tracings can elucidate which component is necessary. It is suggested that if INTEM MA is low (<45 mm) in the setting of normal FIBTEM MA, then platelets be given versus fibrinogen replacement (**Box 1**).[40,42]

As mentioned, viscoelastic testing, when paired with the use of factor concentrates, has resulted in significant decreases in blood product requirements. Görlinger and colleagues[43] have developed algorithms for the safe administration of factor

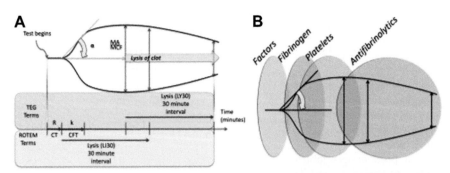

Fig. 2. (*A*, *B*) Thromboelastography and correlation with clotting components. CT, clotting time; CFT, clot formation time; Li30, lysis index 30 minutes after CT; MCF, maximum clot firmness; ROTEM, rotational thromboelastometry; TEG, thromboelastograph; TEG terms are: α, alpha angle; k, kinetics; LY30, lysis 30 minutes after MA; MA, maximum amplitude; R, reaction time. (*From* Pierce A, Pittet JF. Practical understanding of hemostasis and approach to the bleeding patient in the OR. Adv Anesth 2014;32(1):1–21; with permission.)

Box 1
Adapted guidelines for transfusion

1. If FIBTEM-A10 less than 10 mm, transfuse cryoprecipitate to treat fibrinogen deficiency; if greater than 10 mm, proceed to #2.

2. If EXTEM-A10 less than 40 mm, transfuse platelets if greater than 40 mm, proceed to #3.

3. If EXTEM-CT greater than 80 seconds, transfuse plasma or, if prior warfarin therapy, prothrombin complex concentrate.

Abbreviations: EXTEM, tissue factor activated clot formation and corresponds with the extrinsic pathway; FIBTEM, fibrinogen deficiency.
From Williams B, McNeil J, Crabbe A, et al. Practical use of thromboelastometry in the management of perioperative coagulopathy and bleeding. Transfus Med Rev 2017;31(1):13; with permission.

---

concentrates under the guidance of viscoelastic results in cardiac and transplant operations. Therapy was targeted to CT prolongation in the setting of heparin reversal and adequate fibrinogen levels. This was not associated with increased risk of thrombotic complications. Other investigators have adapted algorithms for use in trauma patients (**Fig. 3**). Until more specific protocols become widely available, many have used this protocol to manage massive hemorrhage.

Liver

Perhaps the most complex transfusion issues in organ transplantation are seen with liver transplants. Coagulopathy is quite common, and patients often present to the operating room with anemia; however, patients with end-stage liver disease are often hypercoagulable at the same time owing to increased levels of factor VIII. Physiologic stresses, whether it is an operation, a gastrointestinal bleed, or the development of renal insufficiency, can tip the balance of coagulation in either direction, rendering the patient more prone to bleeding on one end or at risk for thrombosis at the other. The nature and timing of these cases does not often present opportunities for optimization before surgery. Bleeding management and transfusion can be an ongoing challenge from the moment the patient enters the operating room. Blood loss during the case is variable and often depends on surgical technique and experience, with significant variability seen even between different surgeons in the same center. Center-to-center variability in blood product use in liver transplantation has also been noted.[17,44] Nonetheless, the assumption that massive hemorrhage is imminent is the safest and preparation of blood products in anticipation of significant bleeding is standard practice.

In many centers, it is commonly accepted that 10 units of RPBC and 10 units of FFP will be immediately available upon arrival to the operating room. Patients with severe cardiac disease are generally not considered good candidates for liver transplantation; thus, more liberal hemoglobin levels are tolerated and transfusion of chronically anemic patients at onset of surgery is targeted to maintain and hemoglobin of 7 to 8 g/dL. Replacement of coagulation factors may even precede red blood cell infusion if preoperative laboratory values indicate a need. However, aggressive correction of fibrinogen and thrombocytopenia should be approached with caution, particularly during the preanhepatic and anhepatic phases, because the risk for thromboembolic complications may be increased. Given the large volume shifts anticipated during the intraoperative period, crystalloid is usually minimized in favor of blood products and colloid solutions (primarily albumin). It may be preferable to use blood products that have a lower storage age. For high transfusion cases, using higher

Algorithm for Treating Bleeding Patients with Trauma-induced Coagulopathy

• Temperature • BGA • Electrolytes • Hematocrit	*Optimize preconditions*	Temperature >34°C pH >7.2 Calcium >1 mmol/L Hematocrit >24%
Severe trauma (ISS>16) and/or severe shock	*Treat (hyper)fibrinolysis*	TXA: 15–20 mg/kg BW

Run ROTEM (EXTEM, INTEM, FIBTEM, APTEM)*

① Focus on:
fibrin deficit

FIBTEM CA$_{10}$<7 mm

Reassess after treatment

Increase FIBTEM CA$_{10}$ to 10–12 mm
FC: FIBTEM CA$_{10}$ 0–3 mm: 6 g
   FIBTEM CA$_{10}$ 4–6 mm: 3–4 g

② Focus on:
thrombin generation deficit

EXTEM CT>80 s

Reassess after treatment

Treat coagulation factor deficiency
PCC: CT 81–100 s: 500–600 U
   CT 101–120 s: 1000–1200 U
   CT >120 s: 1500–1800 U
and/or
FFP: 15–30 mL/kg BW

③ Focus on:
platelet deficit

EXTEM CA$_{10}$<40 mm
(while FIBTEM CA$_{10}$ >12 mm
and platelet count <50,000/μL)†

Reassess after treatment

Increase EXTEM CA$_{10}$
Platelet concentrate

Severe clot deficiency

EXTEM CA$_{10}$<30 mm

Reassess after treatment

Treat immediately
TXA: 15–20 mg/kg BW
FC: 6–8 g
PCC: 20–30 U/kg BW
or FPP: 30 mL/kg BW
Platelet concentrate: 2 U

ROTEM may also identify:

Potential **heparin exposure** (e.g. cell-saver blood)	HEPTEM CT<INTEM CT	**Treat heparin effect** Protamine: 1000–2000 U
Clot instability not related to hyperfibrinolysis	both **EXTEM ML >15%** and **APTEM ML >15%**	**Consider** Factor XIII: 1250 U

Fig. 3. Rotational thromboelastometry (ROTEM)-guided treatment algorithm for trauma-induced coagulopathy. BGA, blood gas analysis; BW, body weight; CT, clotting time; EXTEM, tissue factor activated clot formation and corresponds with the extrinsic pathway; FC, fibrinogen concentrate; FFP, fresh frozen plasma; FIBTEM, fibrinogen deficiency; INTEM, contact activated and corresponds with the intrinsic pathway; ISS, Injury Severity Score; PCC, prothrombin complex concentrate; TXA, tranexamic acid. (*From* Grottke O, Levy JH. Prothrombin complex concentrates in trauma and perioperative bleeding. Anesthesiology 2015;122(4):925; with permission.)

storage age product may increase the risk for malignant arrhythmias owing to hyper-kalemia on reperfusion.[45] Discussion with surgeons and vigilance over conditions in the surgical field is key to decision making. It is not uncommon for technical difficulty with the portal vein or tension on the inferior vena cava to present with brisk bleeding requiring response during explantation. A difficult and bloody hepatectomy may also be anticipated if portal hypertension is severe and/or the patient has a significant history of prior abdominal surgeries. Regardless of predisposing conditions, the degree of transfusion therapy should always be linked to the results of laboratory testing and, most of all, the state of the surgical field.[46]

In the appropriate—that is, low Model for End-stage Liver Disease—patient population, attempts to reduce blood loss have been advocated in an effort to conserve products. As is commonly practiced in liver resection, some support the maintenance of a low central venous pressure (CVP; <10 mm Hg). If the patient can tolerate it, a CVP below 5 mm Hg is often a goal. Significant reduction in blood transfusion has been shown with low CVP maintenance during recipient explantation; however, other comorbidities have been shown to increase with this technique.[47] It is also prudent to note that the value of CVP monitoring has increasingly been called into question in the last decade. Multiple studies have suggested that CVP values have little correlation with actual circulating blood volume. As a result, many have moved away from relying on CVP values as a reflection of volume status.[48,49] Reevaluation of a low-volume methodology for blood conservation with other metrics for volume status, such as stroke volume variation, may be more informative.

Complex coagulopathy of liver disease is a well-known phenomenon,[33,50] with variable amounts of clinically significant bleeding and clotting dysfunction seen in patients regardless of their actual numerical laboratory values. For instance, patients with elevated International Normalized Ratio/partial thromboplastin time values may often present with thrombotic complications, making the picture unclear with respect to attempts at correction. As such, guidelines for management of patients with end-stage liver disease do not call for the routine correction of abnormal coagulation studies preoperatively, except in cases of significant active hemorrhage. Standard venous access for these cases can itself cause significant bleeding, because these patients are cannulated for jugular and/or subclavian access as well as large-bore peripheral intravenous and arterial lines. Intraoperatively, ongoing clinical assessment during dissection and laboratory analysis dictates transfusion strategy during the case. Significant blood loss can occur throughout the explant portion of the case, with transfusions in the 50 to 100 PRBC unit range possible. Given the complex nature of coagulopathy in these patients, ROTEM has become the standard point-of-care monitoring method at many institutions. Although guidelines for PCC use in liver transplantation have not been clearly delineated, we have seen positive anecdotal results with PCC use in patients who receive it. These patients receive fewer allogeneic blood products and have fewer postoperative complications overall.[51]

The anhepatic and reperfusion phases of liver transplantation present unique issues with coagulopathy. During the anhepatic phase, coagulation factor synthesis and clearance are lost. Fibrinolysis is likely to develop in this phase as tissue plasminogen activator is not cleared and plasminogen activator inhibitor levels remain.[50] A heparin-like effect has been identified during reperfusion. The donor graft can sequester platelets, whereas residual heparin from preservation solution is released systemically. Plasminogen activator inhibitor levels decrease and tissue plasminogen activator production increases, leading to an increased risk for of fibrinolysis.[50,52] These derangements require frequent testing and vigilance. Point-of-care testing should be used to target transfusion and direct antifibrinolytic therapy, should it be necessary (**Box 2**).

Box 2
Key points for liver transplant management

- Adequate blood products in the operating room.
- Watch the field.
- Communicate goals with surgeons.
- Baseline and ongoing laboratory analysis incorporating point-of-care coagulation testing.
- Avoid aggressive correction.

CARDIOTHORACIC

Heart and lung transplantation has increased worldwide,[53] with significant advances in ventricular assist device and extracorporeal membrane oxygenation technologies bridging more end-stage patients to the transplant phase. Blood product conservation in native organ cardiac surgery has been studied extensively with clear advantages shown for patients receiving fewer products.[10,54,55] The use of cardiopulmonary bypass helps with conservation by presenting a bloodless field, although patients often present with significant anemia as well as effects of standard anticoagulation necessary in the use of ventricular assist device and extracorporeal membrane oxygenation therapies.

Significant research and initiatives to reduce blood product use in cardiac surgery have yielded valuable results. This includes the implementation of bleeding management protocols guided by point-of-care testing as well as using a multidisciplinary approach to blood conservation.[10,43,54] Administration of drugs that increase blood volume preoperatively (erythropoietin) or decrease postoperative bleeding (antifibrinolytics), increased use of cell salvage, practicing normovolemic hemodilution, and the routine use of retrograde autologous priming of the cardiopulmonary bypass circuit are all valuable tools in conjunction with a clear delineation of transfusion triggers and goals. Not only have these methodologies resulted in decreased blood product use, they have led to improved overall outcomes and reductions in costs.[55]

KIDNEY

Renal transplantation remains the most commonly performed solid organ transplant in the United States.[53] Anemia is commonly encountered in these patients, leading to the need for frequent preoperative transfusions; however, routine transfusion during kidney transplantation remains rare in most practices. Most often, patients with end-stage renal failure are at risk for multiple transfusions in the pretransplant phase. Concern for alloimmunization from blood transfusion and its later effects of renal graft rejection has traditionally been a concern. However, a recent large metaanalysis sustains that pretransplant blood transfusions did not increase the risk of renal allograft rejection. In fact, many studies have found that the risk for allograft rejection was decreased in patients who received blood transfusions preoperatively. Likewise, the effects of transfusions on patient and graft survival were negligible. Along the same vein, the use of leukoreduced product has also not been shown to have a significant effect on allograft function, patient, or graft survival[56]

SMALL BOWEL

Many often assume that transplantation of the small bowel in isolation should not present as significant a risk of bleeding. Inherent coagulopathy is less likely to be seen without concomitant liver disease, and general hemostasis through control of major vessels is technically more likely to be feasible. However, these patients often present with a history of multiple prior abdominal surgeries, rendering their abdominal dissection surgically challenging and potentially bloody. Also, patients with long-standing intestinal failure requiring transplantation have often developed intestinal failure-associated liver disease. In many instances, the concomitant liver disease is severe enough to warrant a combined liver and intestinal transplant. Further complicating the bowel transplant population is that, more often than not, bowel transplants are performed in the pediatric population.

In 2015, a total of 141 intestinal transplants were performed. This group is composed of almost equal numbers of intestine-only and intestine-liver transplants. A recent study that compared matched groups of liver transplant versus combined liver and intestinal transplant patients found that the combined transplant group presented many more challenges than the isolated liver transplant group. The cold ischemia time, warm ischemia time, and surgical times were naturally longer in the combined transplant group. All of these factors can lead to an increased need for blood transfusion. In fact, the combined transplant group exhibited nearly double the incidence of massive transfusion (62%) when compared with the liver transplant only group (33%). This was accompanied by much higher rates of postreperfusion syndrome, hyperkalemia, and acidemia.[57,58]

COMPOSITE TISSUE ALLOTRANSPLANTATION

Face, hand, penis, and other organs are emerging as options for patients seeking composite tissue allotransplantation. These transplants involve multiple types of tissue, including bone, muscle, blood vessels, and nerves. Often, these transplants involve highly vascular areas that can result in massive hemorrhage and transfusion. A case report describing a face transplant, for instance, aptly points out that osteotomies and dissection of the midface may lead to severe blood loss. The face itself is a highly vascular organ, leading to massive bleeding during both dissection and reperfusion.[59]

Similar experiences have been described for hand transplantation. Centers often establish large-bore access in preparation for potential massive hemorrhage. Rapid infusion systems are recommended, because major bleeding can be anticipated when tourniquets are deflated. Unlike with abdominal organ transplantation, the liberal use of vasopressors is discouraged in composite tissue allotransplantation because perfusion through often tenuous microvascular anastomoses must be preserved. Thus, appropriate fluid resuscitation is of even more vital importance.[60]

REFERENCES

1. World Health Organization (WHO). Blood safety and availability. Geneva: World Health Organization. Available at: http://www.who.int/mediacentre/factsheets/fs279/en/. Accessed January 10, 2017.
2. Ramos E, Dalmau A, Sabate A, et al. Intraoperative red blood cell transfusion in liver transplantation: influence on patient outcome, prediction of requirements, and measures to reduce them. Liver Transpl 2003;9:1320–7.
3. de Boer MT, Christensen MC, Asmussen M, et al. The impact of intraoperative transfusion of platelets and red blood cells on survival after liver transplantation. Anesth Analg 2008;106:32–44 [Table of contents].
4. Cacciarelli TV, Keeffe EB, Moore DH, et al. Effect of intraoperative blood transfusion on patient outcome in Hepatic transplantation. Arch Surg 1999;134(1):25.

5. Weber D, Cottini SR, Locher P, et al. Association of intraoperative transfusion of blood products with mortality in lung transplant recipients. Perioper Med (Lond) 2013;2(1):20.
6. Goldaracena N, Méndez P, Quiñonez E, et al. Liver transplantation without perioperative transfusions single-center experience showing better early outcome and shorter hospital stay. J Transplant 2013;2013:649209.
7. Benson AB, Burton JR, Austin GL, et al. Differential effects of plasma and red blood cell transfusions on acute lung injury and infection risk following liver transplantation. Liver Transpl 2011;17(2):149–58.
8. Boin IFSF, Leonardi MI, Luzo AC, et al. Intraoperative massive transfusion decreases survival after liver transplantation. Transplant Proc 2008;40(3):789–91.
9. Real C, Sobreira Fernandes D, Sá Couto P, et al. Survival predictors in liver transplantation: time-varying effect of red blood cell transfusion. Transplant Proc 2016; 48(10):3303–6.
10. Ad N, Holmes SD, Patel J, et al. The impact of a multidisciplinary blood conservation protocol on patient outcomes and cost after cardiac surgery. J Thorac Cardiovasc Surg 2017;153(3):597–605.e1.
11. Donohue CI, Mallett SV. Reducing transfusion requirements in liver transplantation. World J Transplant 2015;5(4):165–82.
12. Whitaker B, Rajbhandary S, Kleinman S, et al. Trends in United States blood collection and transfusion: results from the 2013 AABB blood collection, utilization, and patient blood management survey. Transfusion 2016;56(9):2173–83.
13. Weber CF, Görlinger K, Meininger D, et al. Point-of-care testing. Anesthesiology 2012;117(3):531–47.
14. Pierce A, Pittet JF. Practical understanding of hemostasis and approach to the bleeding patient in the operating room. Adv Anesth 2014;32(1):1–21.
15. Borgman MA, Spinella PC, Perkins JG, et al. The ratio of blood products transfused affects mortality in patients receiving massive transfusion at a combat support hospital. J Trauma 2007;63:805–13.
16. Spiess BD. Blood transfusion: the silent epidemic. Ann Thorac Surg 2001;72(5): S1832–7.
17. Ozier Y, Pessione F, Samain E, et al. Institutional variability in transfusion practice for liver transplantation. Anesth Analg 2003;97:671–9.
18. Ferraris VA, Brown JR, Despotis GJ, et al. 2011 update to the society of Thoracic surgeons and the society of cardiovascular anesthesiologists blood conservation clinical practice guidelines. Ann Thorac Surg 2011;91(3):944–82.
19. Sihler KC, Napolitano LM. Massive transfusion: new insights. Chest 2009;136: 1654–67.
20. Wojciechowski PJ, Samol N, Walker J. Coagulopathy in massive transfusion. Int Anesthesiol Clin 2005;43(4):1–20.
21. Hess JR, Dutton RB, Holcomb JB, et al. Giving plasma at a 1:1 ratio with red cells in resuscitation: who might benefit? Transfusion 2008;48:1763–5.
22. Riskin DJ, Tsai TC, Riskin L, et al. Massive transfusion protocols: the role of aggressive resuscitation versus product ratio in mortality reduction. J Am Coll Surg 2009;209:198–205.
23. Brohi K, Singh J, Heron M, et al. Acute traumatic coagulopathy. J Trauma 2003; 54:1127–30.
24. Franchini M, Lippi G. Prothrombin complex concentrates: an update. Blood Transfus 2010;8(3):149–54.
25. Grottke O, Levy JH. Prothrombin complex concentrates in trauma and perioperative bleeding. Anesthesiology 2015;122(4):923–31.

26. Schöchl H, Nienaber U, Maegele M, et al. Transfusion in trauma: thromboelastometry-guided coagulation factor concentrate-based therapy versus standard fresh frozen plasma-based therapy. Crit Care 2011;15(2):R83.
27. Kirchner C, Dirkmann D, Treckmann JW, et al. Coagulation management with factor concentrates in liver transplantation: a single-center experience. Transfusion 2014;54(10):2760–8.
28. Görlinger K, Dirkmann D, Hanke AA, et al. First-line therapy with coagulation factor concentrates combined with point-of-care coagulation testing is associated with decreased allogeneic blood transfusion in cardiovascular surgery: a retrospective, single-center cohort study. Anesthesiology 2011;115(6):1179–91.
29. Enter D, Marsh M, Cool N, et al. Prothrombin complex concentrate reduces intraoperative blood product utilization in heart transplantation. J Heart Lung Transpl 2016;35(4):S293.
30. Nuckles KB, Pratt JH, Cameron CM, et al. Case series of four-factor prothrombin complex concentrate for warfarin reversal before heart transplantation. Transplant Proc 2015;47(3):841–3.
31. Rahe-Meyer N, Solomon C, Hanke A, et al. Effects of fibrinogen concentrate as first-line therapy during major aortic replacement surgery: a randomized, placebo-controlled trial. Anesthesiology 2013;118(1):40–50.
32. Noval-Padillo JA, León-Justel A, Mellado-Miras P, et al. Introduction of fibrinogen in the treatment of hemostatic disorders during orthotopic liver transplantation: implications in the use of allogenic blood. Transplant Proc 2010;42(8):2973–4.
33. Kang YG, Martin DJ, Marquez J, et al. Intraoperative changes in blood coagulation and thrombelastographic monitoring in liver transplantation. Anesth Analg 1985;64(9):888–96.
34. Ganter MT, Hofer CK. Coagulation monitoring: current techniques and clinical use of viscoelastic point-of-care coagulation devices. Anesth Analg 2008;106(5):1366–75.
35. Bolliger D, Seeberger MD, Tanaka KA. Principles and practice of thromboelstography in clinical coagulation management and transfusion practice. Transfus Med Rev 2012;26(1):1–13.
36. Cammerer U, Dietrich W, Rampf T, et al. The predictive value of modified computerized thromboelastography and platelet function analysis for postoperative blood loss in routine cardiac surgery. Anesth Analg 2003;96:51–7.
37. Sankaranutty A, Nascimento B, Teodoro da Luz L, et al. TEG and ROTEM in trauma: similar test but different results? World J Emerg Surg 2012;7(Suppl 1):S3.
38. Cacciarelli TV, Keeffe EB, Moore DH, et al. Primary liver transplantation without transfusion of red blood cells. Surgery 1996;120(4):698–705.
39. Williams B, McNeil J, Crabbe A, et al. Practical use of thromboelastometry in the management of perioperative coagulopathy and bleeding. Transfus Med Rev 2017;31(1):11–25.
40. Coakley M, Reddy K, Mackie I, et al. Transfusion triggers in orthotopic liver transplantation: a comparison of the thromboelastometry analyzer, the thromboelastogram, and conventional coagulation tests. J Cardiothorac Vasc Anesth 2006;20(4):548–53.
41. Mazzeffi MA, Chriss E, Davis K, et al. Optimal plasma transfusion in patients undergoing cardiac operations with massive transfusion. Ann Thorac Surg 2016. http://dx.doi.org/10.1016/j.athoracsur.2016.09.071.
42. Roullet S, Pillot J, Freyburger G, et al. Rotation thromboelastometry detects thrombocytopenia and hypofibrinogenaemia during ortho- topic liver transplantation. Br J Anaesth 2010;104:422–8.

43. Görlinger K, Dirkmann D, Hanke AA. Potential value of transfusion protocols in cardiac surgery. Curr Opin Anaesthesiol 2013;26(2):230–43.
44. Feltracco P, Brezzi M, Barbieri S, et al. Blood loss, predictors of bleeding, transfusion practice and strategies of blood cell salvaging during liver transplantation. World J Hepatol 2013;5(1):1–15.
45. Chen J, Singhapricha T, Memarzadeh M, et al. Storage age of transfused red blood cells during liver transplantation and its intraoperative and postoperative effects. World J Surg 2012;36(10):2436–42.
46. Cleland S, Corredor C, Ye JJ, et al. Massive haemorrhage in liver transplantation: consequences, prediction and management. World J Transplant 2016;6(2):291.
47. Massicotte L, Lenis S, Thibeault L, et al. Effect of low central venous pressure and phlebotomy on blood product transfusion requirements during liver transplantations. Liver Transpl 2005;12(1):117–23.
48. Marik PE, Baram M, Vahid B. Does central venous pressure predict fluid responsiveness? A systematic review of the literature and the tale of seven mares. Chest 2008;134(1):172–8.
49. Marik PE, Cavallazzi R. Does the central venous pressure predict fluid responsiveness? An updated meta-analysis and a plea for some common sense. Crit Care Med 2013;41(7):1774–81.
50. Clevenger B, Mallett SV. Transfusion and coagulation management in liver transplantation. World J Gastroenterol 2014;20(20):6146.
51. Wang, Cynthia. "Beyond blood products: prothrombin complex concentrate". 2015. ILTS perioperative care in liver transplantation. San Diego, October 23, 2015.
52. Agarwal S, Senzolo M, Melikian C, et al. The prevalence of a heparin-like effect shown on the thromboelastograph in patients undergoing liver transplantation. Liver Transpl 2008;14(6):855–60.
53. United Network for Organ Sharing (UNOS). Annual report. Available at: https://www.unos.org/about/annual-report/. Accessed January 10, 2017.
54. Pearse BL, Smith I, Faulke D, et al. Protocol guided bleeding management improves cardiac surgery patient outcomes. Vox Sang 2015;109(3):267–9.
55. Society of Thoracic Surgeons Blood Conservation Guideline Task Force, Ferraris VA, Ferraris SP, et al. Perioperative blood transfusion and blood conservation in cardiac surgery: the society of thoracic surgeons and the society of cardiovascular anesthesiologists clinical practice guideline. Ann Thorac Surg 2007; 83(5):S27–86.
56. Chen W, Lee S, Colby J, et al. The impact of pre-transplant red blood cell transfusions in renal allograft rejection. AHRQ technology assessments. Agency for Healthcare Research and Quality; 2012. Available at: https://www.ncbi.nlm.nih.gov/books/NBK253163/.
57. Song X, Farmer DG, Xia VW. Intraoperative management and postoperative outcome in intestine-inclusive liver transplantation versus liver transplantation. Transplant Proc 2015;47(8):2473–7.
58. Smith JM, Skeans MA, Horslen SP, et al. OPTN/SRTR 2015 annual data report: intestine. Am J Transplant 2017;17(Suppl 1):252–85.
59. Dalal A. Face transplantation: anesthetic challenges. World J Transplant 2016; 6(4):646–9.
60. Lang RS, Gorantla VS, Esper S, et al. Anesthetic management in upper extremity transplantation: the Pittsburgh experience. Anesth Analg 2012;115(3):678–88.

Anesthetic Management of Pediatric Liver and Kidney Transplantation

 CrossMark

Nicholas R. Wasson, MD[a],*, Jeremy D. Deer, MD[b],
Santhanam Suresh, MD[c]

KEYWORDS

- Liver • Kidney • Anesthesia • Pediatric transplantation • End-stage liver disease
- End-stage renal disease • Pediatric liver transplantation
- Pediatric renal transplantation

KEY POINTS

- Indications for pediatric liver transplantation may be due to not only to liver failure of varying causes but also due to an underlying metabolic or genetic syndrome, each of which may carry its own set of comorbidities.
- Each phase of the liver transplant procedure has its own unique risks, so careful preoperative planning and vigilant intraoperative management are crucial to the success of the procedure in a child.
- Renal dysfunction exhibits a profound effect on the body's ability to maintain homeostasis and associated comorbidities significantly affect quality of life and survival.
- Anesthetic management of the pediatric patient undergoing renal transplantation is centered on adequate fluid management, adhering to hemodynamic goals, and managing associated comorbidities.

 Video content accompanies this article at www.anesthesiology.theclinics.com.

INTRODUCTION

For the child undergoing organ transplantation, no one individual alone can provide the care sufficient for a successful outcome. It requires a multidisciplinary team to

---

Disclosure Statement: None.
[a] Pediatric Transplant Anesthesia, Pediatric Anesthesiology, Ann & Robert H. Lurie Children's Hospital of Chicago, Northwestern University Feinberg School of Medicine, 225 East Chicago Avenue, Box 19, Chicago, IL 60611, USA; [b] Pediatric Anesthesiology, Ann & Robert H. Lurie Children's Hospital of Chicago, Feinberg School of Medicine, Northwestern University, 225 East Chicago Avenue, Box 19, Chicago, IL 60611-2605, USA; [c] Department of Pediatric Anesthesiology, Ann & Robert H. Lurie Children's Hospital of Chicago, Northwestern University's Feinberg School of Medicine, 225 East Chicago Avenue, Box 19, Chicago, IL 60611-2605, USA
* Corresponding author.
E-mail address: nwasson@luriechildrens.org

Anesthesiology Clin 35 (2017) 421–438
http://dx.doi.org/10.1016/j.anclin.2017.05.001
1932-2275/17/© 2017 Elsevier Inc. All rights reserved.

be involved in the care of these often challenging patients. Multidisciplinary teams, consisting of surgeons, anesthesiologists, nephrologists, hepatologists, cardiologists, operating room staff, and pediatric intensivists, among many others, are all important for ensuring good outcomes in this population. Anesthesiologists play an integral part of this perioperative transplant team. One must take into account the complex anatomy, physiology, and special drug pharmacology of these patients when devising an anesthetic plan for these procedures. Careful preoperative evaluation, close intraoperative monitoring, and frequent communication with the surgeon and other medical specialties are all vital to ensuring excellent care in these medically complex and often challenging pediatric transplant recipients.

PEDIATRIC LIVER TRANSPLANTATION
Introduction

Dr Thomas E. Starzl and colleagues[1] performed the first pediatric liver transplant in 1963 in Denver, Colorado, on a baby with biliary atresia. There are now more than 140 transplant centers in the United States alone. Of those, more than 60 centers in the United States perform pediatric liver transplants. Based on Organ Procurement Transplant Network (OPTN) data, since 1988, there have been more than 15,000 pediatric liver transplants and, currently, about 500 pediatric liver transplants are performed every year in the United States (based on OPTN data as of September 9, 2016) (**Fig. 1**).

Indications

There are several unique indications for pediatric liver transplantation, with biliary atresia being the most common. This is followed by those related to toxin or infection, and genetic or metabolic disease (based on OPTN data as of September 9, 2016) (**Fig. 2**).

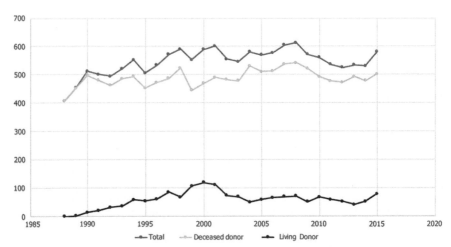

Fig. 1. Pediatric liver transplants (1988–2015). (*Data from* Organ Procurement and Transplantation Network (OPTN). Health Resources and Services Administration, US Department of Health & Human Services. Available at: https://optn.transplant.hrsa.gov/. Accessed September 9, 2016.)

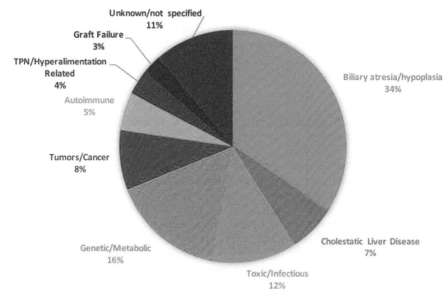

Fig. 2. Pediatric liver transplants by diagnosis (2015). TPN, total parenteral nutrition. (*Data from* Organ Procurement and Transplantation Network (OPTN). Health Resources and Services Administration, US Department of Health & Human Services. Available at: https://optn.transplant.hrsa.gov/. Accessed September 9, 2016.)

Absolute Contraindications

There are few published absolute contraindications to pediatric liver transplantation (**Box 1**).[2] However, when considering liver transplantation in a child, a multidisciplinary discussion must be had between all providers involved with the child's care and perioperative transplant specialists to determine if the child is well enough for

---

Box 1
Absolute contraindications to pediatric liver transplantation

Rapidly progressing hepatocellular carcinoma with metastasis

Extrahepatic malignancy

Uncontrolled systemic infection

Severe multisystem mitochondrial disease

Niemann-Pick type C

Severe portopulmonary hypertension not responsive to medical therapy

Mean pulmonary artery pressure (MPAP) greater than 35 mm Hg despite therapy

Adapted from Squires RH, Ng V, Romero R, et al. Evaluation of the pediatric patient for liver transplantation: 2014 practice guideline by the American Association for the Study of Liver Diseases, American Society of Transplantation and the North American Society for Pediatric Gastroenterology, Hepatology and Nutrition. Hepatology 2014;60(1):385; with permission.

transplantation. This is especially important when a liver transplant may not improve a child's long-term outcome or may put the child at significantly increased risk in light of other existing comorbidities. This includes cases of major cardiopulmonary disease, multiorgan system dysfunction, or severe neurologic impairment. They should also decide if any tests or procedures are necessary (eg, laboratory tests, echocardiogram, cardiac catheterization, cardiac surgery in cases of congenital heart disease) before proceeding to transplant.

Preoperative Evaluation

It is imperative that a careful preoperative assessment be performed when a child presents for liver transplantation, starting with a focused history and physical examination (**Box 2**).

Although some children coming for liver transplant may show classic signs of liver failure (eg, coagulopathy, ascites, varices) others may look perfectly normal with the indication being an underlying metabolic defect or genetic syndrome. These children may also have otherwise normal liver function and coagulation status. However, they may still have other coexisting organ dysfunction related to their underlying disease process, which must be taken into account (**Table 1**).

In addition to a preoperative evaluation, a discussion should take place with the child's family regarding the perioperative plan, including the risks and benefits of anesthesia.

This may be a difficult conversation because liver transplantation is a very high-risk surgery. The complications discussed should include the risks of massive hemorrhage and death; risks of blood transfusion; and other major neurologic, cardiac, pulmonary complications; along with the high likelihood of postoperative intensive care unit (ICU) admission with mechanical ventilation, and the need for reoperation. A discussion should also be had with the patient and should be tailored to developmental level of the child.

Box 2
Preoperative evaluation

Cause of liver failure and reason for transplant

Coagulation status (PT, PTT, international normalized ratio [INR], fibrinogen, platelets)

Sequelae of portal hypertension (eg, esophageal varices, significant ascites)

Current liver and renal function

Cardiopulmonary comorbidities
• Review of recent cardiology evaluation and any imaging studies (eg, echocardiography, stress test)

Acid or base status

Electrolytes and blood glucose (eg, Na+/K+)

Temperature irregularities

Prior surgeries or procedures

Any other existing comorbidities and their anesthetic implications

Data from Bhananker SM, Ramamoorthy C, Geiduschek JM, et al. Anesthesia-related cardiac arrest in children: update from the Pediatric Perioperative Cardiac Arrest Registry. Anesth Analg 2007;105(2):344–50.

Table 1
Anesthetic considerations for coexisting organ dysfunction related to underlying disease process

Diagnosis	Anesthetic Considerations
Autoimmune hepatitis	Preoperative immunosuppression
Alagille syndrome	Congenital heart disease
Hyperoxaluria	Hypertension, renal failure, heart failure
Alpha-1-antitrypsin	Pulmonary disease
Wilson disease	Increased sensitivity to neuromuscular blockade
Hemochromatosis	Diabetes, cardiomyopathy, anemia
Familial intrahepatic cholestasis	Malnutrition
Cystic fibrosis	Lung disease, malnutrition

Induction and Maintenance of Anesthesia

The use of induction agent and technique should be individualized for each patient after careful consideration of underlying liver pathology, coexisting cardiac disease, hemodynamic instability, electrolyte abnormalities, presence of ascites, and any history of gastrointestinal bleeding from any gastric varices, and so forth. Types of induction include

- Sevoflurane mask induction for induction of younger and healthy vigorous patients with no intravenous (IV) access who do not have severe ascites, vomiting, or other aspiration risks
- IV induction for children with existing IV access for whom aspiration concerns exist.

Succinylcholine is acceptable for rapid-sequence induction, unless there are concerns regarding hyperkalemia. High-dose rocuronium may be used as an alternative.

Orotracheal intubation with a cuffed tube is used for most pediatric patients because it is safe, even in small infants.[3] Isoflurane is used for anesthetic maintenance because this has been shown to preserve splanchnic blood flow[4] and vasodilate hepatic vasculature for improved perfusion.[5]

Additional intraoperative analgesia is provided by narcotics, usually by infusion. Fentanyl is often chosen because its metabolism is mostly unchanged in liver disease.[6] For muscle relaxants, cisatracurium is often chosen via infusion as the mode of muscle relaxation because it is metabolized independent of liver metabolism.[7]

Lines and Monitoring

Lines

The establishment of large-bore venous access is critical for liver transplantation because sudden massive hemorrhage necessitating rapid blood product administration can occur. Usually, 2 or more large-bore peripheral IVs are placed in the upper extremities. The inferior vena cava (IVC) is clamped during the anhepatic phase, thus blood or drugs given intravenously through lower extremities may be delayed from reaching central circulation. In regard to central blood administration, unlike adults, there is a higher risk of hyperkalemic cardiac arrest from large-volume central blood product administration in infants and children, so peripheral blood administration is preferred.[8] When attempting to place suitable IVs, ultrasonography or infrared vein finding adjuncts may be used, in addition to interventional radiology for IV access if necessary.

Once IV access is obtained, it is then attached to a rapid transfusion device for most patients and tested for line patency and pressure. It is easy to overtransfuse in this population, so extreme vigilance is especially required when using a rapid transfusion device in small children and infants.[9] There are several risk factors of cardiac arrest related to blood transfusion of large volumes in pediatrics, which must be taken into account during this procedure (**Box 3**).

Arterial access

Invasive monitoring for real-time blood pressure monitoring is extremely useful and advisable.[10] The radial artery is usually the preferred site for cannulation, mainly due to ease of placement and because of the risk possible aortic clamping during procedure. Alternative sites include the posterior tibial and dorsalis pedis arteries. Femoral artery cannulation may be used; however, in pediatrics this can be associated with limb ischemia,[11] so caution is advised. Two arterial lines may be placed for the procedure because they may be useful due to mechanical interference and dampening that may occur during the procedure, as well as for the ability to sample blood gases while monitoring blood pressure.

Central access

Central access is strongly recommended for central venous pressure (CVP) monitoring and vasoactive infusions.[12] The authors' institution routinely has interventional radiology place peripherally inserted central catheters before transplant in preparation for the procedure. Internal jugular or subclavian sites may be used, although caution is advised in the presence of existing coagulopathy.

Monitoring

Standard American Society of Anesthesiologists (ASA) monitors are used for this procedure, along with arterial blood pressure, urine output, and CVP measurements. Defibrillation pads are also attached and checked before the procedure due to risks of severe arrhythmias during the procedure, especially during organ reperfusion.

Additional monitors and devices

Transesophageal echocardiography Transesophageal echocardiography (TEE) is not used routinely in this patient population but is used in several adult centers.[13] However, at the authors' institutions, it can be used to evaluate unstable hemodynamics not explained by blood loss (Videos 1 and 2). It also may be useful for cases in which there is pre-existing congenital heart disease or cardiac dysfunction. Its use in children has been recognized as safe, with minimal complications.[14]

Continuous renal replacement therapy

Continuous renal replacement therapy (CRRT) can be safe and useful in adult patients if planned ahead of time.[15] In pediatrics, however, multiple complications are seen

---

Box 3
Risk factors for transfusion-associated cardiac arrest in children[8,25]

- Young infants or neonates (<1 year old)
- Faster rates of blood transfusion
- Old, unwashed, blood products (>7 days old)
- Electrolyte abnormalities (hypocalcemia, hyperkalemia)
- Central blood administration

when initiating CRRT,[16] including acute hypotension and electrolyte disturbances. From the authors' experiences, renal failure can be managed medically until the patient arrives in the ICU. We recommend dialysis be performed preoperatively and be immediately available postoperatively if needed.

Pulmonary artery catheter
Controversy exists regarding use of pulmonary artery catheters (PACs) in pediatrics.[17] Some studies have noted life-threatening complications, especially in high-risk populations.[18,19] Although helpful in measuring pulmonary artery pressures, temperature, and cardiac output, PACs are not used routinely at the authors' institution during liver transplantation, unlike adult centers.

Intraoperative Management

Stages of liver transplantation
The surgical stages of the pediatric liver transplant operation are the same as they are in adults, with several important caveats for pediatrics in each stage will be discussed (see Dieter Adelmann and colleagues, "Anesthesia for Liver Transplantation," in this issue).

Preanhepatic phase The main problems and goals during the preanhepatic phase are outlined in **Table 2** and **Box 4**. Massive bleeding and hypotension can occur during this time,[20] especially in patients with impaired synthetic liver function, ascites, or prior abdominal surgery, such as the Kasai procedure in patients with biliary atresia. Blood losses are replaced as necessary, with care to avoid overtransfusion. It should be noted that there is a wide range of clinical practice among institutions and anesthesiologists[21] regarding blood transfusions, and it is the authors' practice to use our clinical judgment along with close communication with the surgical team to guide blood product management.

Anhepatic phase During the anhepatic period, once the IVC is cross-clamped, hypotension due to loss of preload is expected.[12] This is worse in patients without portal hypertension and thus few venous collaterals, and is often seen in children with relatively normal hepatic function whose transplant indication is for metabolic disease or hepatoblastoma. One may also see ongoing acidosis, hyperkalemia, and hypoglycemia due to lack of gluconeogenesis, as well as hypothermia as a cold graft is sewn into the patient. **Table 3** outlines goals during the anhepatic phase.

If hypotension occurs during this time, it is the authors' practice to maintain blood pressure with judicious vasopressor use via bolus or infusion. Hypotension from loss of preload due to the IVC clamp is restored once the clamp is released, so it is important during this phase to avoid overtransfusion. Administration of large volumes of IV fluid and blood products may lead to congestion of the graft, so a low-normal CVP technique (6–10 mm Hg) and hemoglobin target of 8 to 9 gm/dL is often used. This has been shown to be safe in a study of pediatric subjects receiving live donor grafts.[22]

Table 2
Common complications during preanhepatic period

Problem	Risk Factors	Treatment
Massive hemorrhage	• Impaired synthetic function • Prior abdominal surgery	• Transfuse as necessary • Vasopressors
Hypotension	• Bleeding • Large-volume ascites drained • Acidosis	• 5% Albumin for ascites • May need vasopressor infusions

> **Box 4**
> **Goal during preanhepatic phase**
>
> Maintenance of hemodynamic stability
>
> Replacement blood or volume losses
>
> Avoidance of significant acidosis
>
> Avoid electrolyte derangements (K+ or Ca+)
>
> Normothermia and normoglycemia

Reperfusion On reperfusion of the donor graft, a bolus of cold fluid, potassium, other ischemic factors,[23] and possibly venous air emboli are released into the recipient patient's circulation from the donor liver. This may result in what is known as postreperfusion syndrome,[24] which results in hypotension; arrhythmias; and, if not treated effectively, cardiac arrest.

Before organ reperfusion, it is important to understand the risks during this period and how to mitigate them (**Table 4**). Treatment of any resulting hyperkalemia includes hyperventilation, calcium chloride boluses for cardiac protection, sodium bicarbonate, insulin or dextrose, inhaled albuterol, and furosemide.[25] Usually, in pediatric patients, dopamine and/or epinephrine is chosen initially to maintain blood pressure and perfusion during this time. Also during this period, patient temperature can be expected to drop more than a degree or more centigrade.[26] Right before the vascular clamps are removed, it is common to administer boluses of calcium, lidocaine, sodium bicarbonate, and/or IV epinephrine, with repeated boluses as necessary. Oxygen at 100% and transiently decreasing volatile anesthetic agent are other measures used to mitigate any hypotension and hyperkalemia that may occur with reperfusion.

Vigilance and close communication among the perioperative team are imperative during this period, as is the readiness and ability to treat any life-threatening arrhythmias that may ensue with CPR or defibrillation.

Neohepatic phase Following reperfusion, the neohepatic phase is marked by ongoing blood loss due to ongoing coagulopathy, bleeding from vascular anastomoses, and bleeding from a partial graft cut surface area if a partial donor graft was used. Cross-clamping of the aorta may occur during this phase if the graft requires a direct

Table 3
Goals during anhepatic phase

Goal	Target or Treatment
Maintenance of intravascular volume and hemodynamic stability	Hct 24%–27% (Hgb 8–9 mg/dL)[22] CVP 6–10 mm Hg Use vasopressor infusions as necessary
Maintain normoglycemia	May need dextrose bolus or infusion
Maintain normothermia	Bair hugger, warmed fluids, HME, low-flow anesthesia
Maintenance of acid-base balance	Hyperventilation Sodium bicarbonate boluses (1–2 mEq/kg)
Maintain normal calcium and low-normal potassium levels	Replace Ca+ as necessary *Treat any hyperkalemia

Abbreviations: Ca+, calcium; Hct, hematocrit; Hgb, hemoglobin; HME, heat moisture exchanger.
Data from Chen CL, Concejero A, Wang CC, et al. Living donor liver transplantation for biliary atresia: a single-center experience with first 100 cases. Am J Transplant 2006;6(11):2672–9.

Table 4
Reperfusion goals

Goal	Treatment
Correct calcium	Calcium chloride (central) • 10–20 mg/kg IV
Prevent or treat hyperkalemia • Low-normal (K+ 3.5–4.0)	• Hyperventilation • Calcium chloride boluses • Sodium bicarbonate • Insulin or dextrose • Inhaled albuterol • Furosemide • Epinephrine
Normothermia • Expect ~1° drop centigrade[26]	• Warm room • Bair hugger • Warm fluids
Normotensive	Vasoactive infusions ready as needed • Dopamine and/or epinephrine
Normal heart rhythm	• Treat as above • Defibrillation pads attached to defibrillator

aortic conduit, resulting in further hemodynamic instability. Also of note during this phase, unlike most adult patients, children receive either a Roux hepaticojejunostomy (bile duct to jejunum) or the usual choledochocholedochostomy (duct to duct) anastomoses following the hepatic arterial anastomosis. This phase ends with abdominal closure and conclusion of the procedure. When the graft begins to function, the acid-base status and electrolyte abnormalities will begin to reverse, and oliguria due to any preexisting hepatorenal syndrome may start to improve.

Following reperfusion, there are other considerations the anesthesiologist must be aware of during a pediatric liver transplant, relating to vascular thrombosis. It has been shown that compared with adults children are more hypercoagulable after liver transplant. This is thought to be due to decreased proteins C and S, plasminogen, and antithrombin III.[27] This is in addition to the elevated levels of factor VIII seen in liver failure.[28] According to a 2009 Cochrane review, children have a much higher incidence of early hepatic artery thrombosis compared with adults (8.3% vs 2.9%) with a 25% mortality rate.[29] Risk factors in that review included arterial size variants, lower weight patients, retransplantation, and prolonged operative times. However, higher blood viscosity and higher hematocrit levels may predispose. Prevention can first include targeting lower hemoglobin targets (8–9 gm/dL shown to be safe).[22] At the authors' institution, we try to avoid over-correcting the prothrombin time (PT) and partial thromboplastin time (PTT) to normal levels and use platelets and cryoprecipitate with caution. Aspirin, alprostadil, and heparin have been used as prophylaxis with some success.[30,31]

At the conclusion of the procedure, care must be taken to ensure adequate oxygenation and ventilation as the abdomen is closed while monitoring for continued bleeding and hemodynamic instability. This vigilance must be continued as the patient is transported to the ICU.

Perioperative extubation A few recent studies have shown that hemodynamically stable patients whose surgical procedures were short and not complicated by intraoperative blood loss may be extubated in the operating room.[32,33] A recent retrospective single-center review of 84 pediatric patients who were extubated in the operating room recommended to attempt extubation if the patients met usual extubation criteria for general surgery cases.[33] There was a 65% extubation rate, with a low rate of reintubation, and a trend toward shorter ICU and hospital stay. They did continue to avoid extubation in patients with an open abdomen, planned return to the operating room within 24 hours, escalating hemodynamic instability, preoperative encephalopathy, airway compromise, or ventilator dependence. Extubation in the operating room often depends on the transplant center, surgeon, and anesthesiologist, as well as on a variety of patient, surgical, and graft factors. However, it likely may safely be done in this patient population, and should be considered.

PEDIATRIC KIDNEY TRANSPLANTATION
Epidemiology and Overview

The prevalence of end-stage renal disease (ESRD) in children of all races and ethnicities is projected to be 4 to 6 per million.[34] The North American Pediatric Renal Trials and Collaborative Studies (NAPRTCS) was founded in 1987 as a collaborative to capture information on current practice and trends to improve the care of pediatric renal transplant recipients. As of the NAPRTCS annual report in 2014, 11,186 renal transplants have been reported.[34] The most common diagnosis for pediatric renal transplantation is aplastic, hypoplastic, or dysplastic kidneys (15.8%). Obstructive uropathy and focal segmental glomerulosclerosis are the second and third most common causes leading to renal transplant at 15.3% and 11.7%, respectively.[34] The 5 most frequent diagnoses constitute more than 50% of transplant cases, indicating that there are several other causes that contribute to pediatric ESRD and subsequent transplantation (**Fig. 3**). The distribution of these diagnoses varies between ethnicities.

Pathophysiology of End-Stage Renal Disease and Preoperative Evaluation

Renal dysfunction has a profound effect on the body's ability to maintain homeostasis. Morbidity and mortality are increased in children in renal failure, particularly in younger children. Growth and development are dramatically affected by renal disease. Intellectual and neurocognitive development are also negatively affected in renal failure. However, in children with ESRD, intelligence quotient measured during dialysis therapy improved after transplantation.[35] Cardiovascular disease remains a significant contributor to morbidity and mortality in pediatric ESRD. From a third to a half of deaths in children with chronic renal failure have been attributed to a cardiac cause.[36]

Coronary artery calcifications and intimal-medial thickening, as well as hyperhomocystemia and dyslipidemia, have demonstrated a greater prevalence in children with ESRD and on renal replacement therapy. Hypertension and left ventricular hypertrophy (LVH) are common and should be expected in children who are on dialysis. Although the risk of cardiac death does decrease after transplantation, these associated pretransplant risk factors seem to persist even after transplantation.[37] In preparation for kidney transplantation, the anesthesiologist should be aware that antihypertensive medications are likely a part of the child's regimen. A thorough review should be implemented given the risk for hemodynamic perturbations during anesthetic management. Some medications, such as beta-blockers, have been recommended to continue in the perioperative period, whereas others, such as angiotensin-converting-enzyme inhibitor-I and angiotensin II receptor blockers should be withheld because of the risk of severe and refractory hypotension after anesthetic induction.[38,39]

Coagulation can be altered in the ESRD patient. Anemia is common both before and after transplant due to a decrease in erythropoietin production and iron deficiency.

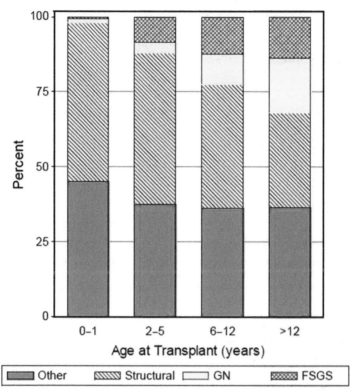

Fig. 3. Primary ESRD diagnosis by age. FSGS, focal segmental glomerulosclerosis; GN, glomerulonephritis. (*From* North American Pediatric Renal Trials and Collaborative Studies (NAPRTCS) 2014 Annual Transplant Report. Available at: https://web.emmes.com/study/ped/annlrept/annualrept2014.pdf. Accessed January 10, 2017; with permission.)

Treatment of anemia has been shown to decrease the progression of renal disease and other comorbidities, such as LVH.[40] Correction of anemia to a hematocrit of at least 30% has been shown to decrease the progression to ESRD and reduce the bleeding time.[41] Uremia contributes to platelet dysfunction, hindering appropriate clot formation.

Electrolyte disturbances are expected in ESRD, particularly potassium levels. Caution should be taken in patients with preoperative potassium levels greater than 6 mmol/L. Recent dialysis history should be obtained before proceeding to transplantation to evaluate intravascular fluid status and the potential for electrolyte imbalances.

Surgical Considerations and Techniques

There is no minimum age for pediatric kidney transplant; success has been reported in children younger than age of one. However, age-matching does seem to influence graft survival. Studies have supported improved transplanted kidney function from donors younger than 16 years old when improved graft function is evaluated based on postoperative glomerular filtration rate in the recipient.[42] Additionally, living donors exhibit better long-term graft survival than deceased donors **(Fig. 4)**.[34] Despite evidence that living donors portend better survival, there continues to be a paucity of

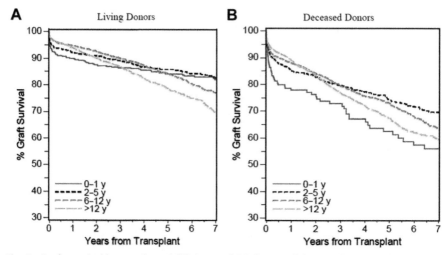

Fig. 4. Graft survival by age from (*A*) living and (*B*) deceased donors. (*From* North American Pediatric Renal Trials and Collaborative Studies (NAPRTCS) 2014 Annual Transplant Report. Available at: https://web.emmes.com/study/ped/annlrept/annualrept2014.pdf. Accessed January 10, 2017; with permission.)

living donors of corresponding age to potential recipients. In lieu of the potential complications of cadaveric donors (graft thrombosis, acute rejection, and primary nonfunction), living related adult donors in pediatric patients have improved graft and patient survival rates.[43] The surgical technique has been modified to accommodate the larger adult kidney in the pediatric patient. Older children can still benefit from the extraperitoneal approach and placement of the donor kidney in the iliac fossa; however, young children often require an intraperitoneal approach where the adult-sized donor kidney may occupy a significant portion of the peritoneum.[44] Vascular anastomosis depends on the size of the recipients' vessels; anastomosis can be made via the common iliac artery and vein, external iliac artery and vein, or directly to the aorta and vena cava.[44,45]

Anesthetic Management

Anesthetic choice

Regional techniques, including epidural anesthesia, have been reported with good outcomes in renal transplantation.[46] Given the proposed risk of coagulopathy and anticoagulation, many centers defer to a regional approach. General endotracheal intubation is more commonly adopted, with maintenance described with both volatile anesthetics and a total intravenous technique, with no difference in outcomes.[47,48] Concerns regarding the use of sevoflurane and the development of potentially nephrotoxic compound A, even during low gas flow anesthetics, has not been shown to demonstrate a clinically significant risk.[48,49]

Monitoring and vascular access

Standard ASA monitors should be used for renal transplantation. Central line insertion with the routine monitoring of CVP for targeting a specific venous pressure or fluid management has not demonstrated any benefit in graft function.[50] However, central venous placement should be reserved for those patients with specific indications, such as poor peripheral IV access or comorbidities that necessitate monitoring of cardiac filling pressures. Central venous access may be considered beneficial in younger or smaller children who are receiving adult-sized kidneys such that adult-sized organ may sequester a significant amount of the younger child's blood volume during reperfusion, resulting in severe hypotension and graft hypoperfusion (**Fig. 5**). In older children in whom adequate large-bore venous access can be attained, central venous access may be deferred. Arterial line catheterization is only truly indicated for patients who are anticipated to have significant cardiovascular instability under anesthesia, such as patients with associated cardiac disease. Vascular access, in general, may be challenging in the ESRD patient.

Induction

Premedication can be safely administered to facilitate parenteral separation. A rapid sequence induction should be considered if the child is at risk for aspiration, such as in the setting of gastroparesis secondary to diabetes or a suspected full stomach. Succinylcholine can be safely administered in the absence of contraindications such as hyperkalemia; an increase in serum potassium of at least 0.5 mmol/L should be expected with its use. High-dose rocuronium (1.2 mg/kg) has been safely used in renal failure with an expected prolonged neuromuscular blockade effect due to its reduced renal elimination. Even after graft transplantation, immediate return of renal function should not be assumed and a prolonged effect of blockade may exist. In general, in the setting of renal failure, the anesthesia provider should avoid any medications that are primarily metabolized and/or excreted by the kidney. Renal function affects both protein-binding and volume of distribution, so medication administration should be adjusted accordingly. Consideration for use of those medications that are preferentially metabolized and/or excreted by any organ-independent mechanism could be advantageous.[48,51] Atracurium or cisatracurium may be preferential in this regard. Medications with active metabolites that are renally excreted, such as morphine, should be used cautiously. Drugs with toxic metabolites, such as meperidine, should be avoided.

Maintenance

Fluid management The exact volume and selection of IV fluid administration remains controversial. The patient should be assumed to be volume-depleted due to perioperative starvation coupled with possible preoperative dialysis. Adequate fluid

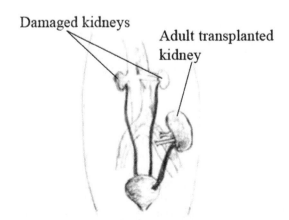

Fig. 5. Adult transplanted kidney into infant. Note comparatively larger size prompting significant hemodynamic variation during reperfusion.

administration has been advised to improve graft function, with some studies advocating for a blood volume of 70 mL/kg to improve immediate graft function.[52] As previously stated, CVPs have not been specifically correlated to graft function; however, a target CVP of 10 to 15 mm Hg has been demonstrated to optimize organ perfusion.[53] Potassium-depleted fluids, such as 0.9% saline or Normosol, have been historically used but recent studies have shown a potential increase in metabolic acidosis with aggressive hydration with 0.9% saline.[54] Colloids, such as albumin, can help improve graft function due to the benefit of enhanced volume expansion and subsequent graft perfusion. Blood is rarely needed but should be available due to preexisting anemia and potential for surgical blood loss.

Hemodynamic goals In considering maintenance anesthetic agents, judicious use of drugs that have negative inotropic and vasodilatory effects should be used. Opiates are considered safe but should be titrated to mitigate a vasodilatory effect. Reperfusion of the grafted kidney will likely demonstrate the most dramatic hemodynamic response. Depending on the size discrepancy of the donor organ to the size of the child, blood sequestration may be dramatic and can reach levels that constitute the total blood volume of the recipient patient. Additionally, reperfusion injury may occur, resulting in significant lactic acidosis and hyperkalemia. Management of reperfusion includes optimizing preload with crystalloid and colloid, and using vasoactive agents to augment cardiac output may be required. Various studies have advocated for CVP goals between 10 and 16 mm Hg, systolic blood pressures greater than 120 mm Hg, and a mean arterial pressure above 65 to 70 mm Hg before reperfusion.[53] The surgeon may also clamp and then unclamp the aorta after the anastomosis to diminish the response. Potent vasoconstrictors with alpha-adrenergic activity, such as phenylephrine, should be avoided because of the risk of vasoconstriction in the graft. The use of drugs such as phenylephrine should be considered only when other measures have failed. The use of dopamine at purposed renal doses (2–3 mcg/kg/min) to promote renal blood flow has been questioned. Studies have shown that transplanted and denervated kidney does not respond in the same manner as native kidneys and that no improvement in graft function has been demonstrated.[55] There has been some promising evidence that a fenoldopam infusion (a DA-1 receptor selective agonist) in comparison to dopamine has resulted in better graft function (diuresis and electrolyte excretion).[56]

Diuretics At the completion of the vascular anastomosis, mannitol and furosemide are frequently administered to facilitate diuresis. Mannitol exerts an osmotic effect after being freely filtered in the renal tubule and its use may help prevent ischemic injury. Furosemide as a sodium-potassium (Na+/K+) pump inhibitor in the ascending loop of Henle promotes urine formation and may prevent oliguria.

Emergence

At the conclusion of surgery, neuromuscular block should be reversed. Assumption of normal renal function and adequate excretion of metabolized paralytics should not be anticipated even after the graft has been successfully placed. Extubation is appropriate if all parameters are met. Postoperative pain is usually of at least moderate intensity and many institutions use patient-controlled analgesia to adequate control pain. Fentanyl is often a good choice given its limited renal excretion. Any regional or neuraxial anesthesia techniques that are used may significantly help augment pain control in the immediate perioperative period.[46] Postoperatively, most patients do not require an ICU admission; however, an ICU admission may be warranted for a higher acuity of care in the immediate postoperative setting, particularly if there are stringent hemodynamic goals.

OUTCOMES

Since the most recent NAPRTCS annual report in 2014, 3-year graft survival for living and deceased donors is 93.4% and 90.4%, respectively.[34] Pediatric kidney transplant recipients experience a significant improvement in the quality of life in comparison with ESRD patients. However, pre-existing comorbidities, such as cardiovascular disease, continue to contribute to long-term morbidity.[36] With the advent of advanced immunosuppression, transplant recipients are increasingly at risk for opportunistic infections, particularly viral infections. In addition to administration of antiviral medications, some transplant specialists will reduce immunosuppression to initiate a reinstated host immune response.[42] Viruses of particular concern in this population are cytomegalovirus and Ebstein-Barr virus, which can lead to the development of post-transplant lymphoproliferative disorder, which is the most common malignancy that develops in the transplanted kidney cohort. The development of a malignant disease in the renal transplanted population has increased threefold over the past 20 years, likely due to more intensified immunosuppressive agents.[51]

SUPPLEMENTARY DATA

Supplementary videos related to this article can be found at http://dx.doi.org/10.1016/j.anclin.2017.05.001.

REFERENCES

1. Starzl TE, Marchioro TL, Vonkaulla KN, et al. Homotransplantation of the liver in humans. Surg Gynecol Obstet 1963;117:659–76.
2. Squires RH, Ng V, Romero R, et al. Evaluation of the pediatric patient for liver transplantation: 2014 practice guideline by the American Association for the Study of Liver Diseases, American Society of Transplantation and the North American Society for Pediatric Gastroenterology, Hepatology and Nutrition. Hepatology 2014;60(1):362–98.
3. Taylor C, Subaiya L, Corsino D. Pediatric cuffed endotracheal tubes: An evolution of care. Ochsner J 2011;11:52–6.
4. O'Riordan J, O'Beirne HA, Young Y, et al. Effects of desflurane and isoflurane on splanchnic microcirculation during major surgery. Br J Anaesth 1997;78(1):95–6.
5. Gatecel C, Losser MR, Payen D. The postoperative effects of halothane versus isoflurane on hepatic artery and portal vein blood flow in humans. Anesth Analg 2003;96(3):740–5.
6. Tegeder I, Lotsch J, Geisslinger G. Pharmacokinetics of opioids in liver disease. Clin Pharmacokinet 1999;37(1):17–40.
7. De Wolf AM, Freeman JA, Scott VL, et al. Pharmacokinetics and pharmacodynamics of cisatracurium in patients with end-stage liver disease undergoing liver transplantation. Br J Anaesth 1996;76(5):624–8.
8. Bhananker SM, Ramamoorthy C, Geiduschek JM, et al. Anesthesia-related cardiac arrest in children: update from the Pediatric Perioperative Cardiac Arrest Registry. Anesth Analg 2007;105:344–50.
9. Greene N, Bhananker S, Ramaiah R. Vascular access, fluid resuscitation, and blood transfusion in pediatric trauma. Int J Crit Illn Inj Sci 2012;2(3):135–42.

10. Uejima T. Anesthetic management of the pediatric patient undergoing solid organ transplantation. Anesthesiol Clin North America 2004;22:809–26.
11. Lin PH, Dodson TF, Bush RL, et al. Surgical intervention for complications caused by femoral artery catheterization in pediatric patients. J Vasc Surg 2001;34: 1071–8.
12. Chen CL, Concejero A, Wang CC, et al. Living donor liver transplantation for biliary atresia: a single-center experience with first 100 cases. Am J Transplant 2006;6:2672–9.
13. Burtanshaw A. The role of tranesophageal echocardiography for perioperative cardiovascular monitoring during orthotopic liver transplantation. Liver Transpl 2006;12:1577–83.
14. Stevenson JG. Incidence of complications in pediatric transesophageal echocardiography: experience in 1650 cases. J Am Soc Echocardiogr 1999;12:527–32.
15. Agopian VG, Dhillon A, Baber J, et al. Liver transplantation in recipients receiving renal replacement therapy: outcomes analysis and the role of intraoperative hemodialysis. Am J Transplant 2014;14(7):1638–47.
16. Santiago MJ, López-Herce J, Urbano J, et al. Complications of continuous renal replacement therapy in critically ill children: a prospective observational evaluation study. Crit Care 2009;13:R184.
17. Perkin RM, Anas N. Pulmonary artery catheters. Pediatri Crit Care Med 2011; 12(Suppl.):S12–20.
18. Carmosino MJ, Friesen RH, Doran A, et al. Perioperative complications in children with pulmonary hypertension undergoing non-cardiac surgery or cardiac catheterization. Anesth Analg 2007;204:521–7.
19. Taylor CJ, Derrick G, McEwen A. Risk of cardiac catheterization under anesthesia in children with pulmonary hypertension. Br J Anaesth 2007;98:657–61.
20. Bechstein WO, Neuhaus P. Bleeding problems in liver surgery and liver transplantation. Chirurg 2000;71(4):363–8.
21. Ozier Y, Pessione F, Samain E, et al. Institutional variability in transfusion practice for liver transplantation. Anesth Analg 2003;97(3):671–9.
22. Jawan B, De Villa V, Luk HN, et al. Perioperative normovolemic anemia is safe in pediatric living donor liver transplantation. Transplantation 2004;77:1394–8.
23. Bulkley GB. Reactive oxygen metabolites and reperfusion injury: aberrant triggering of reticuloendothelial function. Lancet 1994;344(8927):934–6.
24. Bukowicka B, Akar RA, Olszewska A, et al. The occurrence of postreperfusion syndrome in orthotopic liver transplantation and its significance in terms of complications and short-term survival. Ann Transplant 2011;16(2):26–30.
25. Tyler DC. The Pediatric Anesthesia Quality Improvement Initiative Wake Up Safe. Hyperkalemic statement. Wake up Safe, a component of The Society for Pediatric Anesthesia; 2015.
26. Huang C-J, Chen C-L, Tseng C-C, et al. Maintenance of normothermia at operation room temperature of 24°C in adult and pediatric patients undergoing liver transplantation. Transpl Int 2005;18:396–400.
27. Harper PL, Edgar PF, Luddington RJ, et al. Protein C deficiency and portal thrombosis in liver transplantation in children. Lancet 1988;2:924–7.
28. Hugenholtz GC, Northup PG, Porte RJ, et al. Is there a rationale for treatment of chronic liver disease with antithrombotic therapy? Blood Rev 2014;29:127–36.
29. Bekker J, Ploem S, De Jong KP. Early hepatic artery thrombosis after liver transplantation: a systematic review of the incidence, outcome and risk factors. Am J Transplant 2009;9:746–57.

30. Heaton ND. Hepatic artery thrombosis: conservative management or retransplantation? Liver Transpl 2013;19:S14–6.
31. Heffron TG, Welch D, Pillen T, et al. Low incidence of hepatic artery thrombosis after pediatric liver transplantation without the use of intraoperative microscope or parenteral anticoagulation. Pediatr Transplant 2005;9:486–90.
32. O'Meara ME, Whiteley SM. Immediate extubation of children following liver transplantation is safe and may be beneficial. Transplantation 2005;80(7):959–63.
33. Fullington NM, Cauley RP, Potanos KM, et al. Immediate extubation after pediatric liver transplantation: a single-center experience. Liver Transpl 2015;21:57–62.
34. NAPRTCS 2014 Annual Transplant Report. North American Pediatric Renal Trials and Collaborative Studies. 2014. Available at: www.naprtcs.org. Accessed December 15, 2016.
35. Moser J, Veale P, McAllister D, et al. A systematic review and quantitative analysis of neurocognitive outcomes in children with four chronic illnesses. Paediatr Anaesth 2013;23:1084–96.
36. McDonald SP, Craig JC. Long-term survival of children with end-stage renal disease. N Engl J Med 2004;350:2654–62.
37. El-Husseini AA, Sheashaa HA, Hassan NA, et al. Echocardiographic changes and risk factors for left ventricular hypertrophy in children and adolescents after renal transplantation. Pediatr Transplant 2004;8:249–54.
38. Group PS, Devereaus PJ, Yang H, et al. Effects of extended-release metoprolol succinate in patients undergoing non-cardiac surgery (POISE trial): a randomized controlled trial. Lancet 2008;371(9627):1839–47.
39. Auron M, Harte B, Kumar A, et al. Renin-angiotensin system antagonists in the perioperative setting: clinical consequences and recommendations for practice. Postgrad Med J 2011;87(1029):472–81.
40. Gouva C, Nikolopoulos P, Ioannidis JPA, et al. Treating anemia early in renal failure patients slows the decline of renal function: a randomized control trial. Kidney Int 2004;66:753–60.
41. Turitto VT, Weiss HJ. Red blood cells: their dual role in thrombus formation. Science 1980;207(4430):541–3.
42. Giessing M, Muller D, Winkelmann B, et al. Kidney transplantation in children and adolescents. Transplant Proc 2007;39:2197–201.
43. Harmon WE, Alexander SR, Tejani A, et al. The effect of donor age on graft survival in pediatric cadaver renal transplant recipients – a report of the North American Pediatric Renal Transplant Cooperative Study. Transplantation 1992;54:232–7.
44. Healy PJ, McDonald R, Waldhausen JH, et al. Transplantation of the adult living donor kidneys into infants and small children. Arch Surg 2000;135:1035–41.
45. Magee JC, Campell D. Renal transplantation. In: Fonkalsrud EW, Coran AD, editors. Pediatric surgery. 6th edition. Philadelphia: Mosby; 2006. p. 699–716.
46. Coupe N, O'Brien M, Gibson P, et al. Anesthesia for pediatric renal transplantation with and without epidural analgesia – a review of 7 years experience. Paediatr Anaesth 2005;15:220–8.
47. Modesti C, Sacco T, Morelli G, et al. Balanced anesthesia versus total intravenous anesthesia for kidney transplantation. Minerva Anestesiol 2006;72(7–8):627–35.
48. Cote C, Lerman J, Todres D, editors. A practice of anesthesia for infants and children. 5th edition. Philadelphia: Saunders Elsevier; 2009.
49. Conzen PF, Kharasch ED, Czerner SFA, et al. Low-flow sevoflurane compared with low-flow isoflurane anesthesia in patients with stable renal insufficiency. Anesthesiology 2002;97(3):578–84.

50. Campos L, Parada B, Furriel F, et al. Do intraoperative hemodynamic factors of the recipient influence renal graft function? Transplant Proc 2012;44(6):1800–3.
51. Spiro MD, Eilers H. Intraoperative care of the transplant patient. Anesthesiol Clin 2013;31:705–21.
52. Dawidson I, Berglin E, Brynger H, et al. Intravascular volumes and colloid dynamics in relation to fluid management in living related kidney donors and recipients. Crit Care Med 1987;15(7):631–6.
53. Rianthavorn P, Al-Akash S, Ettenger RB. Kidney transplantation in children. In: Weir MR, editor. Medical management of kidney transplantation. Philadelphia: Lippincott Williams & Wilkins; 2005. p. 198–230.
54. O'Malley CM, Frumento RJ, Hardy MA, et al. A randomized, double-blinded comparison of lactated Ringer's solution and 0.9% NaCl during renal transplantation. Anesth Analg 2005;100(5):1518–24.
55. Ciapetti M, Di Valvasone S, Di Filippo A, et al. Low-dose dopamine in kidney transplantation. Transplant Proc 2009;41(10):4165–8.
56. Sorbello M, Morello G, Paratore A, et al. Fenoldopam vs dopamine as a nephroprotective strategy during living donor kidney transplantation: preliminary data. Transplant Proc 2007;39(6):1794–6.

Anesthesia for Kidney and Pancreas Transplantation

Aaron M. Mittel, MD, Gebhard Wagener, MD*

KEYWORDS

- Anesthesia for organ transplant • Kidney transplantation • Pancreas transplantation
- Perioperative management of dialysis • Perioperative management of kidney failure
- Fluid management for organ transplant

KEY POINTS

- There is a high prevalence of cardiovascular disease in the population of patients receiving kidney or pancreas transplants, mandating appropriate vigilance and perioperative screening to limit the risk of major adverse cardiac events during transplant.
- In general, routine dialysis is not necessary immediately before kidney transplant. However, patients with significant volume overload or electrolyte disturbances should be dialyzed before transplant to avoid perioperative complications.
- Graft perfusion is of critical importance during abdominal organ transplant. Particular attention should be paid to fluid management to ensure adequate cardiac output. In the case of renal transplant, balanced crystalloids are the preferred resuscitation fluid.
- Use of vasoactive drugs during transplant is associated with poor outcomes. However, the anesthesiologist must ensure adequate graft perfusion before withholding vasoactive agents.
- Simultaneous kidney and pancreas transplant procedures are associated with better outcomes than isolated kidney or isolated pancreas transplants. However, organ availability is low, thus alternative transplantation approaches are often performed.

INTRODUCTION

Transplantation is often the most effective treatment of end-stage organ dysfunction. End-stage renal disease (ESRD) is relatively common and can be managed for many years with hemodialysis. Thus, a large number of patients are potentially eligible for transplant. Accordingly, kidney transplantation is the most commonly performed solid organ transplant and is occasionally performed simultaneously with pancreas

Disclosure Statement: The authors have no disclosures of any relationships with a commercial company that has a direct financial interest in subject matter or materials discussed in article or with a company making a competing product.
Department of Anesthesiology, Columbia University Medical Center, College of Physicians & Surgeons, Columbia University, PH 527-B, 630 West 168th Street, New York, NY 10032, USA
* Corresponding author.
E-mail address: gw72@cumc.columbia.edu

Anesthesiology Clin 35 (2017) 439–452
http://dx.doi.org/10.1016/j.anclin.2017.04.005
anesthesiology.theclinics.com
1932-2275/17/© 2017 Elsevier Inc. All rights reserved.

transplantation due to shared underlying pathophysiology. Like other organs, the demand for kidney and pancreas transplants outpaces supply, and a complex process is necessary to ensure appropriate resource utilization. In the United States, this process is governed by the Organ Procurement Transplant Network (OPTN), which uses the nonprofit United Network for Organ Sharing (UNOS) to coordinate nationwide organ allocation. UNOS works closely with local organ procurement organizations to match donor organs with regionally appropriate recipients. Once a match is found, time becomes a constraining factor, which is an important consideration in perioperative management of the transplantation process. This article outlines the anesthetic approach to adult kidney and pancreas transplantation procedures with an emphasis on modern perioperative practice.

RENAL TRANSPLANTATION
Epidemiology

According to the OPTN, more than 400,000 kidney transplants have been performed in the United States following the first successful attempt in 1954, with just over 19,000 completed in 2016. Of these, approximately 70% came from deceased donors. There are currently approximately 100,000 patients on the United States waiting list; approximately 5000 patients die each year awaiting transplant. Although the overall number of patients listed has actually slowly decreased from 2005, the number of candidates who have completed work-up and are actively listed has continued to climb, as has the total waiting time, percentage of patients on dialysis, and percentage of elderly patients on the waitlist. Ultimately, these factors reflect a progressively worsening mismatch of supply and demand.[1]

Eligibility for Transplant

For all patients with ESRD, transplantation is the treatment of choice. Diabetes, chronic glomerulonephritis, and polycystic kidney disease are the most common indications, though hypertensive nephrosclerosis is the most common in blacks. Additionally, retransplant following graft failure is an occasional reason for placing a patient on the transplant waiting list. Typically, the glomerular filtration rate must progressively deteriorate without expected improvement to less than 20 mL/min/1.73 m^2 until transplant is considered necessary.[2,3]

Absolute contraindications to transplant include active infection, active malignancy, active substance abuse, reversible renal failure, uncontrolled psychiatric disease and/or treatment nonadherence, and short life expectancy. Relative contraindications include systemic conditions associated with poor graft and patient survival, such as some autoimmune diseases (eg, systemic lupus erythematosus) and cardiac amyloidosis. To this end, patients are screened before transplant with age-appropriate oncologic screens, imaging examinations, laboratory studies to evaluate end-organ function, and laboratory analysis of potential viral infections. Particular attention is paid to human leukocyte antigen typing and reactive antibody assays to reduce risk of graft rejection. Typically, this work-up is performed well in advance of the perioperative period.[4]

Preoperative Evaluation

Patients awaiting kidney transplant generally have a variety of comorbidities that warrant consideration perioperatively. Of particular importance to the anesthesiologist, there is a high prevalence of cardiovascular disease in the renal failure population; cardiac complications are the most frequent cause of death following kidney transplant.[5]

There is wide variability between preoperative cardiovascular screening practices between centers, particularly among patients deemed to be low risk for cardiac disease. In general, preoperative evaluation of patients awaiting renal transplant should be performed according to American College of Cardiology and American Heart Association (ACC/AHA) 2014 guidelines for patients undergoing noncardiac surgery. For example, patients with high functional capacity may not need formal cardiac testing. However, renal dysfunction has been associated with occurrence of adverse perioperative events during noncardiac procedures. Thus, a low threshold for additional testing should be held.[6] Indeed, ACC/AHA 2012 guidelines focusing specifically on renal transplant suggest every patient awaiting renal transplant receive a resting 12-lead electrocardiogram and that consideration should be given to noninvasive stress testing in patients without known cardiac conditions but with multiple coronary artery disease risk factors, regardless of functional status. Diabetes, prior cardiovascular disease, more than 1 year on dialysis, known left ventricular hypertrophy, age older than 60 years, smoking, hypertension, and dyslipidemia are all considered to be relevant risk factors. Furthermore, independent of the results of these studies, it is reasonable to perform preoperative echocardiography to evaluate ventricular function. Patients with ventricular dysfunction or abnormal stress test results should be referred to a cardiologist for consideration of revascularization.[7]

It is often difficult to precisely estimate the timeline to eventual transplantation of a waitlisted patient, which can complicate the decision to revascularize patients who have obstructive coronary artery disease. For patients in whom transplantation is anticipated within 12 months, balloon angioplasty or bare metal stenting is preferred (followed by 4–12 weeks of antiplatelet therapy). Transplantation within 4 weeks of balloon angioplasty, 3 months of bare metal stenting, or 12 months of drug-eluting stenting should be avoided if possible. In patients who have undergone drug-eluting stenting and are taking a thienopyridine as part of dual antiplatelet therapy, the decision to stop the thienopyridine should be a multidisciplinary discussion. It may be reasonable to continue the thienopyridine if the anticipated risk of bleeding is low. However, if necessary, thienopyridines should be stopped 5 days before surgery with a plan to restart as soon as possible. Aspirin monotherapy should be continued perioperatively.[7]

No guidelines specifically address management of pulmonary function of the renal transplant recipient, though routine evaluation should be performed preoperatively. Type I diabetics, in particular, may have reduced lung volumes and diminished diffusion capacity without overt signs of pulmonary dysfunction on examination.[8] Patients with severe pulmonary limitations, such as an oxygen requirement at home, uncontrolled asthma, cor pulmonale, or severe obstructive or restrictive disease, should not undergo renal transplant. Active smokers should be encouraged to quit preoperatively.[3]

Noncardiopulmonary conditions are also very prevalent in the renal transplant population. Diabetes, obesity, peripheral vascular disease, cerebrovascular disease, psychosocial issues, gastrointestinal disease, and other systemic disease may complicate peritransplant operative management. These should be managed in conjunction with preoperative outpatient work-up, focusing especially on documentation of baseline end-organ function and overall functional capacity.[3,4]

Preoperative Dialysis

Preoperative evaluation immediately before transplant especially focuses on the potential need for and timing of dialysis. Some patients, particularly those who are scheduled for living donor transplant, may have yet to start dialysis. In these patients, preemptive transplantation (ie, before initiation of chronic dialysis) is usually preferred because it is associated with improved post-transplant graft function and long-term patient survival, putatively secondary to the avoidance of accumulation of toxic metabolites that promote development of cardiovascular disease.[9,10]

Given the limited supply of donor organs, many patients spend significant time waiting for an organ. Ultimately, most patients on the renal transplant waiting list have already begun dialysis. Unfortunately, chronic dialysis of prolonged duration is associated with decreased graft function. However, if transplant occurs within 6 months of starting dialysis then there is no detrimental effect on graft and patient survival, thus dialysis should be started if necessary.[11]

In the immediate preoperative period, it can be challenging to decide whether to perform routinely scheduled dialysis. Certainly, the implicit risks of hyperkalemia and volume overload must be considered. Chronic hyperkalemia is common in ESRD patients, and has less risk of arrhythmia compared with acute hyperkalemia. Furthermore, most patients demonstrate a rapid improvement in renal function immediately following transplant, thus the risks associated with each dialysis session can potentially be avoided. Older literature suggested that dialysis may be associated with delayed graft function if performed in the 24 hours immediately before transplant. However, this effect is likely ameliorated by modern techniques, and dialysis in the immediate preoperative period probably does not confer harm.[12] Nevertheless, given the frequent uncertainties regarding organ suitability and recipient tolerance of electrolyte derangement, the decision to perform dialysis before transplant should be made on a case-by-case basis.

Living Versus Deceased Organ Donation

Living donor donation is less common than deceased organ donation, and has become increasingly less frequent over the past decade. In general, graft function is superior for living compared with deceased donor transplants. Ten-year graft failure rates approach 50% for deceased donors but only 37% for living donor organs. Although patient survival outcomes remain relatively robust for each group, more than 90% of patients who received a live donor kidney were alive 5 years post-transplant, compared with approximately 85% of patients who received a deceased donor kidney.[1]

Preoperative evaluation of the living kidney donor should follow typical ACC/AHA guidelines for noncardiac surgery while also focusing especially on the baseline renal function and psychosocial needs of the organ donor. Per OPTN policies, similar to the recipient, donors are screened for the presence of malignancy, end-organ dysfunction, and viral infections that may compromise graft function (eg, human immunodeficiency virus [HIV], hepatitis, cytomegalovirus, Epstein-Barr virus). Blood type and crossmatch compatibility are of paramount importance to ensure nonrejection. Human leukocyte antigen typing is also performed to recognize the likely longevity of graft survival, though modern immunosuppressive regimens are usually sufficient for long-term survival.

Organ Acceptance and Retrieval Considerations

For most patients awaiting kidney transplant, finding a living donor is not a feasible option. Instead, they must rely on the limited pool of deceased donor organs in their geographic region. To increase the supply of suitable organs for transplant and reduce waiting time, some patients may elect to receive an expanded criteria donor (ECD) graft. Kidneys are classified as ECD if they are obtained from a deceased donor older than 59 years or aged 50 to 59 years with a serum creatinine greater than 1.5 mg/dL, death due to cerebrovascular accident, or history of hypertension. ECD kidneys confer an increased risk of graft dysfunction and can be a challenging choice to make when considering organ allocation. The kidney donor risk index (KDRI), determined on the basis of 14 donor and transplant factors, is a metric used to calculate the risk of graft failure following transplantation and can inform this decision. The KDRI is converted into a kidney donor profile index (KDPI), which is a percentage risk of graft failure as compared with an ideal organ.[13] Thus, when a potential organ donor is identified by the regional organ procurement organization, a KDPI is calculated, and the decision to transplant is considered.

However, the KDPI does not incorporate factors such as distance between the donor and the recipient's transplant center, graft retrieval timing, and preservation technique. Thus, it is important the donor be optimally supported to limit the risk of post-transplant graft dysfunction. Traditionally, donor kidneys have been retrieved under normothermic conditions. However, a recent trial demonstrated a reduction in the risk of graft dysfunction if therapeutic hypothermia (34°–35°C) was used.[14] Immediately before retrieval, when aortic cross-clamping is necessary, low-dose dopamine can be useful to reduce the risk of graft dysfunction.[15] Following retrieval, the kidneys are preserved in an intracellular type of preservative solution, such as University of Wisconsin solution. Following organ retrieval, cryopreservation is used to mitigate the effects of ischemia. Although static preservation on ice during transport is usually used, there is some evidence that hypothermic machine perfusion may reduce the risk of graft dysfunction.[16]

Intraoperative Anesthetic Considerations

Transplantation of the renal graft is usually performed heterotopically with arteriovenous anastomoses to the external iliac artery and vein after exposure through the lower quadrant of the abdomen, followed by uretero-bladder anastomosis. **Fig. 1** demonstrates the intraoperative visualization from the surgeon's perspective. General anesthesia is usually used, although use of regional and neuraxial approaches have been described.[17] Theoretically, sevoflurane-associated nephrotoxicity could be a concern. However sevoflurane has not been shown to be harmful in patients with chronic renal disease, and rapid improvement in renal function is anticipated following transplant, thus this should not influence the choice of inhalational anesthetic.[18,19] Routine intraoperative monitoring should be used with appropriate modifications for

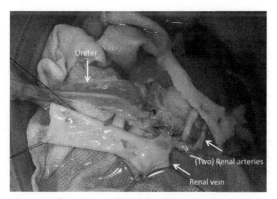

Fig. 1. Cadaveric kidney graft with renal arteries and veins and ureter. This donor had 2 renal arteries.

fluid management (see later discussion). Although therapeutic hypothermia of the donor has been shown to be beneficial, the recipient should be kept normothermic. The recipient should be positioned to avoid possible compression of the extremity through which the patient is routinely dialyzed.

Particularly for patients who have not been recently dialyzed, volume of distribution may be large. This fact, and the patient's cardiovascular reserve, should prompt the anesthesiologist to tailor induction dosing appropriately. Care must be taken to avoid nephrotoxic agents, which is usually not a concern intraoperatively. However, many antibiotics are renally eliminated and thus should be dosed appropriately based on the patient's current renal function. Additionally, some commonly used opioids, such as codeine, meperidine, and morphine, have metabolically active metabolites that are renally eliminated and require judicious dosing.

When choosing agents for induction and maintenance of anesthesia, neuromuscular blocking drugs (NBMDs) are of special importance. Diabetic patients with gastroparesis, or those who have a full stomach, may warrant rapid sequence induction. Succinylcholine will lead to an increase in serum potassium levels comparable to that of the non-ESRD population (approximately 0.5–1.0 mEq/L). Although many patients with ESRD have chronic hyperkalemia and thus can tolerate a transient increase in potassium concentration. The patient who has not been recently dialyzed may require use of a nondepolarizing NBMD instead, such as the commonly used rocuronium. Of note, rocuronium is partially renally eliminated and thus its effects may be prolonged.[20] Likewise, the effect of succinylcholine may also be prolonged because ESRD patients have reduced levels of pseudocholinesterase.[21] Thus, many practitioners favor the use of cisatracurium instead, unless rapid sequence induction is required.

Sugammadex, a relatively novel agent that selectively complexes rocuronium and vecuronium, has recently been approved for use in the United States The binding of sugammadex with rocuronium (or vecuronium) reduces the free concentration of NBMD available for action at the neuromuscular junction, rapidly reversing blockade. This complex is eventually eliminated by the kidneys and thus problematic in ESRD patients.[22] Fortunately, sugammadex-rocuronium is removed by hemodialysis.[23] However, in an anuric patient, it may be prudent to avoid sugammadex administration until renal recovery is evident.

Stress-induced hyperglycemia is a common intraoperative problem during kidney transplants, particularly in patients who are diabetic. Intensive glucose control (serum glucose concentrations between 70–110 mg/dL) theoretically may reduce the sequelae of ischemia-reperfusion. However, this has not been found to have meaningful clinical benefits, does not affect the risk of delayed graft function, and may actually increase the risk of rejection. Instead, anesthesiologists should titrate insulin as necessary to achieve concentrations of 70 to 180 mg/dL to avoid complications of hypoglycemia, as well as unnecessary osmotic diuresis.[7,24]

Intraoperative Fluid Management

Perhaps the most important goal of the intraoperative period is to ensure adequate graft perfusion in an attempt to limit the sequelae of ischemia-reperfusion. To this end, management of both hemodynamics and fluid administration is of critical importance. Autoregulatory mechanisms that ensure renal blood flow in the normal kidney are absent in the recently donated renal graft. Thus, flow through the glomerulus becomes pressure dependent, and systemic pressure is transmitted more directly to the renal parenchyma. In this delicate setting, both hypertension and hypotension can be detrimental because they are associated with acute rejection and delayed graft function, respectively.[25] Importantly, the anesthesia provider should ensure adequate cardiac output by correcting hypovolemia before reperfusion of the transplanted kidney. Failure to do so may result in an inadequately perfused graft and subsequent renal dysfunction.[26,27]

Historically, estimation of intravascular volume status has been inferred via the use of static hemodynamic metrics, such as pulmonary artery pressure and central venous pressure. However, this approach has more recently been discredited by a large body of evidence.[28] Instead, dynamic parameters, which incorporate the influence of juxtacardiac pressures on hemodynamics over time, are better able to identify the potentially hypovolemic patient. These dynamic metrics, such as pulse pressure variation, stroke volume variation, and others, are well-validated and easily calculated in real-time.[29] Most of these dynamic indices require continuous arterial pressure monitoring, thus it is reasonable to place an arterial line in the recipient should fluid responsiveness be uncertain. Many centers advocate the use of central venous catheter insertion during kidney transplants as well. For the purpose of volume assessment, this has little benefit; however, it may be necessary for administration of immunosuppressive or vasoactive drugs.

Traditionally, volume replacement of the hypovolemic kidney transplant recipient has been performed with 0.9% sodium chloride (normal saline) in an effort to avoid potential hyperkalemia with balanced salt solutions.[30] However, normal saline carries the risk of delivering a large chloride load to the patient, creating a hyperchloremic metabolic acidosis that may impair kidney function. Recent randomized trials in which a balanced crystalloid, such as lactated Ringer's or acetated Ringer's (PlasmaLyte) solution is used in lieu of normal saline, have found improved acid-base profiles in the balanced solution groups. Furthermore, serum potassium levels in these studies were actually lower in patients who did not receive normal saline, suggesting improved renal function in the balanced solutions.[31–33] Thus, in patients who are expected to have reasonable graft function postoperatively, it is prudent to use PlasmaLyte or lactated Ringer's instead of normal saline.

Alternatively, some clinicians have advocated use of colloid solutions in an effort to avoid excessive volume overload with the assumption a colloid will expand the intravascular space more effectively than crystalloid. However, this has also proven to be of little benefit. In broad populations needing resuscitation, no proven benefit has been found for using albumin-based colloids over saline.[34,35] Consideration has been given to using alternative, nonalbumin based, synthetic colloids, such as starches, dextrans, or gelatins. These too, however, have largely been shown to be harmful or ineffective compared with crystalloids. Hydroxyethyl starches, specifically, have been associated with both delayed graft function and a high incidence of native kidney injury.[36,37] Dextrans, composed of carbohydrate polymers, and gelatins, polypeptides derived from bovine collagen, have not been studied as well as other colloids but typically provide only short-lasting benefit for volume expansion, are known to cause osmotic diuresis, and may be associated with acute kidney injury.[38,39]

Intraoperative Vasoactive Drugs

Most kidney transplant procedures are not marked by significant hemodynamic instability. However, the high incidence of cardiovascular disease in this population coupled with possible large fluid shifts may necessitate the use of vasoactive agents. This is of particular importance because the newly transplanted graft lacks autoregulatory capabilities. Unfortunately, use of adrenergic agonists, particularly alpha-adrenergic receptor agonists, is associated with renal vasoconstriction and deterioration of graft function. However, this must be counterbalanced by the need to maintain appropriate arterial pressure to drive flow through the glomerular apparatus and reduce risk of delayed graft function.[40] If necessary, an agent with beta-adrenergic activity, such as norepinephrine, may be preferential. When compared with alternative agents, norepinephrine led to less of an increase in renal resistive index, suggesting it may be a more preferable alternative if hypotension is encountered intraoperatively.[41] Certainly, the need for vasoactive agents suggests a more acutely ill patient and in a patient who requires vasoactive substances long-term outcomes are worse.[42]

Intraoperative Renal Protection

Several studies have investigated the use of dopamine, both intraoperatively and postoperatively, in an effort to enhance renal blood flow and thus improve graft function. Unfortunately, these have largely been conflicting. Part of this discrepancy is probably attributable to the variable vascular resistance with the graft itself combined with the individual patient's unpredictable physiologic response to dopamine. Patients whose renal resistance decreases with dopamine probably benefit, whereas others may suffer harm if their resistive index rises.[41,43,44] Thus, empiric use of dopamine is not recommended.

Fortunately, other pharmacologic agents are more successful at preventing graft dysfunction. Mannitol is frequently used intraoperatively to provide some degree of protection from ischemia-reperfusion injury. When administered immediately before arterial clamping when retrieving a live donor organ, 12.5 to 25 g of mannitol has been associated with a decrease in delayed graft function.[45] Similarly, when transplanting a deceased donor kidney, mannitol blousing can reduce postoperative renal failure if administered immediately before clamp removal.[46] In both of these instances, mannitol presumably acts as an osmotic agent to reduce the unavoidable cellular edema that occurs with both ischemia and reperfusion, thus encouraging normal intracellular homeostasis. Occasionally, the transplant surgeon may request an intraoperative bolus of furosemide following graft reperfusion in an effort to increase diuresis. Presumably, this may help more rapidly return the patient's overall volume status toward normal, assuming rapidly improving renal function. However, this practice varies widely and does not correlate with graft survival.[47]

Complications

Intraoperative complications during kidney transplant are uncommon. Certainly, large volume hemorrhage is possible during anastomosis to the iliac vessels but occurs infrequently. Occasionally, ureteral obstructions or fistulae develop, but these are often not recognized until the postoperative period. Vascular complications, including thrombosis, are rare but devastating and can lead to graft loss. To prevent this, heparin is often administered immediately before vessel clamping.[48]

Graft function in the immediate postoperative period is influenced by a combination of donor, recipient, and intraoperative factors. Almost 50% of transplants are complicated by delayed graft function, which is ultimately secondary to ischemia-reperfusion injury. There a several different definitions of delayed graft function but most commonly it is defined as the need for dialysis within the first week after transplant. It is more common in ECD transplants, younger patients receiving comparatively older kidneys, donation after cardiac death, higher KDPI, prolonged ischemia time, intraoperative hypovolemia, and in situations in which the recipient immune response is difficult to suppress. It is generally treated supportively.[49,50] Graft failure, in which patients return to a state of renal dysfunction requiring dialysis, is fortunately uncommon but does occur. Graft failure tends to occur in sicker patients, in those who receive ECD organs, in those who have immunologic mismatch, or suffer a surgical complication.

Ultimately, they may need to be retransplanted or managed chronically with dialysis alone.[51]

PANCREAS TRANSPLANTATION
Epidemiology

Similar to kidney transplantation, end-stage pancreatic failure can be chronically pacified with medical management, creating a persistent mismatch between organ supply and demand. Isolated pancreas transplantation is much less common than kidney transplantation. To date, more than 8000 have been performed in the United States since the first successful operations in the 1960s. According to the OPTN, 215 isolated pancreas transplants were performed in 2016, which is actually slightly lower than preceding years. However, a larger number of patients receive a simultaneous pancreas-kidney (SPK) transplant due to renal failure associated with diabetes. These patients tend to have better outcomes than isolated transplants. In total, more than 22,000 SPK procedures have been performed; nearly 800 were completed in 2016. Additionally, patients may also receive a planned pancreas-after-kidney (PAK) transplant, particularly those with ESRD and chronic pancreatic insufficiency.

There are currently slightly more than 900 patients on the pancreas transplant waiting list, and nearly 1800 on the SPK waiting list. Although the total number of patients waiting has actually declined in the past few years, the number of actively listed candidates has remained constant. In recent years, the proportion of patients removed from the waiting list because they were too sick to transplant has exceeded the proportion of patients who have received a transplant, reflecting a growing trend to avoid transplanting in nonideal patients.[52]

Eligibility for Transplant

In general, isolated pancreas transplant is performed in young patients with type I diabetes who have challenging glycemic control, despite strict adherence to their medical regimen, but preserved renal function. SPK transplants, being much more common, have more stringently defined eligibility criteria and are limited to diabetic patients who have developed nephropathy and renal insufficiency. Absolute contraindications are similar to those for solitary kidney transplant, including active infection, malignancy, and (in some centers) HIV infection. Relative contraindications include morbid obesity, significant cardiovascular disease, advanced age, limited life expectancy, or poor psychosocial status.[53]

Preoperative Evaluation

Patients awaiting pancreas transplant are usually young and thus may have fewer comorbidities than their older, renal transplant counterparts. Nevertheless, microcirculatory dysfunction may manifest as cardiovascular disease and particular attention should be paid to the candidate's functional status. Atypical angina is a common problem in diabetics, thus the perioperative physician should maintain a high index of suspicion for the possibility of unrecognized coronary artery disease. There are no formal guidelines for preoperative cardiovascular evaluation of the SPK or isolated pancreas transplant candidate but it is reasonable to perform 12-lead electrocardiogram and noninvasive stress testing if it has not already been performed during the patient's workup for transplant.[53] Further evaluation should focus on the likelihood of end-organ dysfunction typical in diabetes, including gastroparesis, peripheral vascular disease, peripheral neuropathy, and, of course, nephropathy.

Intraoperative Management

The pancreas is transplanted heterotopically; exposure is accomplished through laparotomy. The exact location depends on surgeon preference and if SPK is being performed but, ultimately, function depends on effective perfusion and limiting total ischemic time. Historically, the bladder was the most frequent site of exocrine duct anastomosis due to technical feasibility. However, this can result in chronic metabolic acidosis from loss of bicarbonate-rich secretions, thus some surgeons now prefer an enteric exocrine anastomosis. When bladder drainage is performed, anatomic limitations reduce vascular anastomotic options and pancreatic venous outflow must occur via anastomosis at a systemic vessel. This results in high systemic concentrations of insulin, which can complicate the postoperative period. Instead, if enteric exocrine drainage can be performed, the venous vessels can be anastomosed to the portal circulation, and long-term peripheral insulin concentrations are closer to the normal, nondiabetic, population.[54] The surgical perspective during enteric anastomosis can be seen in **Fig. 2**.

Perhaps the most critical component of intraoperative care focuses on the need for strict observance of glycemic variation. Monitoring of serum glucose is of extreme importance both intraoperatively and postoperatively because it reflects the graft's viability. Perioperative delayed onset of normoglycemia can reflect a dysfunctional graft, pancreatitis, acute rejection, or insufficient graft size for recipient's needs, and should be communicated to the surgeon promptly.[54]

In terms of outcomes, SPK offers a greater chance of long-term graft survival than isolated pancreas or PAK procedures. However, SPK procedures are limited by the availability of organs, thus the trade-off between more rapid organ transplant with a nonsimultaneous procedure and long-term graft may favor a PAK approach. Generally, isolated pancreas procedures yield an 80% 1-year graft survival compared with 82% in PAK procedures and greater than 90% in SPK.[54]

Complications

Complications following pancreas transplant occur more frequently than in other abdominal solid organ transplants. Although major complications following pancreas transplant are uncommon, several, including pancreatitis, exocrine duct leaks, and pancreatic pseudocysts, are unique to this transplant. The pancreas presents a notoriously difficult operative substrate; technical complications do occasionally occur.

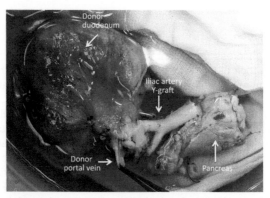

Fig. 2. Intraoperative appearance of deceased donor pancreas graft before enteric anastomosis of exocrine graft.

These are least frequent if combined with renal transplant. Technical failure rates occur with exocrine duct bladder anastomoses less frequently than with enteric anastomoses. Vascular thrombosis may be the result of technical issues or may be a symptom of rejection; it is the most common reason for graft failure. If vascular compromise is severe, graft failure may occur, which may mandate necrosectomy to minimize the risk of abscess and systemic infection.[54]

Early pancreatic graft failure rates have slowly improved over the last 10 years; 7.8% of grafts failed early in 2014 to 2015. Of note, kidney graft failure after SPK is lower than that of solitary kidney transplants, attributable to the higher quality of kidney grafts used for SPK recipients. Kidney graft failure rates after PAK transplant are comparable to those of solitary kidney transplant.[52]

Islet Cell Transplantation

Although outcomes following pancreas transplantation are generally good, the dearth of organs limits the number of patients who can be treated. Islet cell transplantation is an alternative, increasingly prevalent, less invasive, and potentially curative option for the type I diabetic who lacks significant renal dysfunction. Adult patients are eligible if they have frequent, unrecognized hypoglycemic episodes despite aggressive medical management. Donor islet cells are obtained from deceased donors but the requirements for donation are less stringent than that for pancreas transplant itself (eg, obese donors are suitable). Organ procurement for islet cell harvest is similar to that for total pancreas transplant with the exception that less attention needs to be given to ensuring vascular integrity because no anastomosis will be performed. Following resection of the graft, the pancreas is mechanically and enzymatically digested; the islet cell fraction is then obtained via centrifugal purification and then placed in culture for 24 to 72 hours to allow for quality assurance testing and identification of a suitable recipient. This process obtains hundreds of thousands of cell clusters; generally, more than 5000 islet equivalents per kilogram of recipient body weight are desired to achieve benefit.

The final pellet of islet cells is ultimately suspended in heparin and then transfused following cannulation of the portal vein, which can be performed under fluoroscopic or ultrasonographic guidance. The islets then become wedged in portal venules where they may initiate an immune response and trigger a nonspecific prothrombotic inflammatory state, which mandates systemic anticoagulation for 2 weeks following transplant. Islet cells can be obtained from multiple donors, potentially increasing the risk of immunologic activation. Although the risk is lower if a single donor is used, patients receiving islet cell transplants still require induction and maintenance of immunosuppression.

Outcomes following islet cell transplantation are generally good with few complications. The procedure may be performed under moderate sedation (eg, fluoroscopic guidance), or may occur during laparotomy, possibly following kidney transplant, which mandates general anesthesia. Up to 70% of patients achieve durable independence from insulin.[55]

REFERENCES

1. Hart A, Smith JM, Skeans MA, et al. OPTN/SRTR 2015 annual data report: kidney. Am J Transplant 2017;17(Suppl 1):21–116.
2. Suthanthiran M, Strom TB. Renal transplantation. N Engl J Med 1994;331:365–76.
3. Knoll G, Cockfield S, Blydt-Hansen T, et al. Canadian Society of Transplantation: consensus guidelines on eligibility for kidney transplantation. CMAJ 2005;173: S1–25.

4. Abbud-Filho M, Adams PL, Alberú J, et al. A report of the Lisbon Conference on the care of the kidney transplant recipient. Transplantation 2007;83:S1–22.
5. Pilmore H, Dent H, Chang S, et al. Reduction in cardiovascular death after kidney transplantation. Transplantation 2010;89:851–7.
6. Fleisher LA, Fleischmann KE, Auerbach AD, et al. 2014 ACC/AHA guideline on perioperative cardiovascular evaluation and management of patients undergoing noncardiac surgery: a report of the American College of Cardiology/American Heart Association task force on practice guidelines. J Am Coll Cardiol 2014;64: 77–137.
7. Lentine KL, Costa SP, Weir MR, et al. Cardiac disease evaluation and management among kidney and liver transplantation candidates: a scientific statement from the American Heart Association and the American College of Cardiology foundation. J Am Coll Cardiol 2012;60:434–80.
8. Dieterle CD, Schmauss S, Arbogast H, et al. Pulmonary function in patients with type 1 diabetes before and after simultaneous pancreas and kidney transplantation. Transplantation 2007;83:566–9.
9. Kasiske BL, Synder JJ, Matas AJ, et al. Preemptive kidney transplantation: the advantage and the advantaged. J Am Soc Nephrol 2002;13:1358–64.
10. Meier-Kriesche H, Schold JD. The impact of pretransplant dialysis on outcomes in renal transplantation. Semin Dial 2005;18:499–504.
11. Goldfarb-Rumyantzev A, Hurdle JF, Scandling J, et al. Duration of end-stage renal disease and kidney transplant outcome. Nephrol Dial Transplant 2005;20: 167–75.
12. Kikić Z, Lorenz M, Sunder-Plassmann G, et al. Effect of hemodialysis before transplant surgery on renal allograft function–a pair of randomized controlled trials. Transplantation 2009;88:1377–85.
13. Rao PS, Schaubel DE, Guidinger MK, et al. A comprehensive risk quantification score for deceased donor kidneys: the kidney donor risk index. Transplantation 2009;88:231–6.
14. Niemann CU, Feiner J, Swain S, et al. Therapeutic hypothermia in deceased organ donors and kidney-graft function. N Engl J Med 2015;373:405–14.
15. Schnuelle P, Gottmann U, Hoeger S, et al. Effects of donor pretreatment with dopamine on graft function after kidney transplantation: a randomized controlled trial. JAMA 2009;302:1067–75.
16. Moers C, Smits JM, Maathuis MH, et al. Machine perfusion or cold storage in deceased-donor kidney transplantation. N Engl J Med 2009;360:7–19.
17. Akpek EA, Kayhan Z, Donmez A, et al. Eary postoperative renal function following renal transplantation surgery: effect of anesthetic technique. J Anesth 2002;16: 114–8.
18. Higuchi H, Adachi Y, Wada H, et al. The effects of low-flow sevoflurane and isoflurane anesthesia on renal function in patients with stable moderate renal insufficiency. Anesth Analg 2001;92:650–5.
19. Teixeira S, Costa G, Costa F, et al. Sevoflurane versus isoflurane: does it matter in renal transplantation? Transplant Proc 2007;39:2486–8.
20. Cooper RA, Maddineni VR, Mirakhur RK, et al. Time course of neuromuscular effects and pharmacokinetics of rocuronium bromide (Org 9426) during isoflurane anaesthesia in patients with and without renal failure. Br J Anaesth 1993;71: 222–6.
21. Ryan DW. Preoperative serum cholinesterase concentration in chronic renal failure. Clinical experience of suxamethonium in 81 patients undergoing renal transplant. Br J Anaesth 1977;49:945–9.

22. Staals LM, Snoeck MM, Driessen JJ, et al. Reduced clearance of rocuronium and sugammadex in patients with severe to end-stage renal failure: a pharmacokinetic study. Br J Anaesth 2010;104:31–9.

23. Cammu G, Van Vlem B, van den Heuvel M, et al. Dialysability of sugammadex and its complex with rocuronium in intensive care patients with severe renal impairment. Br J Anaesth 2012;109:382–90.

24. Hermayer KL, Egidi MF, Finch NJ, et al. A randomized controlled trial to evaluate the effect of glycemic control on renal transplantation outcomes. J Clin Endocrinol Metab 2012;97:4399–406.

25. Thomas MC, Mathew TH, Russ GR, et al. Perioperative blood pressure control, delayed graft function, and acute rejection after renal transplantation. Transplantation 2003;75:1989–95.

26. Carlier M, Squifflet JP, Pirson Y, et al. Maximal hydration during anesthesia increases pulmonary arterial pressures and improves early function of human renal transplants. Transplantation 1982;34:201–4.

27. Othman MM, Ismael AZ, Hammouda GE. The impact of timing of maximal crystalloid hydration on early graft function during kidney transplantation. Anesth Analg 2010;110:1440–6.

28. Marik PE, Cavallazzi R. Does the central venous pressure predict fluid responsiveness? An updated meta-analysis and a plea for some common sense. Crit Care Med 2013;41:1774–81.

29. Durairaj L, Schmidt GA. Fluid therapy in resuscitated sepsis: less is more. Chest 2008;133:252–63.

30. O'Malley CM, Frumento RJ, Bennett-Guerrero E. Intravenous fluid therapy in renal transplant recipients: results of a US survey. Transplant Proc 2002;34:3142–5.

31. O'Malley CM, Frumento RJ, Hardy MA, et al. A randomized, double-blind comparison of lactated Ringer's solution and 0.9% NaCl during renal transplantation. Anesth Analg 2005;100:1518–24.

32. Hadimioglu N, Saadawy I, Saglam T, et al. The effect of different crystalloid solutions on acid-base balance and early kidney function after kidney transplantation. Anesth Analg 2008;107:264–9.

33. Wan S, Roberts MA, Mount P. Normal saline versus lower-chloride solutions for kidney transplantation. Cochrane Database Syst Rev 2016;(8):CD010741.

34. Cochrane Injuries Group Albumin Reviewers. Human albumin administration in critically ill patients: systematic review of randomised controlled trials. BMJ 1998;317:235–40.

35. Finfer S, Bellomo R, Boyce N, et al. A comparison of albumin and saline for fluid resuscitation in the intensive care unit. N Engl J Med 2004;350:2247–56.

36. Cittanova ML, Leblanc I, Legendre C, et al. Effect of hydroxyethylstarch in brain-dead kidney donors on renal function in kidney-transplant recipients. Lancet 1996;348:1620–2.

37. Perner A, Haase N, Guttormsen AB, et al. Hydroxyethyl starch 130/0.42 versus Ringer's acetate in severe sepsis. N Engl J Med 2012;367:124–34.

38. Mårtensson J, Bellomo R. Are all fluids bad for the kidney? Curr Opin Crit Care 2015;21:292–301.

39. Bayer O, Reinhart K, Kohl M, et al. Effects of fluid resuscitation with synthetic colloids or crystalloids alone on shock reversal, fluid balance, and patient outcomes in patients with severe sepsis: a prospective sequential analysis. Crit Care Med 2012;40:2543–51.

40. Morita K, Seki T, Nonomura K, et al. Changes in renal blood flow in response to sympathomimetics in the rat transplanted and denervated kidney. Int J Urol 1999;6:24–32.
41. Lauschke A, Teichgräber UK, Frei U, et al. 'Low-dose' dopamine worsens renal perfusion in patients with acute renal failure. Kidney Int 2006;69:1669–74.
42. Choi JM, Jo JY, Baik JW, et al. Risk factors and outcomes associated with a higher use of inotropes in kidney transplant recipients. Medicine (Baltimore) 2017;96:e5820.
43. Dalton RS, Webber JN, Cameron C, et al. Physiologic impact of low-dose dopamine on renal function in the early post renal transplant period. Transplantation 2005;79:1561–7.
44. Ciapetti M, di Valvasone S, di Filippo A, et al. Low-dose dopamine in kidney transplantation. Transplant Proc 2009;41:4165–8.
45. Andrews PM, Cooper M, Verbesey J, et al. Mannitol infusion within 15 min of cross-clamp improves living donor kidney preservation. Transplantation 2014; 98:893–7.
46. van Valenberg PL, Hoitsma AJ, Tiggeler RG, et al. Mannitol as an indispensable constituent of an intraoperative hydration protocol for the prevention of acute renal failure after renal cadaveric transplantation. Transplantation 1987;44:784–8.
47. Hanif F, Macrae AN, Littlejohn MG, et al. Outcome of renal transplantation with and without intra-operative diuretics. Int J Surg 2011;9:460–3.
48. Parada B, Figueiredo A, Mota A, et al. Surgical complications in 1000 renal transplants. Transplant Proc 2003;35:1085–6.
49. Siedlecki A, Irish W, Brennan DC. Delayed graft function in the kidney transplant. Am J Transplant 2011;11:2279–96.
50. Schröppel B, Legendre C. Delayed kidney graft function: from mechanism to translation. Kidney Int 2014;86:251–8.
51. Weiss-Salz I, Mandel M, Galai N, et al. Factors associated with primary and secondary graft failure following cadaveric kidney transplant. Clin Transplant 2004; 18:571–5.
52. Kandaswamy R, Stock PG, Gustafson SK, et al. OPTN/SRTR 2015 annual data report: pancreas. Am J Transplant 2017;17(Suppl 1):117–73.
53. Freise CE, Narumi S, Stock PG, et al. Simultaneous pancreas-kidney transplantation: an overview of indications, complications, and outcomes. West J Med 1999; 170:11–8.
54. Larsen JL. Pancreas transplantation: indications and consequences. Endocr Rev 2004;25:919–46.
55. Shapiro AM, Pokrywczynska M, Ricordi C. Clinical pancreatic islet transplantation. Nat Rev Endocrinol 2017;13(5):268–77.

Anesthesia for Heart Transplantation

Davinder Ramsingh, MD[a],*, Reed Harvey, MD[b], Alec Runyon, MD[a],
Michael Benggon, MD[a]

KEYWORDS

- Heart transplantation • Criteria for heart transplantation • Right heart failure
- Circulatory support

KEY POINTS

- The common primary diagnosis for patients undergoing heart transplantation has shifted over time along with an increase in bridge therapy with mechanical circulatory support.
- Donor age, gender, size, and presence of panel-reactive antibodies remain important factors for successful transplantation.
- Coordination of donor and receipt procedures, along with the appreciation for patients with end-stage heart failure having "fixed" stroke volumes are key for intraoperative management.
- Rapid assessment of cardiac function, in particular right ventricular function, and preparation for treatment strategies is crucial for posttransplantation management.
- Both short-term and long-term survival of heart transplant recipients has gradually improved over time.

INTRODUCTION AND HISTORY

With advances in the pharmacologic and surgical treatment options for heart failure (HF) coupled with an aging population, the number of people with HF in the United States is expected to rise significantly. However, mortality for these patients remains at nearly 50% within 5 years of diagnosis.[1] Although left ventricular assist devices (LVADs) are able to prolong and improve quality of life for those with American College of Cardiology Foundation/American Heart Association (AHA)

Disclosure Statement: No author reports any relevant conflicts of interest.
[a] Department of Anesthesiology, Loma Linda Medical Center, 11234 Anderson Street, MC-2532-D, Loma Linda, CA 92354, USA; [b] Department of Anesthesiology, Ronald Reagan UCLA Medical Center, University of California at Los Angeles, 757 Westwood Plaza, Suite 3325, Los Angeles, CA 90095-7403, USA
* Corresponding author.
E-mail address: dramsingh@llu.edu

Key points

- The number of patients with heart failure qualifying for cardiac transplantation is growing
- Immunosuppressive agents have dramatically improved success of heart transplantation
- The most common primary diagnosis has shifted over time from ischemic cardiomyopathy (ICM) to non-ICM
- The use of bridge therapy with mechanical circulatory support now exceeds 50%
- Both short-term and long-term survival of heart transplant recipients has gradually improved over time

---

stage D refractory HF (**Box 1**), heart transplantation (HT) remains the definitive treatment.[2,3]

The first successful human-to-human HT occurred in 1967.[4] In the year following, 102 HTs were attempted worldwide, with consistently poor results due to acute organ rejection and surgical inexperience. Two advancements in the detection and treatment of rejection in the 1970s transformed the landscape of HT. In 1973, Caves and colleagues[5] described the technique for transvenous endomyocardial biopsy for the diagnosis of immune rejection. Although this technique provided the means for identification of rejection, Jean-Francois Borel's[6] 1976 description of the immunosuppressive effects of cyclosporin A finally identified an effective preventive treatment.[7] This success translated to a worldwide exponential increase in the use of HT for the treatment of end-stage HF. Although HT volumes have been stable for years, with recent liberalization of donor criteria, HT volumes are increasing once again.[8]

Box 1
Definition of advanced heart failure

1. Severe symptoms of HR with dyspnea and/or fatigue at rest or with minimal exertion (NYHA class III or IV).

2. Episodes of fluid retention and/or reduced cardiac output at rest (peripheral hypoperfusion).

3. Objective evidence of severe cardiac dysfunction shown by at least 1 of the following: (1) LVEF <30%, (2) pseudonormal or restrictive mitral inflow pattern, (3) mean PCWP >16 mm Hg and/or RAP >12 mm Hg by PA catheterization, (4) high BNP or NT-proBNP plasma levels in the absence of noncardiac causes.

4. Severe impairment of functional capacity shown by any 1 of the following: (1) inability to exercise, (2) 6-minute walk distance 300 m, (3) peak Vo_2 12 to 14 mL/kg per minute.

5. History of at least 1 heart failure hospitalization in the past 6 months.

6. Presence of all the previous features despite "attempts to optimize" therapy, including diuretics and GDMT, unless these are poorly tolerated or contraindicated, and CRT when indicated.

Abbreviations: BNP, B-type natriuretic peptide; CRT, cardiac resynchronization therapy; GDMT, guideline-directed medical therapy; HR, heart rate; LVEF, left ventricular ejection fraction; NT-proBNP, N-terminal pro-B-type natriuretic peptide; NYHA, New York Heart Association; PA, pulmonary artery; PCWP, pulmonary capillary wedge pressure; RAP, right atrial pressure; Vo_2, peak exercise oxygen consumption.

Adapted from Metra M, Ponikowski P, Dickstein K, et al. Advanced chronic heart failure: a position statement from the Study Group on Advanced Heart Failure of the Heart Failure Association of the European Society of Cardiology. Eur J Heart Fail 2007;9(6–7):685; with permission.

Through June 30, 2015, there have been 118,788 HTs performed worldwide. According to the Organ Procurement and Transplantation Network (OPTN), there were a record high 2924 HTs performed in the United States in 2016 (optn. transplant.hrsa.gov). The number of adult candidates on the waiting list for HT in the United States increased by 34.2% from 2003 to 2013.[9] Mortality for these patients, however, has reduced over the past decade (14.8 deaths per 100 waitlist-years in 2002 to 10.7 in 2013).[9] This has manifested as an increase in the number of high-urgency candidates (United Network of Organ Sharing [UNOS] status 1A or 1B). Median waiting time for patients of status 1A has increased from 64 days in 2003 to 2006, to 87 days in 2011 to 2014, and from 79 to 253 days for patients of status 1B in the same time frame.[10] This increase in high-urgency candidates, waiting times, and survival is most likely due to the increasing number of ventricular assist devices being implanted in patients with end-stage HF. In fact, the number of HT recipients bridged with mechanical circulatory support (MCS) now exceeds 50%.[8]

The International Society for Heart and Lung Transplantation (ISHLT) identifies 8 primary diagnoses for adult HT recipients (**Table 1**). The most common primary diagnosis has shifted over time from ischemic cardiomyopathy (ICM) to non-ICM (NICM), with NICM now representing 49.2% of all HT recipients. ICM remains the most prevalent diagnosis in patients older than 59 years.[8] This trend continues even though older patients now represent an increasing proportion of the transplant population.[9]

Both short-term and long-term survival of HT recipients has gradually improved over time. The 2013 OPTN Annual Data Report reported a 1-year, 3-year, and 5-year survival of 88.1%, 81.3%, and 75.3%, respectively.[9] Data from the most recent ISHLT registry continues to show improvement in unadjusted survival for adult HT recipients, particularly in the short-term, with the median survival now reported at 11.9 years overall, and 13.2 years conditional on survival to 1 year.[8] As HF is a heterogeneous disorder with significant differences in underlying etiology and baseline risk characteristics, survival for HT recipients varies significantly based on underlying diagnosis. One-year survival is highest for patients with NICM, and lowest for patients with congenital heart disease and those undergoing retransplantation. Importantly, posttransplant survival decreases with increasing recipient and donor age.

Table 1
Primary underlying diagnosis for adult heart transplant recipients

	Frequency, %
Non-ischemic cardiomyopathy	49.2
Ischemic cardiomyopathy	34.6
Restrictive cardiomyopathy	3.3
Congenital heart disease	3.2
Retransplantation	3.0
Hypertrophic cardiomyopathy	3.0
Valvular cardiomyopathy	2.7
Other	1.1

Adapted from Lund LH, Edwards LB, Dipchand AI, et al. The Registry of the International Society for Heart and Lung Transplantation: thirty-third adult heart transplantation report-2016; focus theme: primary diagnostic indications for transplant. J Heart Lung Transplant 2016;35(10):1159; with permission.

Even with improvements in immunosuppression and a decreased incidence of identified and treated rejection, the first year after transplantation continues to be the time with highest mortality. Primary graft failure is common after HT and its incidence seems to be increasing.[11] Graft failure remains the leading cause of death in the first 30 days after transplantation, accounting for 40.2% of all deaths, and cumulatively remains the leading cause of mortality in the long-term as well. Non-cytomegalovirus (CMV) infection and multiple organ failure also are additional major contributors to mortality within the first year, accounting for 31.1% and 15.9% of deaths from 31 days to 1-year posttransplant, respectively. Although primary graft failure, infection, and organ failure limit survival in the short-term, side effects from chronic immunosuppressive therapy and the development of coronary allograft vasculopathy (CAV) seem to limit long-term survival. Development of malignancy becomes the leading cause of death in years 5 through 10 after transplantation, and the prevalence of malignancy in HT recipients at 10 years is 27.4%.[8] CAV is a diffuse process of concentric longitudinal intimal hyperplasia of the large epicardial coronary arteries as well as microcirculation. Although multifactorial in nature, the panarterial involvement of the graft vasculature with sparing of the recipient's vasculature suggests a primarily immune-mediated etiology. The prevalence on CAV in transplant survivors increases from 8% at 1 year to 50% by 10 years,[12] and it becomes 1 of the 3 leading causes of death by 5 years after transplantation.

RECIPIENT SELECTION

Key points

- The time to receive a transplant is increasing
- UNOS has a priority allocation algorithm
- Fixed pulmonary hypertension remains an absolute contraindication

---

Although the number of HTs performed in the United States in 2016 reached a record high, the number of patients added to the waiting list continues to outpace organ availability.

Selection of HT candidates requires a multidisciplinary approach to identify patients with end-stage HF who remain symptomatic despite optimal medical therapy. Patients with a primary indication for HT (**Box 2**) should be referred to a transplant center for evaluation. Identification of patients with absolute or relative contraindications to transplantation (**Box 3**), as well as identification of potentially reversible medical conditions, is paramount to ensure appropriate organ allocation to those who will benefit most.[13] Listing for transplantation focuses on patients requiring continuous inotropic support or MCS, or those with severe functional impairments despite optimal medical therapy.

Efforts to prioritize organ allocation to those patients with the highest mortality were first introduced by UNOS in 1989 with the introduction of a high-priority UNOS status 1 listing. This status was further divided into tiers, status 1A and 1B, in 1999.[14] Data from OPTN shows that of the patients currently listed for HT, 54.1% are currently either status 1A or 1B, with status 1A candidates increasing from 21.6% to 43.9% over the preceding decade.[9] This increase in high-urgency candidates has led to longer waiting times for transplantation. Status 1A patient criteria are listed in **Box 4**.

Box 2
Primary indications for heart transplantation

- Cardiogenic shock requiring either continuous intravenous inotropic support or MCS with an intra-aortic balloon pump
- Persistent NYHA class IV congestive heart failure symptoms refractory to maximal medical therapy (LVEF <20%; peak Vo_2 <12 mL/kg per minute)
- Intractable or severe angina symptoms in patients with coronary artery disease not amenable to percutaneous or surgical revascularization
- Intractable life-threatening arrhythmias unresponsive to medical therapy, catheter ablation, and/or implantation of intracardiac defibrillator

Abbreviation: MCS, mechanical circulatory support.
Adapted from Mancini D, Lietz K. Selection of cardiac transplantation candidates in 2010. Circulation 2010;122(2):174; with permission.

Box 3
Contraindications to heart transplantation

Absolute Contraindications

Systemic illness with a life expectancy <2 years despite heart transplant, including the following:
- Active or recent solid organ or blood malignancy within 5 years
- AIDS with frequent opportunistic infection
- Systemic lupus erythematosus, sarcoid, or amyloidosis that has multisystem involvement and is still active
- Irreversible renal or hepatic dysfunction in patients considered for only heart transplantation
- Significant obstructive pulmonary disease (FEV1 <1 L/min)

Fixed pulmonary hypertension
- Pulmonary artery systolic pressure >60 mm Hg
- Mean transpulmonary gradient >15 mm Hg
- Pulmonary vascular resistance >6 wood units

Relative Contraindications

Age >72 years

Any active infection (with exception of device-related infection in ventricular assist device recipients)

Active peptic ulcer disease

Diabetes with end-organ damage

Severe peripheral vascular or cerebrovascular disease

Morbid obesity (BMI >35 kg/m²) or cachexia (BMI <18 kg/m²)

Creatinine >2.5 mg/dL or creatinine clearance <25 mL/min

Bilirubin >2.5 mg/dL, serum transaminases >3 times normal, or INR >1.5 off warfarin

Severe pulmonary dysfunction with FEV1 <40% expected

Active mental illness or psychosocial instability

Drug, tobacco, or alcohol abuse within 6 months

Recent pulmonary infarction within 6 to 8 weeks

Irreversible neurologic or neuromuscular disorder

Adapted from Mancini D, Lietz K. Selection of cardiac transplantation candidates in 2010. Circulation 2010;122(2):174; with permission.

Box 4
United Network of Organ Sharing Status 1A Criteria

1. Currently hospitalized patients who meet any 1 of the following criteria:
   a. Mechanical circulatory support with total artificial heart, intra-aortic balloon pump, or extracorporeal membrane oxygenation (must be renewed every 14 days)
   b. Requires continuous mechanical ventilation (must be renewed every 14 days)
   c. Requires continuous infusion of high-dose inotropes and continuous monitoring of left ventricular filling pressures (must be renewed every 7 days)

2. Current hospitalization not required for the following:
   a. Mechanical circulatory support with left ventricular assist device, right ventricular assist device, or biventricular assist device (30 days allocated)
   b. Mechanical circulatory support for more than 30 days with evidence of device-related complication

Adapted from Organ Procurement and Transplantation Network (OPTN). Health Resources and Services Administration, U.S. Department of Health & Human Services. Available at: https://optn.transplant.hrsa.gov/. Accessed May 9, 2017.

Patients of status 1B are those with MCS or continuous intravenous inotropic dependence who do not meet status 1A criteria. Status 1 B listing does not require recertification and the patient may be listed indefinitely as long as criteria are met. The full UNOS criteria and exceptions for assignments are available via the OPTN Web site (optn.transplant.hrsa.gov).

In 2016, the ISHLT published updated guidelines for HT listing criteria.[15] For the cohort of patients who do not require continuous inotropic support or MCS, these guidelines focus on the prognostic value of clinical indices, HF prognosis scores, and identification of unacceptably high-risk comorbid conditions to guide listing for transplantation. Additionally, the guidelines focus on evolving areas of importance in candidacy selection that were not addressed fully in the 2006 guidelines, such as congenital heart disease, restrictive cardiomyopathy, and candidates with infectious diseases.

Cardiopulmonary stress testing and determination of peak exercise oxygen consumption (Vo_2) remains the cornerstone in establishing patients who would benefit from HT. A Vo_2 cutoff of ≤ 12 mL/kg per minute for patients on beta-blocker therapy and $Vo_2 \leq 14$ mL/kg per minute for those intolerant of beta-blocker therapy are suggested to guide listing (class I recommendation). The new guidelines recommend that HF prognosis scores, such as the Seattle Heart Failure Model[16,17] or Heart Failure Survival Score, should be performed along with cardiopulmonary exercise testing to guide listing in ambulatory patients (class IIb).

Fixed pulmonary hypertension remains an absolute contraindication to HT and there is a close relationship between pulmonary vascular resistance (PVR) and mortality after HT.[11] New guidelines recommend right heart catheterization in all adults undergoing transplant evaluation and at 3-month to 6-month intervals in listed patients.[15]

HT is relatively contraindicated for patients with the following pulmonary artery (PA) pressure values:

a. Systolic PA pressure greater than 60 mm Hg
b. PVR >6 wood units
c. Transpulmonary gradient (TPG) = mean PA pressure − mean pulmonary capillary wedge pressure >16 to 20 mm Hg[18]

Additionally, a TPG ≥ 12 mm Hg has been associated with a fivefold increase in mortality at 6 months and a 7 times greater mortality at 1 year after HT.[19] Patients with elevated PVR (systolic PA pressure >50 mm Hg, transpulmonary gradient >15 mm Hg, or PVR >3 wood units) should undergo a vasodilator challenge to determine reversibility. Patients failing the vasodilator challenge may undergo medical therapy (inotropes, diuretics) with continuous invasive monitoring of PVR. MCS with LVAD or intra-aortic balloon pumps (IABPs) for unloading of the left ventricle should be considered in patients failing medical therapy.[15] Reevaluation of hemodynamics after initiation of therapy should be done at 3-month to 6-month intervals to ascertain reversibility of pulmonary hypertension.

The recent ISHLT guidelines also address the impact of comorbid conditions (age, body mass index [BMI], malignancy, diabetes, renal dysfunction, cerebrovascular disease), substance abuse, and psychosocial support in transplant candidacy.[15] A few important changes to the 2006 guidelines include increasing the upper limit of BMI for candidacy from 30 kg/m^2 to 35 kg/m^2 and establishing a cutoff glomerular filtration rate value of 30 mL/min/1.73 m^2 as a relative contraindication to HT alone. Additional recommendations include a thorough evaluation of patient frailty in assessing candidacy, and the use of MCS as a bridge to candidacy in patients with potentially reversible comorbidities.

Although retransplantation still makes up a very small percentage of all transplant recipients, early mortality for these patients is quite high.[20] Listing for retransplantation is now recommended for patients who develop significant CAV with refractory graft dysfunction without evidence of ongoing rejection.

DONOR SELECTION

Key points

- Donor age is an independent risk factor for increased recipient mortality
- Echocardiographic assessment is crucial and coronary angiography may be warranted for older donor candidates
- Successful transplantation depends on matching ABO blood group compatibility, the presence of panel-reactive antibodies (PRA), and size and gender matching

---

The number of donors has begun to increase in recent years to a record high of 3241 in 2016. This increase in donor utilization may be due in part to more widespread adoption of expanded donor criteria that was initially proposed in 2001 as the Crystal City guidelines.[21] Despite donor age being an independent risk factor of increased recipient mortality,[22] the average donor age has increased from 32 years in 1992 to 2003, to 35 years in recent years. Approximately 50% of donors in 2016 were aged 18 to 34 years, and transplantation with donor hearts older than 60 years is still rare. When accepting older donors, it is important to minimize additional risks, such long ischemic times and significant additional comorbidities.

The leading causes of death for donors are head trauma, anoxia, and stroke.[8] On confirmation of brain death in potential donors consented for organ transplantation, a preliminary matching list based on UNOS criteria is generated and communication established between an institutional transplant coordinator and a local organ procurement organization. Initial survey of the potential donor includes donor age, gender, height, weight, ABO blood typing, cause of death, and drug or alcohol abuse history.[23] Specific history relevant to the suitability of a potential cardiac donor includes history of thoracic trauma, cardiopulmonary resuscitation, hemodynamic stability, and pressor/inotropic requirements.[24] Review of pertinent laboratory data and clinical studies should be performed, including viral serologies (CMV, hepatitis B and C, and human immunodeficiency virus) and arterial blood gas analysis.

Quality assessment of the potential donor heart is essential for successful transplantation. All potential donors should have a chest radiograph, electrocardiogram (ECG), serum cardiac enzymes, and echocardiogram. Coronary angiography is recommended in male donors older than 45 years and female donors older than 55 years. Many potential donors have undergone cardiopulmonary bypass (CPB), are on inotropic medications, or have suffered thoracic trauma or neurologic insult, and may display nonspecific ECG changes or elevation in serum cardiac enzymes. These changes may not be indicative of true cardiac injury and always should be correlated with echocardiographic findings.[23] Modest elevations in donor troponin I levels have not been shown to correlate with posttransplant mortality or need for MCS.[25] Echocardiographic assessment should be focused on identification of left ventricular hypertrophy (LVH), regional wall motion abnormalities, physiologically significant valvular dysfunction, and identification of congenital abnormalities. The presence of significant LVH greater than 14 mm has been associated with poor outcomes in HT recipients.[26] Donor contraindications include excessive inotropic support, left ventricular ejection fraction (LVEF) less than 40%, regional wall motion abnormalities, intractable ventricular arrhythmias, congenital heart disease, transmissible disease, and systemic malignancy. Final acceptance of the donor heart is made after direct visual and manual inspection of the organ by the procuring cardiothoracic surgeon.

Beyond the identification of a healthy donor organ, successful transplantation depends on matching the donor organ to the recipient based multiple characteristics, including ABO blood group compatibility, the presence of PRAs, and size and gender matching. Typically, a donor-recipient size mismatch of greater than 30% is considered significant enough to preclude transplantation. Caution should be used in the transplantation of undersized hearts in recipients with pulmonary hypertension because of the risk of posttransplant right ventricular failure. There is improved survival with transplant gender concordance. Male recipients of female donor hearts have increased incidence and severity of graft rejection.[27]

VENTRICULAR ASSIST DEVICES

Key points

- LVAD indications and current use as a bridge to HT has increased
- There are benefits of LVADs compared with medical therapy for HT candidates
- Use of LVADs as a temporizing measure can result in improvement of HF
- MCS national registry development and evolution from pulsatile pumps to continuous flow pumps

---

More than 64% of patients require life support as a bridge to transplantation.[28] Examples of support include IABPs, inotropes, mechanical ventilation, and LVADs. The ISHLT reports that 45% of transplant recipients in 2013 had an LVAD compared with 12% between 1992 and 2000.[29] Benefits of LVADs while awaiting HT include a

45% decrease in intensive care unit hospitalizations before transplant, prolonged survival compared with inotropes and IABPs, and a higher rate of remission from American College of Cardiology/AHA stage D HF.[28,30,31] Indications to LVADs include their use as a bridge to transplantation, rescue therapy, and destination therapy. Between 2012 and 2016, 45% of implants were for destination therapy, whereas 54% were placed for bridge to transplantation.[32] Between 2009 and 2014, 43% of HT candidates were bridged to transplantation with MCS.[29] Initially there was concern about whether the additional sternotomy required for LVAD insertion could worsen posttransplantation outcomes. Fortunately, it has been shown that there is no difference in posttransplant outcomes between patients bridged to transplantation with LVADs compared with those without LVADs.[29,33] Additionally, duration of LVAD use before transplantation does not appear to confer additional risk.[34–36]

In 2006, the Interagency Registry for Mechanically Assisted Circulatory Support (INTERMACS) was developed. INTERMACS data collected between 2006 and 2016 found that 1-year survival rates were 74% for continuous flow pumps versus 60% for pulsatile pumps.[32] Given the improvement in outcomes, nonpulsatile pumps have become more favored and, as of 2011, more than 99% of LVAD implants were continuous flow devices.

PREANESTHETIC CONSIDERATIONS

Key points

- HT is an urgent or emergent procedure
- Preoperative evaluation of recipient
- Preoperative device interrogation
- Approach to perioperative anticoagulation
- Timing of induction and incision
- Venous and arterial access
- Antibiotics and immunosuppression

HT can occur at any time, and is considered an urgent or emergent surgery. Factors that influence the timing of transplantation include the time of donor surgery and organ transport, potential preoperative optimization of recipients, adequate time for induction of anesthesia and line placement, and appropriate recipient surgical timing to minimize ischemic time. It is imperative that the harvesting team, recipient surgical team, and anesthesia team communicate clearly with each other to minimize any delays.

Because of the often-emergent nature of HT, preoperative evaluations must be prompt and efficient. Approximately 64% of patients presenting for HT have some type of cardiovascular support (eg, LVAD, IABP, inotropes); therefore, a clear understanding of their current regimen is necessary.[28] The anesthesiologist should assess any antiarrhythmic devices and evaluate the patency and sterility of monitoring and access lines.

Antiarrhythmic devices should be interrogated preoperatively and reprogrammed to a mode that will not misinterpret electrocautery interference. Implantable cardioverter defibrillators should have the defibrillators inactivated. Magnets should be available, and the effects of a magnet should be verified against each device. In most cases, the antiarrhythmic devices are removed during the HT surgery after the donor heart is successfully transplanted.

The preoperative evaluation should include an assessment of the patient's coagulation status and risk of bleeding. Laboratory studies should be reviewed; preoperative anemia, thrombocytopenia, and an elevated international normalized ratio are all associated with increased perioperative bleeding during cardiac surgery. Redo sternotomies, which are common given the increasing prevalence of ventricular assist devices, also increase the risk of perioperative bleeding. As such, blood should be immediately available before incision. Adequate access, including large-bore peripheral intravenous lines and a central venous catheter, should be accessible in case rapid transfusion of blood products or fluids is required. There is significant variability in intraoperative blood product requirements during HT; a range of 3 to 9 units of packed red blood cells, 3 to 10 units of fresh frozen plasma, and 0 to 13 units of platelets have been reported.[37]

Multiple studies have shown that the duration of ischemic time has an adverse effect on survival.[38–40] In an effort to minimize ischemia, the induction of anesthesia and recipient surgical incision should preferably begin as soon as the harvesting team has evaluated the donor heart and found it to be acceptable. Ideally, CPB should be initiated and the heart excised as soon as the donor heart arrives to the recipient hospital. To improve this timing, the anesthesiologist should communicate his or her anticipated time for induction and line placement with the surgical teams.

Antibiotic selection requires evaluation of the donor and recipient's infection patterns and forthcoming immunosuppressants. Clear, closed-loop communication with the transplant surgery team is imperative, because the timing of immunosuppressant medications is crucial. Aseptic techniques should be maintained during line placement and throughout the case to minimize the risk of line-associated infections.

INDUCTION AND MAINTENANCE

Key points

- Patients with end-stage HF have "fixed" stroke volumes and require adequate preload, maintenance of elevated systemic vascular resistance, and adequate heart rate to maintain cardiac output
- PA catheter is useful to evaluate pressures and right ventricular function
- Coordination of surgical procedures of donor and receipt is key to minimize ischemia time

---

As with preoperative assessment, coordination of care is key regarding timing of induction of anesthesia for the HT recipient. Recent registry data demonstrated a statistically significant increase in acute graft failure in 1-year and 5-year mortality rates with ischemic times longer than 210 minutes.[41] Currently, all efforts should be made to minimize organ ischemic time, with a target goal of less than 4 hours.[41,42] However, recent evidence has demonstrated noninferiority with the use of ex vivo perfusion systems that are designed to increase out of body time.[43]

For determining the appropriate timing of the recipient to undergo general anesthesia, one must factor the time it will take to transport the donor heart with the time it will take to prepare the recipient. Importantly, one must account for the fact that these patients often have experienced multiple punctures of arteries and central veins. Additionally, given the emergency basis of these procedures, it is possible that patients may not be NPO (nil per os) and should be evaluated for the need of rapid sequence intubation.[44]

Monitoring

Standard American Society of Anesthesiologists monitors, including pulse oximetry (bilateral), noninvasive blood pressure monitor, 5-lead electrocardiography, and gas analysis should be established before induction of anesthesia. Additional monitors for patients undergoing HT include invasive arterial blood pressure (ideally before induction), central venous pressure, large-bore intravenous access, PA catheter, and transesophageal echocardiogram. Frequently, a femoral arterial catheter is placed in addition to a radial arterial catheter for congruence and also as a backup monitoring line during surgery. Of note, arterial lines may be more difficult to place by palpation in patients with LVADs. Thus, ultrasound equipment should be readily available. A central line is required for inotrope and vasotropic administration, monitoring, and for volume administration. Many anesthesiologists prefer to place a PA catheter before induction to help guide their hemodynamic management during induction. Given the significantly higher incidence of intraoperative awareness for patients undergoing CPB,[45] use of processed electroencephalogram technologies may be beneficial. Cerebral oximetry has also demonstrated utility for patients undergoing cardiac surgery[46]; however, further research in this area is needed.[47]

Placement of a PA catheter is useful to assess pulmonary artery pressures and assess right-sided cardiac output in both the operating room and the intensive care unit. However, successful positioning of the PA catheter can be difficult in HT recipients secondary to right ventricle (RV) dilation, tricuspid regurgitation, and frequent arrhythmias.[48] Additionally, the utilization of PA catheter has decreased secondary to associated complications from placement, inaccuracy of derived hemodynamic values, and inconsistencies with data interpretation.[49] It is important to note that continuous cardiac output monitoring from a PA catheter averages data from the past 5 to 15 minutes. Average in vivo time delays associated with sudden changes in CO of critically ill patients were reported to be 9.3, 10.5, and 11.8 minutes for a 50%, 75%, and 90% response, respectively.[50] Despite these limitations, the ability to continuously assess PA pressures is often crucial for intraoperative and postoperative management.

Transesophageal Echocardiography

The use of transesophageal echocardiography (TEE) for all patients undergoing HT has been suggested,[51] and it currently has a class II indication by the American Society of Echocardiography.[52] TEE is used before bypass to assess biventricular function, contractility, volume status, pleural effusions, aortic atherosclerosis, and the detection of intracardiac thrombi. TEE is crucial to facilitate separation from CPB. Particular concerns during separation include evaluation of intracardiac air, ventricular function (RV function), valvular function, and absence of intracardiac shunts. TEE guidance also allows for early detection of hemodynamic compromise and facilitates rapid therapeutic intervention to maintain hemodynamic stability.

Induction

The main goal for induction is to minimize hemodynamic instability and prevent cardiovascular collapse. Patients with end-stage HF have "fixed" stroke volumes and require adequate preload, maintenance of elevated systemic vascular resistance, and adequate heart rate to maintain cardiac output. Use of etomidate may offer some advantage in terms of hemodynamic stability. Additionally, a conservative dose of rapid-acting opioids, such that sympathetic activity is not completely suppressed, and a fast-acting muscle relaxant (succinylcholine/rocuronium) are often used. It is important to stress that induction medications result in decreased contractility, increased venous capacitance, and decreased vascular tone. Thus, rather than identifying specific medications, the key to induction of anesthesia involves vigilance as well as early detection and treatment of alterations in cardiovascular function. Continuation of all preoperative inotropic and vasoconstrictive agents is essential. Patients with end-stage HF have downregulation of the beta-adrenergic receptors and will require potentially higher doses of beta-agonist inotrope therapy.[53] Reduced cardiovascular function may not respond to ephedrine or phenylephrine, and rapid escalation to other medications, such as epinephrine, norepinephrine, or dobutamine, should be expected. Of note, vasopressin increases systemic vascular resistance with less impact on PVR.[54]

Preparations also should include immediate availability of blood and blood products. CMV status of the donor and of the recipient is needed to determine whether CMV-negative packed red blood cells should be ordered. Additionally, patients with ventricular assist devices should be placed on a higher risk for post-bypass bleeding. Finally, placement of external defibrillator pads should be routine.

Ventilation

After endotracheal intubation, ventilation should be initiated with a high inspiratory oxygen concentration and small inspiratory tidal volumes (6 mL/kg). Ventilatory management should be focused on its effects on PVR and RV function. Alveolar hypoxia and hypercarbia are potent pulmonary vasoconstrictors, whereas hypocarbia is a pulmonary vasodilator.[55–57] PVR is increased when function residual capacity (FRC) is elevated over closing capacity (CC) secondary to compression of small intra-alveolar vessels.[55–57] However, PVR also increases when FRC is reduced below CC secondary to increased large-vessel resistance from hypoxic pulmonary vasoconstriction.[55–57] Positive end expiratory pressure (PEEP) improves oxygenation by increasing FRC, which is reduced with general anesthesia. However, administration of higher levels of PEEP also may adversely increase FRC above optimal values. Intraoperative use of spirometry via modern anesthesia machines allows one to visualize the PEEP required to optimize the patient's FRC. Specifically, identification of the lower infliction point of the patient's pressure volume loop can identify the PEEP required to increase FRC just above the CC. Thus, ventilation of the HT recipient should involve high concentrations of oxygen, moderate tidal volumes, rates sufficient to achieve hypocarbia, and optimized levels of PEEP.[55–57]

MAINTENANCE

Key points

- Early detection of RV failure is paramount
- TEE is crucial to evaluate hemodynamic status
- Preparation should be made for post-bypass bleeding

Before Cardiopulmonary Bypass

Maintenance of anesthesia before CPB most often involves inhalational agents along with moderate doses of opioids. Nitrous oxide should be avoided secondary to possible increases in PVR. Use of antifibrinolytic therapy should be started before CPB in most cases. Specific antibiotics and immunosuppressive agents should be given before incision. As per standard CPB procedures, heparin is administered before aortic cannulation. Of note, patients with recent exposure to heparin are at risk for heparin-induced thrombocytopenia, with antibodies usually decreasing to negative titers within 3 months.[58] Before superior vena cava cannulation, the PA catheter should be withdrawn from the heart into the superior vena cava.

HT surgery is performed through a median sternotomy incision, using CPB in much the same way as other common cardiac surgical procedures. Cannulation of the aorta is often higher in the aortic arch than traditional cardiac surgery and is followed by individual cannulation of the superior and inferior vena cava. Orthotropic HT has 3 surgical approaches: the biatrial, bicaval, and total transplantation techniques. The biatrial approach involves 4 sites of anastomoses, including the left and right atrial cuffs, pulmonary, and aorta.[59] The bicaval method involves 5 areas of anastomoses, including the left atrial cuff, superior vena cava and inferior vena cava, PA, and aorta.[60] This technique has demonstrated an improvement in perioperative mortality, maintenance of sinus rhythm, improved valvular function, fewer pacemaker insertions, and a small survival advantage.[61,62] However, recent retrospective review between bicaval and biatrial techniques did not demonstrate a difference in survival between groups.[63] The final approach involves total transplantation with 8 anastomoses sites and is rarely used.[64]

Weaning from Cardiopulmonary Bypass

As with all CPB procedures, a protocolized "head to toe" review should be performed to prepare for separation from CPB. The patient should be warm (>35.5°C), have adequate level of sedation, ventilation should be initiated with verification of bilateral lung expansion, arterial blood gas should be reviewed, and electrolytes should be corrected. Identification of vascular resistance can be estimated by mean arterial pressure (MAP) on full-flow CPB and vasoconstrictive agents should be considered for MAP less than 60 mm Hg.[53] Initial TEE evaluation should focus on retention of air in area of anastomosis as well as along the left ventricular (LV) apex. After cross-clamp removal, direct-acting inotropic agents should be started, given the absence of reflex-mediated heart rate responses. Use of chronotropic agents, such as isoproterenol is more common compared with other CPB procedures. Use of atrial and ventricular pacing also is not uncommon, with 4% to 12% of patients requiring a permanent pacemaker from loss of sinus node function.[41] During weaning from CPB, volume within the heart should be restored slowly and the PA catheter should be repositioned.

Of particular concern for the HT recipient is the PVR and RV function. The transplanted heart should be carefully loaded with close monitoring of RV function and PA pressures given that the naïve RV can acutely fail when exposed to pressures higher than 45 mm Hg.[41] To reduce stress on RV function, one must minimize PVR and improve inotropy. Ventilation strategies described previously to reduce PVR should be reinitiated. Beta-adrenergic agents, such as epinephrine (0.05–0.4 μg/kg per minute). or dobutamine (3–8 μg/kg per minute), should be initiated to improve inotropy. Phosphodiesterase inhibitors, such as milrinone, are common medications used to decrease PVR and improve contractility, but these also reduce systemic vascular resistance as well. Levosimendan, a calcium sensitizer, has demonstrated improved RV function in patients with biventricular failure[65]; however, it is currently not approved in North America and is undergoing phase III trials.

Use of inhaled PA vasodilators also should be considered. Finally, to support RV function that is refractory to medical therapy, one should consider the use of a ventricular assist device.[66] Postoperative management strategies of RV dysfunction are discussed as follows.

Before separation from bypass, a full TEE evaluation should be performed. Specific areas of interest include the following:

1. Evaluation of RV size and function
2. Evaluation of tricuspid regurgitation
3. Evaluation for turbulent flow across anastomoses sites
4. Atrial sizes
5. LV size and function
6. Mitral regurgitation
7. Presence of pericardial effusions
8. Diastolic function

Diastolic function has been demonstrated to be negatively altered posttransplantation.[67] Finally, TEE should be used for evaluation for hemodynamic instability, which may be secondary to rejection, RV dysfunction, hypovolemia, vasodilatation, tamponade, RV outflow tract obstruction, or LV outflow tract obstruction.

On successful transition from CPB and removal of venous and aortic cannulae, protamine is given to reverse the heparin. Immediate evaluation of post-bypass coagulopathy should be performed to ensure adequate reversal. Additionally, the utility of point of care testing has been demonstrated for complex cardiac surgery procedures.[68]

MANAGEMENT AFTER CARDIOPULMONARY BYPASS

Key points

- Failure of the donor right heart after transplantation is a common cause of mortality, and therefore post-CPB management is directed at supporting right heart function

- The denervated donor heart is reliant on direct stimulation for chronotropy via electrical pacing or direct ino-chronotropic intravenous infusions

- Acute rejection and primary graft failure are concerns for the postoperative period that may require changes to the immunosuppressive regimen, mechanical support, and possibly even retransplantation

---

Often the transplanted donor heart systolic function is very good for both the LV and RV; however, this may worsen over the next 12 hours depending on several factors, such as total ischemic time, donor LV wall thickness, or acute rejection. As mentioned previously, the right heart function may worsen in minutes depending on, for example, preexisting pulmonary hypertension, pulmonary edema, volume overload, or protamine reaction. Any pathologic increase in right ventricular afterload can be detrimental to an unconditioned heart causing decreased right-sided cardiac output with dilation of the RV, increasing tricuspid regurgitation, and an underfilled LV.

Post-CPB anesthetic and immediate postoperative intensive care unit management may require close monitoring of PVR and pulmonary pressures with a PA catheter or bedside echocardiography. Inodilators, such as milrinone or dobutamine, can be combined with inhaled pulmonary vasodilators to maximize right heart function while decreasing afterload. In instances of severe HF, an RV assist device may be necessary to support the cardiac output until physiologic adaptations are made. Extracorporeal membrane oxygenation has also been used to mechanically support failing transplanted right hearts.[69]

The denervated donor heart is initially paced via temporary wires or direct beta-agonists. A rate of 80 to 100 beats per minute helps to improve cardiac output and contractility after CPB. Damage to the donor sino atrial (SA) node from surgical trauma also may cause arrhythmias or bradycardia that may require long-term pacemaker placement. Prolonged ischemic time also can damage the SA or atrioventricular node, which may prolong the need for chronotropic infusions or necessitate permanent pacing. Permanent pacing is required in 4% to 12% of transplanted hearts due to sinus node dysfunction.[70]

Early rejection is divided into acute and hyperacute based on pathology. Acute rejection occurs within the first 6 months after transplantation. It manifests as general dysfunction from low cardiac output to arrhythmias and is caused by the recipient's immune response to the foreign tissue. Testing includes taking serial endomyocardial biopsies of the transplanted heart, invasive monitoring, and frequent echocardiography. Treatment entails more aggressive immunosuppression therapy. Hyperacute rejection occurs within minutes to hours and is rare.[71] Preformed recipient antibodies to HLA class I on the vascular endothelium of the heart cause complement activation and fixation leading to cell death, thrombosis, ischemia, and HF.[72] The only chance for survival is mechanical support until another heart can be transplanted. Primary graft failure is defined by most as single or biventricular dysfunction within the first 24 hours after transplantation manifesting as severe hemodynamic instability requiring 2 or more inotropes or mechanical support. It is the most common cause of early mortality in the first 30 days after transplantation. The etiology is thought to be from ischemia reperfusion injury with myocardial stunning. Some factors that contribute are increasing age of donor, donor heart dysfunction, increased ischemic time, donor-recipient size mismatch, and recipient factors, such as pulmonary hypertension.[73] Treatment is supportive with inotropic and/or mechanical agents until the heart recovers.

REFERENCES

1. Yancy CW, Jessup M, Bozkurt B, et al. 2013 ACCF/AHA guideline for the management of heart failure: a report of the American College of Cardiology Foundation/American Heart Association Task Force on Practice Guidelines. J Am Coll Cardiol 2013;62(16):e147–239.

2. Metra M, Ponikowski P, Dickstein K, et al. Advanced chronic heart failure: a position statement from the Study Group on Advanced Heart Failure of the Heart Failure Association of the European Society of Cardiology. Eur J Heart Fail 2007;9(6–7):684–94.

3. Lower RR, Shumway NE. Studies on orthotopic homotransplantation of the canine heart. Surg Forum 1960;11:18–9.

4. Barnard CN. The operation. A human cardiac transplant: an interim report of a successful operation performed at Groote Schuur Hospital, Cape Town. S Afr Med J 1967;41(48):1271–4.

5. Caves PK, Stinson EB, Billingham ME, et al. Diagnosis of human cardiac allograft rejection by serial cardiac biopsy. J Thorac Cardiovasc Surg 1973;66(3):461–6.
6. Borel JF. Comparative study of in vitro and in vivo drug effects on cell-mediated cytotoxicity. Immunology 1976;31(4):631–41.
7. DiBardino DJ. The history and development of cardiac transplantation. Tex Heart Inst J 1999;26(3):198–205.
8. Lund LH, Edwards LB, Dipchand AI, et al. The Registry of the International Society for Heart and Lung Transplantation: thirty-third adult HT report-2016; focus theme: primary diagnostic indications for transplant. J Heart Lung Transplant 2016;35(10):1158–69.
9. Colvin-Adams M, Smith JM, Heubner BM, et al. OPTN/SRTR 2011 annual data report: heart. Am J Transplant 2013;13(Suppl 1):119–48.
10. Burchill LJ, Edwards LB, Dipchand AI, et al. Impact of adult congenital heart disease on survival and mortality after HT. J Heart Lung Transplant 2014;33(11):1157–63.
11. Kobashigawa J, Zuckermann A, Macdonald P, et al. Report from a consensus conference on primary graft dysfunction after cardiac transplantation. J Heart Lung Transplant 2014;33(4):327–40.
12. Lund LH, Edwards LB, Kucheryavaya AY, et al. The registry of the International Society for Heart and Lung Transplantation: thirty-first official adult heart transplant report-2014; focus theme: retransplantation. J Heart Lung Transplant 2014;33(10):996–1008.
13. Mancini D, Lietz K. Selection of cardiac transplantation candidates in 2010. Circulation 2010;122(2):173–83.
14. Renlund DG, Taylor DO, Kfoury AG, et al. New UNOS rules: historical background and implications for transplantation management. United Network for Organ Sharing. J Heart Lung Transplant 1999;18(11):1065–70.
15. Mehra MR, Canter CE, Hannan MM, et al. The 2016 International Society for Heart Lung Transplantation listing criteria for HT: a 10-year update. J Heart Lung Transplant 2016;35(1):1–23.
16. Levy WC, Aaronson KD, Dardas TF, et al. Prognostic impact of the addition of peak oxygen consumption to the Seattle Heart Failure Model in a transplant referral population. J Heart Lung Transplant 2012;31(8):817–24.
17. Goda A, Williams P, Mancini D, et al. Selecting patients for HT: comparison of the Heart Failure Survival Score (HFSS) and the Seattle heart failure model (SHFM). J Heart Lung Transplant 2011;30(11):1236–43.
18. Mehra MR, Kobashigawa J, Starling R, et al. Listing criteria for HT: International Society for Heart and Lung Transplantation guidelines for the care of cardiac transplant candidates-2006. J Heart Lung Transplant 2006;25(9):1024–42.
19. Erickson KW, Costanzo-Nordin MR, O'Sullivan EJ, et al. Influence of preoperative transpulmonary gradient on late mortality after orthotopic HT. J Heart Transplant 1990;9(5):526–37.
20. Chih S, Ross HJ, McDonald MA, et al. Highly sensitized patients in cardiac transplantation: early outcomes from the Canadian Prioritized Organ Sharing Program. J Heart Lung Transplant 2012;31(7):780–2.
21. Zaroff JG, Rosengard BR, Armstrong WF, et al. Consensus conference report: maximizing use of organs recovered from the cadaver donor: cardiac recommendations, March 28-29, 2001, Crystal City, Va. Circulation 2002;106(7):836–41.
22. Hong KN, Iribarne A, Worku B, et al. Who is the high-risk recipient? Predicting mortality after heart transplant using pretransplant donor and recipient risk factors. Ann Thorac Surg 2011;92(2):520–7 [discussion: 527].

23. Kilic A, Emani S, Sai-Sudhakar CB, et al. Donor selection in HT. J Thorac Dis 2014;6(8):1097–104.
24. John R. Donor management and selection for HT. Semin Thorac Cardiovasc Surg 2004;16(4):364–9.
25. Khush KK, Menza RL, Babcock WD, et al. Donor cardiac troponin I levels do not predict recipient survival after cardiac transplantation. J Heart Lung Transplant 2007;26(10):1048–53.
26. Kuppahally SS, Valantine HA, Weisshaar D, et al. Outcome in cardiac recipients of donor hearts with increased left ventricular wall thickness. Am J Transplant 2007;7(10):2388–95.
27. Welp H, Spieker T, Erren M, et al. Sex mismatch in HT is associated with increased number of severe rejection episodes and shorter long-term survival. Transplant Proc 2009;41(6):2579–84.
28. Vega JD, Moore J, Murray S, et al. HT in the United States, 1998-2007. Am J Transplant 2009;9(4 Pt 2):932–41.
29. Lund LH, Edwards LB, Kucheryavaya AY, et al. The Registry of the International Society for Heart and Lung Transplantation: thirty-second official adult ht report–2015; focus theme: early graft failure. J Heart Lung Transplant 2015;34(10):1244–54.
30. Rose EA, Gelijns AC, Moskowitz AJ, et al. Long-term use of a left ventricular assist device for end-stage heart failure. N Engl J Med 2001;345(20):1435–43.
31. Ross HJ, Law Y, Book WM, et al. Transplantation and mechanical circulatory support in congenital heart disease: a scientific statement from the American Heart Association. Circulation 2016;133(8):802–20.
32. INTERMACs Quarterly Statistical Report 2016 Q1. Available at: http://www.uab.edu/medicine/intermacs/images/Federal_Quarterly_Report/Federal_Partners_Report_2016_Q1.pdf. Accessed December 19, 2016.
33. Kamdar F, John R, Eckman P, et al. Postcardiac transplant survival in the current era in patients receiving continuous-flow left ventricular assist devices. J Thorac Cardiovasc Surg 2013;145(2):575–81.
34. John R, Pagani FD, Naka Y, et al. Post-cardiac transplant survival after support with a continuous-flow left ventricular assist device: impact of duration of left ventricular assist device support and other variables. J Thorac Cardiovasc Surg 2010;140(1):174–81.
35. Birks EJ, Drakos SG, Selzman CH, et al. Remission from stage D heart failure (RESTAGE-HF): early results from a prospective multi-center study of myocardial recovery. The Journal of Heart and Lung Transplantation 2015;34(4):S40–1.
36. Netuka I, Schmitto JD, Zimpfer D, et al. HeartMate 3 fully magnetically levitated LVAD for the treatment of advanced heart failure: results from the CE Mark Trial. Presented at the 19th Annual Meeting of the Heart Failure Society of America (HFSA). Washington, DC, September 26-29, 2015.
37. Hillyer CD. Blood banking and transfusion medicine: basic principles & practice. 2nd edition. Philadelphia: Churchill Livingstone/Elsevier; 2007.
38. Kilic A, Weiss ES, George TJ, et al. What predicts long-term survival after HT? An analysis of 9,400 ten-year survivors. Ann Thorac Surg 2012;93(3):699–704.
39. Russo MJ, Chen JM, Sorabella RA, et al. The effect of ischemic time on survival after HT varies by donor age: an analysis of the United Network for Organ Sharing database. J Thorac Cardiovasc Surg 2007;133(2):554–9.
40. Russo MJ, Iribarne A, Hong KN, et al. Factors associated with primary graft failure after HT. Transplantation 2010;90(4):444–50.

41. Fischer S, Glas KE. A review of cardiac transplantation. Anesthesiol Clin 2013; 31(2):383–403.
42. Stehlik J, Edwards LB, Kucheryavaya AY, et al. The Registry of the International Society for Heart and Lung Transplantation: twenty-eighth adult heart transplant report–2011. J Heart Lung Transplant 2011;30(10):1078–94.
43. Ardehali A, Esmailian F, Deng M, et al. Ex-vivo perfusion of donor hearts for human HT (PROCEED II): a prospective, open-label, multicentre, randomised non-inferiority trial. Lancet 2015;385(9987):2577–84.
44. Waterman PM, Bjerke R. Rapid-sequence induction technique in patients with severe ventricular dysfunction. J Cardiothorac Anesth 1988;2(5):602–6.
45. Phillips AA, McLean RF, Devitt JH, et al. Recall of intraoperative events after general anaesthesia and cardiopulmonary bypass. Can J Anaesth 1993;40(10): 922–6.
46. Murkin JM, Adams SJ, Novick RJ, et al. Monitoring brain oxygen saturation during coronary bypass surgery: a randomized, prospective study. Anesth Analg 2007; 104(1):51–8.
47. Deschamps A, Hall R, Grocott H, et al. Cerebral oximetry monitoring to maintain normal cerebral oxygen saturation during high-risk cardiac surgery: a randomized controlled feasibility trial. Anesthesiology 2016;124(4):826–36.
48. Ramakrishna H, Jaroszewski DE, Arabia FA. Adult cardiac transplantation: a review of perioperative management Part-I. Ann Card Anaesth 2009;12(1):71–8.
49. Marik PE. Obituary: pulmonary artery catheter 1970 to 2013. Ann Intensive Care 2013;3(1):38.
50. Leibowitz AB, Oropello JM. The pulmonary artery catheter in anesthesia practice in 2007: an historical overview with emphasis on the past 6 years. Semin Cardiothorac Vasc Anesth 2007;11(3):162–76.
51. Hilberath JN, Oakes DA, Shernan SK, et al. Safety of transesophageal echocardiography. J Am Soc Echocardiogr 2010;23(11):1115–27 [quiz: 1220–1].
52. Cheitlin MD, Armstrong WF, Aurigemma GP, et al. ACC/AHA/ASE 2003 Guideline Update for the Clinical Application of Echocardiography: summary article. A report of the American College of Cardiology/American Heart Association Task Force on Practice Guidelines (ACC/AHA/ASE Committee to Update the 1997 Guidelines for the Clinical Application of Echocardiography). J Am Soc Echocardiogr 2003;16(10):1091–110.
53. Shanewise J. Cardiac transplantation. Anesthesiol Clin North America 2004; 22(4):753–65.
54. Holmes CL, Landry DW, Granton JT. Science review: vasopressin and the cardiovascular system part 2-clinical physiology. Crit Care 2004;8(1):15–23.
55. Hill NS, Roberts KR, Preston IR. Postoperative pulmonary hypertension: etiology and treatment of a dangerous complication. Respir Care 2009;54(7):958–68.
56. Pritts CD, Pearl RG. Anesthesia for patients with pulmonary hypertension. Curr Opin Anaesthesiol 2010;23(3):411–6.
57. Satoh D, Kurosawa S, Kirino W, et al. Impact of changes of positive end-expiratory pressure on functional residual capacity at low tidal volume ventilation during general anesthesia. J Anesth 2012;26(5):664–9.
58. Levy JH, Winkler AM. Heparin-induced thrombocytopenia and cardiac surgery. Curr Opin Anaesthesiol 2010;23(1):74–9.
59. Shumway NE, Lower RR, Stofer RC. Transplantation of the heart. Adv Surg 1966; 2:265–84.

60. Sievers HH, Weyand M, Kraatz EG, et al. An alternative technique for orthotopic cardiac transplantation, with preservation of the normal anatomy of the right atrium. Thorac Cardiovasc Surg 1991;39(2):70–2.

61. Davies RR, Russo MJ, Morgan JA, et al. Standard versus bicaval techniques for orthotopic HT: an analysis of the United Network for Organ Sharing database. J Thorac Cardiovasc Surg 2010;140(3):700–8, 708.e1–2.

62. Schnoor M, Schäfer T, Lühmann D, et al. Bicaval versus standard technique in orthotopic HT: a systematic review and meta-analysis. J Thorac Cardiovasc Surg 2007;134(5):1322–31.

63. Dell'Aquila AM, Mastrobuoni S, Bastarrika G, et al. Bicaval versus standard technique in orthotopic heart transplant: assessment of atrial performance at magnetic resonance and transthoracic echocardiography. Interact Cardiovasc Thorac Surg 2012;14(4):457–62.

64. Yacoub M, Mankad P, Ledingham S. Donor procurement and surgical techniques for cardiac transplantation. Semin Thorac Cardiovasc Surg 1990;2(2):153–61.

65. Yilmaz MB, Yontar C, Erdem A, et al. Comparative effects of levosimendan and dobutamine on right ventricular function in patients with biventricular heart failure. Heart Vessels 2009;24(1):16–21.

66. Kavarana MN, Sinha P, Naka Y, et al. Mechanical support for the failing cardiac allograft: a single-center experience. J Heart Lung Transplant 2003;22(5):542–7.

67. StGoar FG, Gibbons R, Schnittger I, et al. Left ventricular diastolic function. Doppler echocardiographic changes soon after cardiac transplantation. Circulation 1990;82(3):872–8.

68. Shore-Lesserson L, Manspeizer HE, DePerio M, et al. Thromboelastography-guided transfusion algorithm reduces transfusions in complex cardiac surgery. Anesth Analg 1999;88(2):312–9.

69. Listijono DR, Watson A, Pye R, et al. Usefulness of extracorporeal membrane oxygenation for early cardiac allograft dysfunction. J Heart Lung Transplant 2011;30(7):783–9.

70. Boilson BA, Raichlin E, Park SJ, et al. Device therapy and cardiac transplantation for end-stage heart failure. Curr Probl Cardiol 2010;35(1):8–64.

71. Weil R 3rd, Clarke DR, Iwaki Y, et al. Hyperacute rejection of a transplanted human heart. Transplantation 1981;32(1):71–2.

72. Lindenfeld J, Miller GG, Shakar SF, et al. Drug therapy in the heart transplant recipient: part II: immunosuppressive drugs. Circulation 2004;110(25):3858–65.

73. Iyer A, Kumarasinghe G, Hicks M, et al. Primary graft failure after HT. J Transpl 2011;2011:175768.

Anesthesia for Lung Transplantation

Alina Nicoara, MD[a],*, John Anderson-Dam, MD[b]

KEYWORDS

- Lung transplantation • Intraoperative management • Graft dysfunction • Anesthesia

KEY POINTS

- The preoperative evaluation of the lung transplant candidate is performed by a multidisciplinary team. Besides usual anesthetic issues of airway assessment, comorbidities, current medications, adverse reactions, and aspiration risk, the evaluation on the day of surgery should focus on the current state of illness, and on aspects that will determine intraoperative ventilatory strategy and hemodynamic optimization.
- Induction of anesthesia is one of the most critical periods. Communication with the surgical, perfusion, and nursing teams should alert them to the potential for hemodynamic instability during induction and should establish plans for deployment of cardiopulmonary bypass, or extracorporeal membrane oxygenation at any time during the procedure.
- Management of mechanical ventilation immediately after lung transplantation is an opportunity to reduce incidence of primary graft dysfunction and influence short-term and long-term outcome of lung transplant recipients. Lung protective strategies should be implemented from the time of allograft reperfusion.
- Transesophageal echocardiography has become part of routine monitoring during lung transplantation. It has well-defined application during all stages of procedure, as well as in the immediate postoperative period in the intensive care unit.

INTRODUCTION

The first human lung transplant was performed in 1962; however, the success of lung transplantations was seen in the 1980s.[1] In 2005, the Organ Procurement and Transplantation Network (OPTN) introduced the lung allocation score (LAS) to change organ allocation from a system that was based on time on the waiting list to a system based on medical urgency.[2]

Disclosure Statement: None of the authors has any conflict of interest.
[a] Division of Cardiothoracic Anesthesia, Department of Anesthesiology, Duke University Medical Center, 2301 Erwin Road, HAFS Building, Box 3094, Durham, NC 27710, USA; [b] Department of Anesthesiology and Perioperative Medicine, Ronald Reagan UCLA Medical Center, David Geffen School of Medicine, University of California, 757 Westwood Boulevard, Suite 3325, Los Angeles, CA 90095, USA
* Corresponding author.
E-mail address: alina.nicoara@duke.edu

Anesthesiology Clin 35 (2017) 473–489
http://dx.doi.org/10.1016/j.anclin.2017.05.003
anesthesiology.theclinics.com

The year after the introduction of the LAS, the number of deaths on the waiting list dropped 40%, from more than 500 per year previously.[2] The increasing severity of illness of patients listed, however, has likely led to a steady increase in the rate of mortality on the waitlist in the decade since the introduction of the LAS. The median LAS score at transplantation has risen over the past decade. The proportion of patients older than 60 years increased every year since 2005. The proportion of patients with restrictive lung disease increased to almost 50%. In 2015, the OPTN introduced its first revision to the LAS (LAS-R).[3] It is yet to be seen what effect this will have, but most likely will increase the proportion of patients with pulmonary hypertension and right ventricular dysfunction.

The number of transplants has increased every year in the United States.[3] Both the utilization of "extended criteria" donors and ex vivo lung perfusion systems have allowed for an increase in the number of recovered donor organs.[2] Despite transplanting more complex patients and a greater acceptance of donor organs, survival has not changed over the past 5 years (84.6% 1-year, 67.8% 3-year, and 55.5% 5-year survival). The increased number of transplants along with stable survival resulted in more lung transplant recipients being alive than ever before.[3] Lung transplantation is a life-saving therapy for end-stage lung disease that requires perioperative physicians versatile in caring for these patients in the preoperative, intraoperative, and postoperative periods.

INDICATIONS FOR LUNG TRANSPLANTATION AND PATIENT SELECTION

Lung transplantation is an established therapy for end-stage lung disease. Largely, the indications for transplantation can be grouped into obstructive (chronic obstructive pulmonary disease and bronchiolitis obliterans), suppurative (cystic fibrosis [CF], ciliary dyskinesia, and bronchiectasis), interstitial (idiopathic pulmonary fibrosis, hypersensitivity pneumonia, and nonspecific pneumonia), and vascular (pulmonary arterial hypertension). The introduction of the LAS caused a shift away from obstructive disease; the largest diagnosis category since 2007 has been restrictive lung disease.[2]

The overarching goal of patient selection for lung transplantation is to select those patients most in need while providing stewardship over a scarce resource. To help guide clinicians in this goal, the International Society of Heart and Lung Transplantation (ISHLT) has published a consensus document for the selection of lung transplant candidates.[4]

To be considered for listing, a patient should have end-stage lung disease, a >50% chance of mortality within 2 years, a >80% chance of survival 90 days after transplantation, and a >80% chance of 5-year survival with preserved graft function.[4] Lung transplantation itself risks morbidity and mortality, so only those with a high chance of disease-related mortality should be considered. Those who are too sick to survive the short-term or long-term should not be listed, as those organs should be given to a patient who has a chance to benefit. Of note, lung transplantation has been unique in that its allocation score has always considered best utilization of donor organs and not just patients' risk without transplantation.

The selection committee proposed global absolute contraindications and relative contraindications (**Box 1**).[4] These act as guidance regardless of underlying diagnosis. Criteria for listing for lung transplantation according to the 2014 ISHLT update consensus document for the selection of lung transplant candidates are summarized in **Table 1**.[4]

Box 1
Contraindications (absolute and relative) to lung transplantation

Absolute Contraindications

- Recent malignancy (5-year disease-free period for any major malignancy)
- Untreatable major organ dysfunction not paired with another transplant
- Uncorrected atherosclerotic disease with end-organ dysfunction and CAD not amenable to revascularization
- Acute medical instability (eg, sepsis, myocardial infarction, liver failure)
- Uncorrectable bleeding diathesis
- Chronic infection with highly virulent and/or resistant microbe that is poorly controlled pretransplant
- Mycobacterium tuberculosis infection
- Significant chest was deformity expected to cause severe restriction
- BMI $\geq$35
- Current or prolonged past medical non-adherence
- Psychiatric or psychological condition that results in an inability to cooperate with medical care
- Absence of an adequate social support system
- Severely limited functional status with poor rehab potential

Relative Contraindications

- Age >65 with low physiologic reserve and age >75 is unlikely to be successful
- BMI 30 to 35
- Progressive or severe malnutrition
- Severe, symptomatic osteoporosis
- Extensive prior chest surgery
- Mechanical ventilation or mechanical circulatory support
- Colonization or infection with highly resistant microbes
- HIV outside of experienced centers or with poorly controlled disease
- Other medical conditions that can be optimized should be before listing (eg, diabetes mellitus, epilepsy, gastroesophageal reflux)

Abbreviations: BMI, body mass index; CAD, coronary artery disease; HIV, human immunodeficiency virus.
Data from Weill D, Benden C, Corris PA, et al. A consensus document for the selection of lung transplant candidates: 2014—an update from the pulmonary transplantation council of the international society for heart and lung transplantation. J Heart Lung Transplant 2015;34(1):1–15.

PERIOPERATIVE CONSIDERATIONS
Preoperative Assessment

The evaluation of a lung transplant candidate is performed by a multidisciplinary team and involves pulmonologists, thoracic surgeons, infectious disease specialists, nurses, nutritionists, physiotherapists, psychologists, and social workers. Standard evaluation with pulmonary, cardiac, and gastrointestinal evaluation, as well as laboratory testing is summarized in **Table 2**.[5] Besides usual anesthetic issues of airway

Table 1 Criteria for listing for lung transplantation for different underlying lung pathologies	
Obstructive diseases	BODE index ≥ 7 FEV1 <15%–20% of predicted Three or more severe exacerbations in the past year Moderate to severe pulmonary hypertension One severe exacerbation with acute hypercapnic respiratory failure
Suppurative diseases	Chronic respiratory failure ($Paco_2$ >50 mm Hg, Pao_2 <60 mm Hg, or a combination of the two) Need for noninvasive ventilation Pulmonary hypertension Frequent hospitalizations Rapid decline in lung function World Health Organization functional status IV
Interstitial diseases	$\geq 10\%$ decline in FVC at 6 mo of follow-up $\geq 15\%$ decline in DLCO at 6 mo of follow-up Desaturation <88%, 6MWD <250 m, or a >50-m decline in the 6MWD at 6-mo follow-up Pulmonary hypertension Hospitalization because of functional deterioration, pneumothorax, or acute exacerbation
Vascular diseases	NYHA class III or IV despite optimal therapy (including prostanoids) Cardiac index <2 L/min/m^2 Mean right atrial pressure >15 mm Hg 6MWD <350 m Hemoptysis, pericardial effusion, or signs of right heart failure

Abbreviations: 6MWD, 6-minute walking distance; BODE, body mass index, airflow obstruction, dyspnea, exercise capacity; DLCO, diffusing capacity of the lungs for carbon monoxide; FEV1, forced expiratory volume in 1 second; FVC, forced vital capacity; NYHA, New York heart association; $Paco_2$, partial pressure of Co_2 in arterial blood; Pao_2, partial pressure of O_2 in arterial blood.

Data from Weill D, Benden C, Corris PA, et al. A consensus document for the selection of lung transplant candidates: 2014—an update from the pulmonary transplantation council of the International Society for Heart and Lung Transplantation. J Heart Lung Transplant 2015;34(1):1–15.

assessment, comorbidities, current medications, adverse reactions, and aspiration risk, the evaluation on the day of surgery should focus on certain aspects of the preoperative workup that will determine the following:

1. Which lung will tolerate better one-lung ventilation (OLV) and strategies of intraoperative ventilation (pulmonary function tests, arterial blood gas on room air)
2. Which lung should be transplanted first (ventilation-perfusion scan)
3. Inotrope and vasopressor support, or need for extracorporeal circulation (right heart catheterization, echocardiography)

Also, because lung transplant recipients may experience variable waiting times after the lung transplant candidacy has been established, the assessment on the day of surgery should also focus on the current state of the illness and the amount of deterioration since the investigations were performed. Certain aspects of the preoperative workup are highlighted as follows.

The ventilation-perfusion (V/Q) scan will determine whether the patient will tolerate OLV and which lung will be transplanted first. A nonoperative lung that receives little perfusion (<40%) based on the V/Q scan may result in hypoxemia during OLV due to shunting, or refractory hemodynamic instability at clamping of the pulmonary artery on the operative side due to severe right heart failure.

Table 2
Standard evaluation for lung transplant candidates

Pulmonary evaluation	Pulmonary function testing
	Arterial blood gas on room air
	Chest radiography
	6-min walk distance test
	Noncontrast computed tomography scan
	Quantitative ventilation and perfusion scan
	Fluoroscopy of the diaphragms
Cardiac evaluation	Electrocardiogram
	Right heart catheterization
	Echocardiogram with bubble study
	Left heart catheterization for age >40 or computed tomography coronary angiography for age >40
	Cardiac MRI (for patients with lung sarcoidosis)
Gastrointestinal evaluation	Barium swallow
	24-h pH probe testing
	Esophageal manometry
	Solid gastric emptying (if concern for gastroparesis)
	Liver ultrasound (age <55)
	Liver computed tomography scan (age >55)
Laboratory testing	Routine hematologic, chemistry and coagulation studies
	Viral serologies for the following:
	Cytomegalovirus
	Herpes simplex virus
	Epstein- Barr virus
	Varicella zoster virus
	Hepatitis B, C
	Human immunodeficiency virus
	Flow cytometry for HLA antibodies

Abbreviation: HLA, human leukocyte antigen.
Data from Gray AL, Mulvihill MS, Hartwig MG. Lung transplantation at Duke. J Thorac Dis 2016;8(3):E185–96.

Right ventricular function and the presence of pulmonary hypertension, most often precapillary (mean pulmonary artery pressure ≥25 mm Hg and pulmonary artery wedge pressure ≤15 mm Hg), warrant particular attention. Patients with idiopathic pulmonary artery hypertension, other indications for lung transplantation associated with severe pulmonary hypertension (eg, pulmonary veno-occlusive disease, pulmonary fibrosis), or secondary pulmonary hypertension associated with right ventricular dysfunction poorly tolerate hypoxemia, hypercapnia, hemodynamic instability associated with surgical manipulation, and pulmonary artery clamping requiring proactive inotropic and vasopressor support, or elective or emergent deployment of extracorporeal mechanical circulatory support.[6,7]

Patients with CF present with comorbidities specific to the underlying disease. They are more likely to have had prior thoracic procedures, such as pleurodesis for pneumothoraces, which will increase the complexity of the recipient pneumonectomy and increase the likelihood of pleural bleeding. They are also likely to be colonized with pan-resistant *Pseudomonas aeruginosa*, different species of *Burkholderia*, fungal pathogens (eg, *Aspergillus fumigatus*), and nontuberculous *Mycobacteria*. The impact of pretransplant colonization on lung transplant outcome may result in increased perioperative morbidity[8] and may require more aggressive, or alternative antibiotic regimens targeted at preventing early infection. Gastrointestinal comorbidities include liver dysfunction, pancreatic exocrine insufficiency, and malnutrition. Patients with liver dysfunction limited to cholestasis are at low risk for perioperative liver decompensation; however, patients with cirrhosis may be considered unsuitable for isolated lung transplantation. The most common comorbidity associated with CF is diabetes, which occurs in 20% of adolescents and 40% to 50% of the adults.[9]

Older patients are now being transplanted for chronic obstructive pulmonary disease (COPD), idiopathic interstitial pneumonia, and other indications, with many centers performing lung transplants on patients beyond the age of 70. Older recipients are more likely to have other comorbidities, such as coronary artery disease and osteoporosis, due to the presence of other risk factors, such as history of smoking, chronic steroid use, and vitamin D deficiency. If significant cardiac disease warrants intervention, pretransplant percutaneous coronary revascularization via stenting is preferred; however, concurrent surgical revascularization with lung transplantation can be considered for selected patients (eg, high functional status, <65 year old).[5]

Preinduction

Communication with the surgical, perfusion, and nursing teams should alert them to the potential for hemodynamic instability during induction and should establish plans for deployment of cardiopulmonary bypass (CPB) or extracorporeal membrane oxygenation (ECMO) at any time during the procedure.

Sedation outside of the operating room, if needed, should be provided with great caution, as it may precipitate hypoxemia, hypercarbia, increase in pulmonary vascular resistance, right ventricular failure, and cardiorespiratory arrest. We establish arterial and large-bore peripheral venous access before induction with minimal or no sedation but with generous administration of local anesthetic and good counseling of the patients.

The immunosuppression and antibiotic regimen should be reviewed with the surgical team. Standard immunosuppression regimen around the period of induction consists of the following:

1. Tacrolimus 1 mg sublingual (or 0.5 mg for patients older than 65 years) before transplantation at the time the donor lungs are deemed acceptable and the decision to proceed with transplant has been made
2. Basiliximab 20 mg administered intraoperatively
3. Mycophenolate mofetil 1000 mg administered intraoperatively

All patients with a calculated panel reactive antibody greater than 25% are treated with an infusion of intravenous immunoglobulin 2 g/kg intraoperatively.[5] Standard intraoperative antibiotic prophylaxis at our institution includes cefepime for gram-negative coverage, vancomycin for gram-positive coverage, and fluconazole for candida prophylaxis. Recipients who are at risk for cytomegalovirus (CMV) (either recipient CMV immunoglobulin [Ig]G positive or donor IgM/IgG positive) are treated intraoperatively with ganciclovir 5 mg/kg.[5]

Induction

Induction of anesthesia is one of the most critical periods. Most patients will have elevated pulmonary artery pressure, preexisting right ventricular dysfunction, and hypercapnia at baseline. Cardiovascular collapse on induction, especially in patients with limited cardiorespiratory reserve can result from hypoxia, hypercapnia, decreased endogenous sympathetic drive, institution of positive pressure ventilation resulting in further increase in right ventricular afterload, and hypotension due to systemic vasodilation or myocardial depression. Irrespective of the induction agents used, they should be administered in judicious titrated doses. In patients with severe pulmonary hypertension and right ventricular dysfunction, hemodynamics may need to be optimized before induction through administration of inhaled pulmonary vasodilators (eg, preoxygenation with inhaled nitric oxide [iNO]) and administration of alpha$_1$ and beta$_1$ agonist infusions. Emphasis should be placed on a thorough air examination and contingency plans for intubation, as these patients will not tolerate prolonged periods of apnea resulting from difficult intubation.

We prefer placing a left-sided double lumen tube (DLT) for all cases, as the position of the bronchial lumen will not interfere with the surgical access to the left main stem and performing the left-sided bronchial anastomosis, irrespective of the type of the procedure performed (single or double-lung transplantation).

Central line and a pulmonary artery catheter are typically placed after induction. Transesophageal echocardiography (TEE) probe for intraoperative TEE monitoring is performed in all cases.

Surgical Aspects and Maintenance of Anesthesia

Bilateral orthotopic lung transplantation (BOLT) is generally performed through bilateral thoracosternotomy with the patient positioned supine with arms abducted, supported, and padded above the head to expose both the chest and the axillary regions. Single orthotopic lung transplantation (SOLT) can be performed through an anterolateral thoracotomy (supine position) or through a posterolateral approach (lateral decubitus position).[5,10]

During the surgical dissection, a particular challenge is management of OLV of the diseased lungs. OLV may not only lead to hypoxia, but also to hypercapnia and acidosis with further increase in pulmonary vascular resistance and spiraling right ventricular failure and hemodynamic instability. Some of the recommendations for OLV are as follows:

1. Tidal volumes 4 to 6 mL/kg ideal body weight
2. Positive end-expiratory pressure (PEEP) 3 to 10 cm H_2O titrated to best lung compliance
3. Titrated inspired oxygen fraction to achieve oxygen saturation 92% to 96%
4. Minimize peak and plateau pressures (ie, peak pressure <30 cm H_2O, and plateau pressure <20 cm H_2O).[11]

Although implementing these recommendations is desirable, underlying pathology in the recipient lungs will impact OLV management. Challenges associated with each pathology and management strategies to overcome them are listed in **Table 3**.

Moderate hypercapnia may be tolerated well in lung transplant recipients, as long as hypoxia and acidosis (pH <7.2) do not ensue. Permissive hypercapnia has been an integral part of lung protective strategy. However, beyond enabling reduced mechanical trauma and stress by avoiding volutrauma and barotrauma, elevated levels of CO2 may have other beneficial effects, such as attenuating the tumor necrosis factor–inflammatory response in alveolar macrophages[12] and reducing interleukin levels both locally in the bronchoalveolar lavage and systemically in the blood serum.[13] Severe hypercapnia, however, may lead to cardiac rhythm disturbances, decreased myocardial contractility, decreased renal blood flow, and increased intracranial pressure.[14]

Maintenance of anesthesia can be achieved with inhalational agents, propofol infusion, or both. Dose-dependent inhibition of hypoxic pulmonary vasoconstriction is well documented with older inhaled anesthetics (eg, halothane), but it has not been shown to occur with newer agents at less than 1 minimum alveolar concentration.[15] A recent systematic review of randomized controlled trials of intravenous (eg, propofol) versus

Table 3
Challenges and intraoperative management strategies for different underlying lung pathologies

Recipient Pathology	Intraoperative Complications	Management Strategies
Obstructive (COPD, BOS)	• Dynamic hyperinflation • Tension pneumothorax	• Use pressure control ventilation to minimize dynamic hyperinflation • Maximum exhalation time (I:E = 1:3–1:4) to minimize auto- PEEP • Check for auto-PEEP: interrupted inspiratory flow on the flow-volume curve • No or low extrinsic PEEP (3–4 cm H_2O)
Suppurative (cystic fibrosis, bronchiectasis)	• Thick, profuse secretions • Severe hypercapnia • Difficult dissection due to prior thoracic procedures	• Initial SLT intubation for BAL and suctioning • May require higher airway pressures • May require higher level of PEEP • Frequent suctioning
Restrictive (pulmonary fibrosis, hypersensitivity pneumonia)	• Severe pulmonary hypertension • May not tolerate OLV	• May need high peak inspiratory pressures (40 cm H_2O) • Maximize inspiratory time (I:E = 1:1–1:2) • Higher extrinsic PEEP (8–10 cm H_2O)
Primary pulmonary hypertension	• Severe hemodynamic instability due to right ventricular failure	• Central venous access before induction • Inotropic/vasopressor/inhaled pulmonary vasodilators on induction • Continue perioperative intravenous prostaglandins • Prepare for extracorporeal mechanical circulatory support

Abbreviations: BAL, bronchoalveolar lavage; BOS, bronchiolitis obliterans syndrome; COPD, chronic obstructive pulmonary disease; I:E, inspiratory time to expiratory time ratio; OLV, one-lung ventilation; PEEP, positive end- expiratory pressure; SLT, single-lumen tube.

inhalational (eg, isoflurane, sevoflurane, desflurane) anesthesia in patients undergoing OLV found that very little evidence is available to show differences in outcomes.[16] However, end-stage lung disease and pneumonectomy of the native lungs may impact the uptake of inhaled agents, making total intravenous anesthesia more reliable. Irrespective of the anesthetic drug used, adequate depth of anesthesia should be monitored, as these patients are at increased risk of intraoperative awareness.

Although many donor and recipient characteristics determine which side is transplanted first during BOLT, generally the side that receives less perfusion is first transplanted.[10] For the pneumonectomy of the native lung, the pulmonary vessels are divided first followed by the bronchus. The bronchial lumen of the DLT should be positioned comfortably away from the division line to avoid damage of the bronchial cuff. Clamping of right pulmonary artery of the operative lung may improve oxygenation by removing intrapulmonary shunt, but it will also divert the entire cardiac output to the contralateral lung with predictable increase of pulmonary artery pressures. This rapid increase in right ventricular afterload will be tolerated well in patients with mild pulmonary hypertension but may lead to hemodynamic instability in patients with pre-existent right ventricular dysfunction and pulmonary hypertension. Preemptive hemo-dynamic optimization with inotropes/vasopressors/inhaled pulmonary vasodilators before clamping of the pulmonary artery and continued efforts to reduce pulmonary vascular resistance, and maintain right ventricle perfusion pressure and contractility after clamping may avoid institution of extracorporeal mechanical support. At this time, continued monitoring by TEE of the right ventricular function, severity of tricuspid regurgitation, and volume status will provide clues into adjusting management strategies.

The implantation of the transplanted lung is conducted sequentially beginning with the most posterior structure, the bronchial anastomosis. The pulmonary artery anas-tomosis is fashioned next, followed by the left atrial anastomosis of the donor upper and lower pulmonary veins surrounded by a cuff of donor atrium to the recipient atrium. Once the posterior aspect of the left atrial anastomosis is completed, intrave-nous methylprednisolone (500 mg) and mannitol (25 g) are administered for each allo-graft. Surgical exposure and access to the atrium and hilum necessitates retraction, resulting in arrhythmias and hypotension, and constant communication between the surgeon and the anesthesiologist is crucial. Before finishing the anterior aspect of the left atrial anastomosis, the left atrial clamp is removed to allow de-airing of the graft and removal of the remaining pneumoplegia. The pulmonary artery is unclamped slowly over 10 to 15 minutes, allowing controlled low-pressure perfusion of the trans-planted lung. Ventilation of the transplanted lung is initiated during this time, initially by hand, with a low Fio_2 (less than 30%) and then by mechanical ventilation. A gentle Val-salva maneuver may allow for alveolar recruitment and expansion of the allograft. Se-vere hypotension may occur with reperfusion of the lung due to possible blood loss through leaks in the vascular anastomosis, wash-out of ischemic metabolites, and pneumoplegia from the allograft, or air entrained in the coronary arteries, most commonly the right coronary artery.

Ventilation Strategies of the Transplanted Lungs

Primary graft dysfunction (PGD) after lung transplantation occurs in the early period following reperfusion of the allograft with incidence reported between 10% and 57%.[17] The ISHLT criteria for diagnosis and grading of PGD are summarized in **Table 4**.[17] Severe (grade 3) PGD is both a risk factor for early mortality following lung transplantation, and a risk factor for the development of bronchiolitis obliterans syndrome, one of the late complications following lung transplantation. PGD is

Table 4
The International Society for Heart and Lung Transplantation primary graft dysfunction definition and grading

Grade	Pao_2/Fio_2	Radiographic Infiltrates
0	>300	Absent
1	>300	Present
2	200–300	Present
3	<200	Present

Abbreviations: Fio_2, fraction of inspired oxygen; Pao_2, partial pressure of oxygen in arterial blood.
Adapted from Oto T, Levvey BJ, Snell GI. Potential refinements of the International Society for Heart and Lung Transplantation primary graft dysfunction grading system. J Heart Lung Transplant 2007;26(5):435; with permission.

clinically and histopathologically similar to acute respiratory distress syndrome (ARDS), with diffuse pulmonary infiltrates and high oxygen requirements in the first 72 hours following transplantation.[18,19] Several risk factors have been identified: donor-related (age >45 years or <21 years, African American race, female gender, history of smoking >10 pack years, head trauma, prolonged mechanical ventilation), recipient-related (female gender, body mass index >25, elevated pulmonary artery pressure at the time of surgery, diagnosis of idiopathic pulmonary arterial hypertension), and operative (prolonged ischemic time, use of CPB, SOLT, blood products transfusion).[20]

Management of mechanical ventilation immediately after lung transplantation is an opportunity to reduce incidence of PGD and influence short-term and long-term outcome of lung transplant recipients. Lung protective strategies with low tidal volumes (6 mL/kg ideal body weight) have been shown to benefit not only patients with ARDS,[21] but also patients at risk for ARDS,[22] surgical patients undergoing short periods of intraoperative mechanical ventilation,[23] and donor management for transplantation.[24] Although not directly studied in lung transplant recipients, principles of lung protective mechanical ventilation are easily generalizable to those patients who have multiple respiratory impairments:

1. Fresh thoracotomy wound
2. Phrenic and pleural dysfunction
3. Allograft airway mucosa and bronchial anastomosis at risk for ischemia and poor healing
4. Ischemia-reperfusion injury of the allograft[18]

A unique aspect to lung transplantation is the situation of lungs undersized to the recipient thoracic cavity size. In this case, ventilation with tidal volumes calculated based on recipient characteristics will lead to higher tidal volumes when compared with matched or oversized allografts.[25] There is a growing body of evidence that undersized allografts are associated with increased rates of PGD, tracheostomy, resource utilization, and risk of first-year mortality.[26–28] Whether overinflation of the undersized graft is associated with higher rates of PGD is unclear, and calls more for more research in this area. In a recent international survey of practices of mechanical ventilation immediately after lung transplantation, 65% of the responders answered that they did not consider donor characteristics when setting the ventilator, and more than half (58%) answered that the team managing the ventilator did not have this information.[29] Several studies have shown a strong association between an increased FiO_2 at reperfusion and higher incidence of PGD.[19] The lowest FiO_2 (preferably <30%) should be used to maintain an appropriate partial pressure of oxygen in the arterial blood (≥70 mm Hg). Recommendations for ventilation strategies after lung transplantation are summarized in **Box 2**.

Inhaled Pulmonary Vasodilators After Lung Transplantation

iNO in the range of 10 to 40 ppm is a staple in the management of patients undergoing lung transplantation for providing pulmonary vasodilation selectively in the ventilated regions of the lung leading to improved ventilation-perfusion match and oxygenation. iNO may also modulate aspects of inflammation, oxidative stress, permeability, and coagulation.[30] Beyond the hemodynamic effects, iNO may mitigate acute lung injury in the transplanted lung by decreasing the hydrostatic forces associated with reperfusion and protecting the allograft from inflammatory insults and apoptosis. Pulmonary reperfusion-ischemia injury is a complex process thought to be initiated by hypoxemia of the endothelial cells and reperfusion stress, ultimately leading to endothelial

---

Box 2
Recommendations for intraoperative mechanical ventilation of the transplanted lungs

- Tidal volume of 6 mL/kg IBW. Adjust for OLV, if needed. Consider using donor body weight if the allograft is undersized

- PEEP 6 to 8 cm H_2O

- PIP less than 30 cm H_2O

- Careful recruitment maneuvers

- Lowest Fio_2 to maintain Pao_2 $\geq$70 mm Hg

- Normocapnia or low levels of permissive hypercapnia (if it allows for low Vt and not associated with acidosis)

- Bronchoscopic airway clearance

Abbreviations: Fio_2, fraction of inspired oxygen; IBW, ideal body weight; OLV, one-lung ventilation; Pao_2, partial pressure of arterial oxygen; PEEP, positive end-expiratory pressure; PIP, peak inspiratory airway pressure; Vt, tidal volume.

Adapted from Barnes L, Reed RM, Parekh KR, et al. Mechanical ventilation for the lung transplant recipient. Curr Pulmonol Rep 2015;4(2):92; with permission.

---

activation and dysfunction, deregulation of pulmonary vasoreactivity, platelet aggregation, inflammation, apoptosis, and impaired gas exchange.[31–34] Several preclinical studies have shown that iNO may have a strong effect on some of the pathways involved in the pathology of lung ischemia-reperfusion injury. Clinical studies, however, have shown little evidence regarding the role of iNO in preventing or attenuating the development of ischemia-reperfusion injury.[34–36] The inability to translate promising preclinical results into the clinical setting may be because genetic mechanisms related to injury and subsequent PGD are already triggered at the donor and cold ischemia stage, with little opportunity for iNO to modulate events at the reperfusion stage. There is, however, consensus about the role of iNO in intraoperative hemodynamic and oxygenation management and more importantly in avoiding the use of CPB,[37] which has emerged as one of the modifiable risk factors associated with the development of PGD in a recent prospective multicenter cohort study by the Lung Transplant Outcomes Group.[19] Several small studies have shown similar results with inhaled prostacyclin[35,38]; however, this is an area of ongoing research.

Transesophageal Echocardiography During Lung Transplantation

Transesophageal echocardiography has become part of routine monitoring and has well-defined application during all stages of procedure (pretransplantation, intratransplantation, and posttransplantation), as well as in the immediate postoperative period in the intensive care unit.

Considering that lung transplantation recipients experience variable times awaiting transplantation, TEE should confirm findings of the preoperative workup regarding ventricular function and valvular lesions, especially with respect to right ventricular function and tricuspid regurgitation. TEE also should evaluate the presence of intracardiac shunts (eg, patent foramen ovale, atrial septal defect), which may warrant surgical closure at the time of transplantation. At all times during lung transplantation, TEE can differentiate among different causes of hemodynamic instability, such as right ventricular failure, hypovolemia, myocardial ischemia with wall motion abnormalities, or pulmonary tamponade in cases of severe emphysema and lung hyperinflation (**Fig. 1**). After transplantation, TEE can assist with de-airing maneuvers and

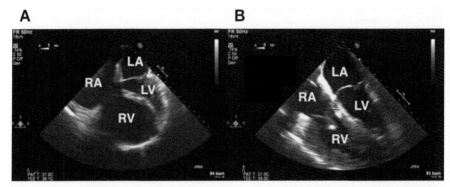

Fig. 1. Midesophageal 4-chamber view shows a severely dilated right ventricle (RV) with shift of the interventricular septum toward the left impinging on the left ventricle (LV) and likely impeding adequate filling and function (A) in a patient with severe pulmonary hypertension. (B) The same echocardiographic view after lung transplantation showing a hypertrophied, dilated RV but with a midline positioned interventricular septum. LA, left atrium; RA, right atrium.

assessment of the vascular anastomotic sites. Because intraoperatively PGD is a diagnosis of exclusion, it is particularly important to rule out problems involving vascular anastomosis, such as stenosis, torsion, or thrombosis, as a cause for hypoxemia. Pulmonary arterial anastomoses are considered normal if the minimal diameter of the anastomosis is at least 75% that of the proximal pulmonary artery and if color flow Doppler shows unobstructed flow through the anastomosis.[39] Although the right pulmonary artery can be imaged easily in the midesophageal short axis ascending aorta view (**Fig. 2**), the left pulmonary artery is difficult to image because of the interposition of the left bronchus but it still can be achieved at the level of the proximal descending aorta as it passes anteriorly to it. The left and right pulmonary veins can be imaged easily in the midesophageal views (**Fig. 3**). The incidence of abnormalities of pulmonary vein anastomoses has been reported as high as 29%.[40] A venous anastomosis is considered normal when on 2-dimensional imaging the diameter is comparable with the vein upstream, with a diameter of less than 0.5 cm considered acceptable.[40] Peak systolic flow velocities less than 1 m/s are considered

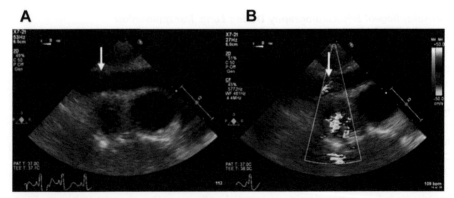

Fig. 2. Midesophageal ascending aorta short axis view with the probe turned toward the right showing (A) the right pulmonary artery and (B) with color flow Doppler. The arrow marks the most likely area of anastomosis.

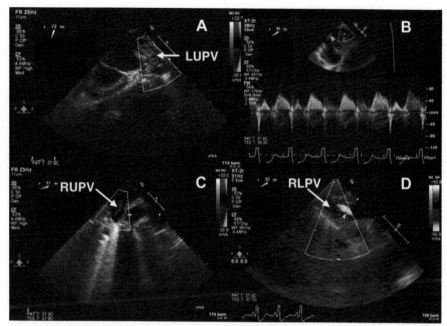

Fig. 3. (*A*) Midesophageal view of the left upper pulmonary vein (LUPV) with color flow Doppler. (*B*) Pulsed-wave Doppler of the LUPV, displaying peak velocities less than 80 cm/s. (*C*) Midesophageal view of the right upper pulmonary vein (RUPV) with color flow Doppler. (*D*) Midesophageal view of the right lower pulmonary vein (RLPV) with color flow Doppler.

acceptable.[41] However, loss of phasic(systolic/diastolic) flow even in the presence of low velocities should raise the suspicion of stenosis and prompt further evaluation. As peak velocities can be influenced by cardiac output, pulmonary blood flow, left atrial pressure, ventricular systolic and diastolic function, the absolute velocity values should be compared with the contralateral side and considered into the hemodynamic context.[42]

Fluid Management During Lung Transplantation

One of the pathophysiological mechanisms of PGD is alveolar decreased fluid clearance due to lymphatic drainage disruption.[43] It is very likely, therefore, that the newly transplanted lungs are sensitive to large volume fluid administration and there is a growing body of literature that intraoperative administration of fluid is a modifiable risk factor for PGD. Geube and colleagues[44] showed that increased intraoperative fluid volume is associated with the most severe form of PGD. In their retrospective study on a cohort of almost 500 patients, the most severe form of PGD (grade 3 PGD) occurred in 25% of patients. Each additional liter of intraoperative fluid was associated with increased odds for grade 3 PGD by approximately 22%. Patients who developed grade 3 PGD also received larger volumes of red blood cell concentrate than patients who did not develop PGD (1.1 vs 0.4, adjusted odds ratio 1.7; 95% confidence interval 1.08–2.7; $P = .002$). There was no association between non-blood components of fluid therapy (colloids and crystalloids) and grade 3 PGD. Similar findings were reported by the Lung Transplant Outcomes Group; transfusing more than 1 L of red blood cell concentrate was associated with a twofold increase in the incidence of PGD,[19] although the investigators state that potential unmeasured procedural characteristics leading to transfusion requirements may confound this relationship. Without being very specific, the ISHLT working group on primary lung graft dysfunction recommends cautious correction of fluid losses while optimizing hemoglobin and coagulation status.[45]

Other Anesthetic Considerations

At the end of the procedure, the DLT must be exchanged for a single-lumen endotracheal tube and a bronchoscopy is performed to inspect the anastomoses and clear secretions. As lung transplantations tend to be lengthy procedures, the stomach should be emptied of gastric secretions with the aid of an orogastric tube before the tube exchange. The exchange should be performed under direct or videolaryngoscopic vision using a soft-tipped exchange catheter, as the airway is likely to be edematous at the end of the procedure. Inability to reintubate the patient and loss of airway may have disastrous consequences.

ROLE OF EXTRACORPOREAL MECHANICAL SUPPORT IN LUNG TRANSPLANTATION

Extracorporeal mechanical circulatory support, either CPB or ECMO, is required in up to 30% to 40% of lung transplant procedures.[46] Intraoperatively, it allows for hemodynamic stability and a larger degree of flexibility in surgical manipulation while performing the surgical anastomoses. These benefits are not without costs. In a recent prospective, multicenter cohort study by the Lung Transplant Outcomes Group, the use of CPB has been associated with a threefold increase in the incidence of PGD, although it was not possible to differentiate between planned or emergent institution of CPB for deteriorating hemodynamics and oxygenation.[19] No randomized trials regarding the use of CPB exist, and in a recent review of the topic, including retrospective analyses and cohort studies, some studies showed significant disadvantages to the use of CPB, some showed no difference, and others showed both, depending on the postoperative outcome assessed.[47] A growing body of evidence suggests that veno-arterial ECMO may be preferable to CPB if mechanical circulatory support is needed. Relative to CPB, ECMO is associated with fewer transfusions, fewer reoperations, less PGD,[48] decreased rates of renal complications,[49] shorter intensive care unit stays, and shorter hospital length of stay.[46] Other benefits of ECMO are lower required heparin dose, less blood air interface with less inflammatory response, and the ability to convert to postoperative support.

Veno-venous ECMO (VV ECMO) can be used as a bridge to lung transplantation with comparable short-term and midterm outcomes, especially in highly experienced centers.[5] Newer cannulation strategies with dual-lumen single cannula allow for ambulatory VV ECMO with patients being able to participate in physical therapy and rehabilitation before transplantation.[5]

Patients with severe forms of PGD after lung transplantation and who are on maximal ventilator support (peak inspiratory pressures 30 cm H_2O, Fio_2 >0.6) should be considered for VV ECMO. VV ECMO should be instituted within 24 hours of onset of severe PGD and the patients can be transitioned back to lung protective ventilator strategies and Fio_2 of 0.21.[5]

POSTOPERATIVE PAIN MANAGEMENT

Thoracic epidural analgesia (TEA) is the cornerstone of pain management in the lung transplantation population as part of a multimodal strategy. We prefer to place the epidural catheters postoperatively in awake or lightly sedated patients immediately before extubation in the intensive care unit. We elect not to place them preoperatively for several reasons: (1) risk of epidural hematoma in the event of need for anticoagulation for extracorporeal mechanical support (ECMO or CPB) or development of significant intraoperative coagulopathy, (2) possible delayed extubation, and (3) need for expeditious preparation for surgery. TEA can be supplemented with a combination of preferably nonopioid analgesics. The use of paravertebral catheters both in single as well as double-lung transplantation has been described.[50]

SUMMARY

Lung transplantation is a continuously evolving field with unique surgical and medical aspects. The perioperative management of the patients undergoing lung transplantation is challenging and requires constant communication among the surgical, anesthesia, perfusion, and nursing teams. Although all aspects of the anesthetic management are import, certain intraoperative strategies (mechanical ventilation, fluid management, extracorporeal mechanical support deployment) have tremendous impact on the subsequent evolution of the lung transplant recipient, especially with respect to allograft function and should be carefully considered.

REFERENCES

1. Nathan SD. The future of lung transplantation. Chest 2015;147(2):309–16.
2. Egan TM, Edwards LB. Effect of the lung allocation score on lung transplantation in the United States. J Heart Lung Transplant 2016;35(4):433–9.
3. Valapour M, Skeans MA, Smith JM, et al. OPTN/SRTR 2015 annual data report: lung. Am J Transplant 2017;17(Suppl 1):357–424.
4. Weill D, Benden C, Corris PA, et al. A consensus document for the selection of lung transplant candidates: 2014–an update from the pulmonary transplantation council of the International Society for Heart and Lung Transplantation. J Heart Lung Transplant 2015;34(1):1–15.
5. Gray AL, Mulvihill MS, Hartwig MG. Lung transplantation at Duke. J Thorac Dis 2016;8(3):E185–96.
6. Ius F, Sommer W, Tudorache I, et al. Five-year experience with intraoperative extracorporeal membrane oxygenation in lung transplantation: indications and midterm results. J Heart Lung Transplant 2016;35(1):49–58.
7. Mohite PN, Sabashnikov A, Patil NP, et al. The role of cardiopulmonary bypass in lung transplantation. Clin Transplant 2016;30(3):202–9.
8. Morrell MR, Pilewski JM. Lung transplantation for cystic fibrosis. Clin Chest Med 2016;37(1):127–38.
9. Moran A, Dunitz J, Nathan B, et al. Cystic fibrosis-related diabetes: current trends in prevalence, incidence, and mortality. Diabetes Care 2009;32(9):1626–31.
10. Hayanga JW, D'Cunha J. The surgical technique of bilateral sequential lung transplantation. J Thorac Dis 2014;6(8):1063–9.
11. Brassard CL, Lohser J, Donati F, et al. Step-by-step clinical management of one-lung ventilation: continuing professional development. Can J Anaesth 2014; 61(12):1103–21.
12. Lang CJ, Barnett EK, Doyle IR. Stretch and CO2 modulate the inflammatory response of alveolar macrophages through independent changes in metabolic activity. Cytokine 2006;33(6):346–51.
13. Gao W, Liu DD, Li D, et al. Effect of therapeutic hypercapnia on inflammatory responses to one-lung ventilation in lobectomy patients. Anesthesiology 2015; 122(6):1235–52.

14. Lohser J. Evidence-based management of one-lung ventilation. Anesthesiol Clin 2008;26(2):241–72, v.

15. Pruszkowski O, Dalibon N, Moutafis M, et al. Effects of propofol vs sevoflurane on arterial oxygenation during one-lung ventilation. Br J Anaesth 2007;98(4):539–44.

16. Modolo NS, Modolo MP, Marton MA, et al. Intravenous versus inhalation anaesthesia for one-lung ventilation. Cochrane Database Syst Rev 2013;(7):CD006313.

17. Oto T, Levvey BJ, Snell GI. Potential refinements of the International Society for Heart and Lung Transplantation primary graft dysfunction grading system. J Heart Lung Transplant 2007;26(5):431–6.

18. Barnes L, Reed RM, Parekh KR, et al. Mechanical ventilation for the lung transplant recipient. Curr Pulmonol Rep 2015;4(2):88–96.

19. Diamond JM, Lee JC, Kawut SM, et al. Clinical risk factors for primary graft dysfunction after lung transplantation. Am J Respir Crit Care Med 2013;187(5): 527–34.

20. Lee JC, Christie JD. Primary graft dysfunction. Clin Chest Med 2011;32(2): 279–93.

21. Needham DM, Yang T, Dinglas VD, et al. Timing of low tidal volume ventilation and intensive care unit mortality in acute respiratory distress syndrome. A prospective cohort study. Am J Respir Crit Care Med 2015;191(2):177–85.

22. Serpa Neto A, Cardoso SO, Manetta JA, et al. Association between use of lung-protective ventilation with lower tidal volumes and clinical outcomes among patients without acute respiratory distress syndrome: a meta-analysis. JAMA 2012;308(16):1651–9.

23. Futier E, Constantin JM, Paugam-Burtz C, et al. A trial of intraoperative low-tidal-volume ventilation in abdominal surgery. N Engl J Med 2013;369(5):428–37.

24. Mascia L, Pasero D, Slutsky AS, et al. Effect of a lung protective strategy for organ donors on eligibility and availability of lungs for transplantation: a randomized controlled trial. JAMA 2010;304(23):2620–7.

25. Dezube R, Arnaoutakis GJ, Reed RM, et al. The effect of lung-size mismatch on mechanical ventilation tidal volumes after bilateral lung transplantation. Interact Cardiovasc Thorac Surg 2013;16(3):275–81.

26. Eberlein M, Arnaoutakis GJ, Yarmus L, et al. The effect of lung size mismatch on complications and resource utilization after bilateral lung transplantation. J Heart Lung Transplant 2012;31(5):492–500.

27. Eberlein M, Reed RM, Bolukbas S, et al. Lung size mismatch and primary graft dysfunction after bilateral lung transplantation. J Heart Lung Transplant 2015; 34(2):233–40.

28. Eberlein M, Reed RM, Maidaa M, et al. Donor-recipient size matching and survival after lung transplantation. A cohort study. Ann Am Thorac Soc 2013;10(5): 418–25.

29. Beer A, Reed RM, Bolukbas S, et al. Mechanical ventilation after lung transplantation. An international survey of practices and preferences. Ann Am Thorac Soc 2014;11(4):546–53.

30. Benedetto M, Romano R, Baca G, et al. Inhaled nitric oxide in cardiac surgery: evidence or tradition? Nitric Oxide 2015;49:67–79.

31. Christie JD, Bavaria JE, Palevsky HI, et al. Primary graft failure following lung transplantation. Chest 1998;114(1):51–60.

32. Fischer S, Cassivi SD, Xavier AM, et al. Cell death in human lung transplantation: apoptosis induction in human lungs during ischemia and after transplantation. Ann Surg 2000;231(3):424–31.

33. Pasero D, Martin EL, Davi A, et al. The effects of inhaled nitric oxide after lung transplantation. Minerva Anestesiol 2010;76(5):353–61.
34. Shah RJ, Bellamy SL, Localio AR, et al. A panel of lung injury biomarkers enhances the definition of primary graft dysfunction (PGD) after lung transplantation. J Heart Lung Transplant 2012;31(9):942–9.
35. Khan TA, Schnickel G, Ross D, et al. A prospective, randomized, crossover pilot study of inhaled nitric oxide versus inhaled prostacyclin in heart transplant and lung transplant recipients. J Thorac Cardiovasc Surg 2009;138(6):1417–24.
36. Moreno I, Vicente R, Mir A, et al. Effects of inhaled nitric oxide on primary graft dysfunction in lung transplantation. Transplant Proc 2009;41(6):2210–2.
37. Germann P, Braschi A, Della Rocca G, et al. Inhaled nitric oxide therapy in adults: European expert recommendations. Intensive Care Med 2005;31(8):1029–41.
38. Della Rocca G, Coccia C, Costa MG, et al. Inhaled areosolized prostacyclin and pulmonary hypertension during anesthesia for lung transplantation. Transplant Proc 2001;33(1–2):1634–6.
39. Hausmann D, Daniel WG, Mugge A, et al. Imaging of pulmonary artery and vein anastomoses by transesophageal echocardiography after lung transplantation. Circulation 1992;86(5 Suppl):II251–8.
40. Leibowitz DW, Smith CR, Michler RE, et al. Incidence of pulmonary vein complications after lung transplantation: a prospective transesophageal echocardiographic study. J Am Coll Cardiol 1994;24(3):671–5.
41. Michel-Cherqui M, Brusset A, Liu N, et al. Intraoperative transesophageal echocardiographic assessment of vascular anastomoses in lung transplantation. A report on 18 cases. Chest 1997;111(5):1229–35.
42. Cartwright BL, Jackson A, Cooper J. Intraoperative pulmonary vein examination by transesophageal echocardiography: an anatomic update and review of utility. J Cardiothorac Vasc Anesth 2013;27(1):111–20.
43. Sugita M, Ferraro P, Dagenais A, et al. Alveolar liquid clearance and sodium channel expression are decreased in transplanted canine lungs. Am J Respir Crit Care Med 2003;167(10):1440–50.
44. Geube MA, Perez-Protto SE, McGrath TL, et al. Increased intraoperative fluid administration is associated with severe primary graft dysfunction after lung transplantation. Anesth Analg 2016;122(4):1081–8.
45. Shargall Y, Guenther G, Ahya VN, et al. Report of the ISHLT working group on primary lung graft dysfunction part VI: treatment. J Heart Lung Transplant 2005; 24(10):1489–500.
46. Machuca TN, Collaud S, Mercier O, et al. Outcomes of intraoperative extracorporeal membrane oxygenation versus cardiopulmonary bypass for lung transplantation. J Thorac Cardiovasc Surg 2015;149(4):1152–7.
47. Nagendran M, Maruthappu M, Sugand K. Should double lung transplant be performed with or without cardiopulmonary bypass? Interact Cardiovasc Thorac Surg 2011;12(5):799–804.
48. Biscotti M, Yang J, Sonett J, et al. Comparison of extracorporeal membrane oxygenation versus cardiopulmonary bypass for lung transplantation. J Thorac Cardiovasc Surg 2014;148(5):2410–5.
49. Bermudez CA, Shiose A, Esper SA, et al. Outcomes of intraoperative venoarterial extracorporeal membrane oxygenation versus cardiopulmonary bypass during lung transplantation. Ann Thorac Surg 2014;98(6):1936–42 [discussion: 1942–3].
50. Hutchins J, Apostolidou I, Shumway S, et al. Paravertebral catheter use for postoperative pain control in patients after lung transplant surgery: a prospective observational study. J Cardiothorac Vasc Anesth 2017;31(1):142–6.

Anesthesia for Liver Transplantation

Dieter Adelmann, MD[a], Kate Kronish, MD[a], Michael A. Ramsay, MD, FRCA[b],*

KEYWORDS

- Liver transplantation • Anesthesia • Liver • Cirrhosis • End stage liver disease
- Coagulopathy

KEY POINTS

- Each program appoints a director of liver transplant anesthesia, who must meet the requirements of the American Society of Anesthesiologists and the United Network for Organ Sharing.
- Liver cirrhosis may cause major dysfunction in all organ systems.
- Cirrhotic cardiomyopathy may be masked by the typical high cardiac output and low peripheral vascular resistance often found in liver failure.
- Portopulmonary hypertension and hepatopulmonary syndrome often found with liver cirrhosis are at opposite ends of a vascular endothelial dysfunction pathway.
- The proper management of the coagulopathy of a failing liver requires an understanding of clot formation in "real time" and routine laboratory coagulation tests.

LIVER: BASIC ANATOMY AND PHYSIOLOGY

The liver is the largest internal organ in the body, receiving 25% to 30% of the cardiac output. It has a dual blood supply. The hepatic artery provides 25% and the portal vein provides 75% of the blood supply. Each vessel provides 50% of oxygen delivery. In liver transplantation (LT), adequate flow through the hepatic artery is essential for the viability of a new liver graft.[1] Terminal branches of both the arterioles and venules drain into sinusoids, where Kupffer cells filter and degrade particulate matter such as endotoxins from the blood. Venous drainage is through hepatic veins into the inferior vena cava. Bile canaliculi, between hepatocytes, form into bile ducts that drain into the intestine.

D. Adelmann and K. Kronish have contributed equally to this article.
Disclosure Statement: None of the authors have financial disclosures related to this article.
[a] Department of Anesthesiology and Perioperative Care, University of California San Francisco, Box O648, 4th Floor MUE, 500 Parnassus Avenue, San Francisco, CA 94143, USA; [b] Department of Anesthesiology, Baylor University Medical Center, 3500 Gaston Avenue, Dallas, TX 75246, USA
* Corresponding author.
E-mail address: docram@baylorhealth.edu

The liver plays a major role in the metabolic pathway of carbohydrates, fats, and proteins. Glucose is stored as glycogen and is converted by the liver to lactate, with the generation of energy. Protein is metabolized to ammonia and urea, which is then excreted in the urine. The liver also produces nearly all the plasma proteins, except immunoglobulins. Notably, the liver produces albumin, which serves as the most abundant plasma protein, the body's primary transport protein and major determinant of oncotic pressure. Another important liver function is drug metabolism, especially via the cytochrome p450 isoenzymes. The liver is also involved in hormone, vitamin, and mineral metabolism.

LIVER DISEASE: PATHOPHYSIOLOGY

A thorough understanding of the pathophysiology of liver disease is required to care for the liver transplant patient. The etiologies of the liver disease that most frequently need transplantation are listed in **Box 1**.

In the United States, hepatitis C virus is currently the number one indication for LT, with hepatic malignancy second. Given the new effective antiviral therapies for hepatitis C virus and the increasing obesity epidemic, nonalcoholic fatty liver disease is likely to become the most common cause of liver disease in the United States in the future.

Liver Cirrhosis

The term liver cirrhosis was coined by Rene Laennec in the 1840s. Hepatocellular death can occur via necrosis or apoptosis, most often owing to ischemia, viruses, and drug and alcohol toxicity. Cirrhosis refers to the damaging effects of inflammation, hepatocellular injury, and the resulting fibrosis and regeneration of the liver, all of which result in loss of normal liver function. Increased resistance to blood flow through the liver leads to portal hypertension and the development of varices. The failing liver is no longer able to clear the toxins that pass through it. Extensive endothelial dysfunction adversely affects all major organs.

Two commonly used scoring systems assess the severity of liver dysfunction. The Child-Turcotte-Pugh (CTP) classification has been used to assess surgical risk in

---

Box 1
Common liver diseases that present at selection committee for possible transplantation

Viral Hepatitis

Alcoholic (Laennec's) cirrhosis

Nonalcoholic steatohepatitis or nonalcoholic fatty liver disease

Hepatocellular cancer

Primary sclerosing cholangitis

Primary biliary cirrhosis

Autoimmune hepatitis

Cryptogenic cirrhosis

Drug induced (acetaminophen, amiodarone)

Acute liver failure

Genetic: amyloidosis, Wilson's disease

cirrhotic patients, and the Model for End-stage Liver Disease (MELD) score is validated to assess survival on the liver transplant waiting list.

The CTP score is calculated from:

Prothrombin time (seconds)

Encephalopathy

Ascites

Bilirubin (mg/dL)

Albumin (g/dL)

International Normalized Ratio (INR)

The MELD score calculation uses:

Serum creatinine (mg/dL)

Bilirubin (mg/dL)

INR

The sickest patients, who are most likely to die awaiting LT, receive highest waitlist priority. The CTP severity score was initially used to allocate livers. In 2002, the MELD score replaced the CTP score for liver allocation. It is a better predictor of 3-month waitlist mortality and is less subjective. In 2016, serum sodium was added to the MELD score for liver allocation, now called the MELD-Sodium. Higher waitlist priority is also given to patients with certain disease processes, such as acute liver failure, primary nonfunction of a recently transplanted liver, and hepatocellular carcinoma. These patients are given exception points because their increased waitlist mortality is not reflected in the MELD score. Rules regarding scoring and exception points are changing to attempt to address inequities in access.

TRANSPLANT SELECTION COMMITTEE

Before patients are accepted on the liver transplant waiting list, their suitability for transplantation must be assessed by a selection committee. This committee includes surgeons, hepatologists, anesthesiologists, and social workers. They focus on medical comorbidities, functional status, and a psychosocial evaluation. In the United States alone, 40,000 patients die of liver disease each year, but only 6000 liver transplants are performed annually. Thus, organ stewardship is extremely important. Selection committees are tasked with choosing patients with the greatest likelihood of successful transplantation and posttransplant survival. The presence of anesthesiologists on selection committees is important to assess the perioperative risk. Contraindications to transplantation include active alcohol and substance abuse, active infection, malignancy outside of the liver, and the lack of social support and finances. Advanced multiorgan system failure may be a contraindication to transplant, or may require multiorgan transplantation. Given that deceased organ availability does not meet waitlist demand, living donation of partial livers has emerged as alternative, particularly for patients with low MELD scores.[2]

PREOPERATIVE ASSESSMENT

The patient admitted for possible LT has often spent many months on the waiting list. At the time of transplantation, their MELD score might have increased significantly. This patient may be significantly sicker than when they were discussed at the selection committee. Therefore, all patients require careful reassessment by the anesthesiologist. If this patient is now too sick to be transplanted, the graft can be used to save another life.

Some conditions that may critically affect the management of the liver recipient are cirrhotic cardiomyopathy (CM), portopulmonary hypertension (POPH), hepatopulmonary syndrome (HPS), acute tubular necrosis of the kidney, cerebral edema, and severe electrolyte derangements. Competency with transesophageal echocardiography (TEE), the availability for renal replacement therapy, and the ready access to consultants are paramount.

CENTRAL NERVOUS SYSTEM: HEPATIC ENCEPHALOPATHY AND ACUTE LIVER FAILURE

Chronic liver dysfunction is associated with the accumulation of neurotoxins such as ammonia, short chain fatty acids, and mercaptans. These toxins can bypass the liver via portosystemic shunts. Their metabolism is impaired in liver dysfunction. In the central nervous system, ammonia is metabolized to glutamine. Glutamine increases intracellular osmolality and can lead to cerebral edema.[3]

Benzodiazepines should be used with care because they may potentiate this encephalopathy and precipitate hepatic coma.

The nonabsorbable disaccharide lactulose and nonabsorbable antibiotics such as rifaximin can reduce bacterial production of ammonia and treat hepatic encephalopathy in chronic liver disease.[4] As liver failure progresses, encephalopathy may deteriorate to hepatic coma and cerebral edema develops (**Box 2**). Acute management of hepatic encephalopathy consists of early intubation for airway protection to prevent

---

Box 2
Classification of hepatic encephalopathy

Unimpaired
- No signs or symptoms
- Normal psychometric or neuropsychological tests

Grades 0 to 1
- Also known as minimal or convert hepatic encephalopathy
- No overt clinical symptoms to mild decrease in attention span, awareness, altered sleep rhythm
- Abnormal psychometric or neuropsychological tests

Grade 2
- Obvious personality change, inappropriate behavior, asterixia, dyspraxia, disorientation, lethargy
- Objectively disoriented to time

Grade 3
- Somnolence, gross disorientation, bizarre behavior
- Objectively disoriented to time and space

Grade 4
- Coma

From Suraweera D, Sundaram V, Saab S. Evaluation and management of hepatic encephalopathy: current status and future directions. Gut Liver 2016;10(4):510; with permission.

aspiration, maintain oxygenation, and prevent hypercarbia. Mild hypocapnia and mild hypothermia may be helpful for neuroprotection.

In patients with cerebral edema, increased intracranial pressure can be managed by the placement of an intracranial pressure monitoring system. The common indications are papilledema, cerebral swelling, cardiovascular instability, and high ammonia levels. Coagulopathy associated with acute liver failure puts patients at increased risk for intracranial hemorrhage from the placement of invasive intracranial pressure monitors. Administration of blood products, factor concentrates, or recombinant activated factor VII can mitigate this risk.[5,6] Some centers use artificial liver support systems as a bridge to LT. Renal replacement therapy may be necessary to treat acidosis, hyperkalemia, volume overload, and elevated ammonia and lactate levels.[3,7]

THE CARDIOVASCULAR SYSTEM

Cardiac dysfunction may be a consequence of liver disease, independent of liver disease or owing to a condition that affects both the heart and the liver. The typical hemodynamic changes associated with cirrhosis are decreased systemic vascular resistance and high cardiac output.[8] Although the left ventricular ejection fraction might be preserved, cardiac function in cirrhosis can be severely impaired. CM is difficult to identify, and clinicians not familiar with liver disease might mischaracterize the heart function as that of a well-trained athlete when in fact it is severely weakened. Therefore, cardiologists consulted should be very familiar with liver disease and its effects on the heart.

Cirrhotic Cardiomyopathy

Cardiomyopathy, characterized by systolic and diastolic dysfunction and electrophysiologic changes, may exist to some degree in all patients with liver cirrhosis.[8–10] It initially presents as a blunted response to β-adrenergic receptor agonists, so vasopressor therapy may not be effective in traditional doses. CM is defined as an impaired contractile responsiveness to physiologic or pharmacologic stress, impaired left ventricular relaxation, and electrophysiologic abnormalities with prolonged QT interval.[8,11] Diagnostic criteria are presented in **Table 1**. Early onset of atrial fibrillation is also common.[12]

Both systolic and diastolic dysfunction are best evaluated using echocardiography, although a hyperdynamic circulation in the patient with liver cirrhosis can make the echocardiographic examination more difficult. Previously undiagnosed CM can present at the time of LT, with invasive monitoring showing low cardiac output in the presence of high filling pressures. TEE can help to assess for CM that may have developed since the last evaluation.

Cardiac failure may be precipitated by the increased cardiac output that follows transjugular intrahepatic portosystemic shunt placement or LT itself. The presence of diastolic dysfunction has been associated with an increased risk of death in patients with cirrhosis.[13,14] Patients with CM are also at increased risk for graft failure or death during LT.[15,16] This cardiomyopathy is progressive without LT (**Fig. 1**). Successful transplantation can reverse the effects of CM, although physiologic changes may take up to 6 months to resolve.[17]

Primary Cardiac Disease

Coronary artery disease

All liver transplant waitlist patients should be screened for coronary artery disease (CAD). Traditional risk factors include hypertension, smoking, diabetes, hypercholesterolemia,

Table 1
Diagnostic tests for cirrhotic cardiomyopathy

Methods	Signs
Electrocardiogram	• Prolonged QT interval
Exercise test	• Reduced exercise tolerance
Cardiopulmonary exercise test	• Alteration of aerobic capacity (peak V_{O_2}) or ventilatory efficiency (VE/VCO$_2$ or OUES)
Six-minute walk test	• Reduced tolerance
Echocardiography	• Systolic dysfunction (LVEF <55%) • Diastolic dysfunction • Left ventricular hypertrophy • Diastolic dysfunction (mean E/E′ index >10)
Exercise or dobutamine stress echocardiography	• Reduced contractile reserve
Magnetic resonance	• Systolic dysfunction (LVEF <55%) • Diastolic dysfunction (peak filling rate) • Left ventricular hypertrophy
BNP/NT-proBNP	• Elevated levels

Abbreviations: A wave, peak late atrial filling velocity (A, cm s^{-1}); BNP, brain natriuretic peptide; EDT, E wave deceleration time (m/s); E wave, peak early filling velocity (E, cm s^{-1}); LVEF, left ventricular ejection fraction; OUES, oxygen uptake efficiency slope; proBNP, prohormone brain natriuretic peptide; VE, ventilator efficiency; VE/VCO$_2$, minute ventilation/carbon dioxide production; VO$_2$, oxygen volume (oxygen consumption); VCO$_2$, carbon dioxide production.

From Zardi EM, Zardi DM, Chin D et al. Cirrhotic cardiomyopathy in the pre- and post-liver transplantation phase. J Cardiol 2016;67(2):128; with permission.

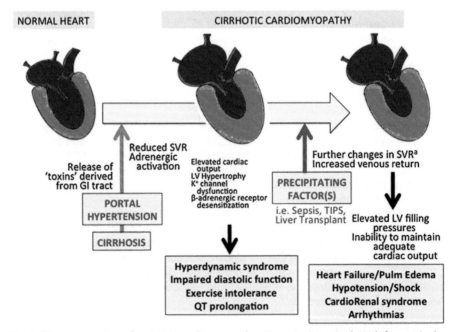

Fig. 1. The progression of cirrhotic cardiomyopathy. GI, gastrointestinal; LV, left ventricular; SVR, systemic vascular resistance; TIPS, transjugular intrahepatic portosystemic shunt. (*From* Zardi EM, Zardi DM, Chin D et al. Cirrhotic cardiomyopathy in the pre- and post-liver transplantation phase. J Cardiol 2016;67(2):127; with permission.)

obesity, and genetic history. These comorbidities are especially likely in patients with nonalcoholic fatty liver disease. The prevalence of CAD in transplant candidates with 2 or more traditional risk factors is 50%.[18–20] In patients who receive adequate treatment for CAD before transplantation, postoperative outcomes are comparable to patients without CAD.[21]

Hypertrophic cardiomyopathy can increase perioperative cardiovascular complications in patients presenting for LT. Strategies for successful management include preoperative alcohol septal ablation, and careful intraoperative management using TEE to optimize contractility and heart rate.[22,23]

Diseases affecting both the liver and the heart include alcoholic disease, amyloid disease, obesity, and hemosiderosis. Combined heart transplantation and LT can be considered if the risk of single organ transplant is high, such as in patients with familial amyloid disease.[24]

Preoperative Cardiac Assessment

Cardiac testing for all patients evaluated for LT should include an electrocardiogram and transthoracic echocardiography.[25] A prolonged QT interval and atrial fibrillation can be detected using an electrocardiogram. Impaired diastolic function can be detected using left ventricular inflow velocities (E:A ratio) and tissue Doppler (E:E′ ratio, velocity of myocardial displacement).[11] Dobutamine stress echocardiography and myocardial perfusion scintigraphy are widely used to assess left ventricular function and screen for ischemic heart disease. In patients with multiple risk factors or when noninvasive testing is suggestive of ischemia, coronary angiography is indicated for diagnosis and possible treatment.[25]

PULMONARY SYSTEM

Pulmonary dysfunction affects up to 50% of patients with liver disease. The major pulmonary concerns are: refractory hepatic hydrothorax, HPS, POPH, hemorrhagic hereditary telangiectasia, interstitial lung disease, and alpha-1-antitrypsin deficiency-related emphysema.

Hepatic Hydrothorax

Cirrhosis can cause a restrictive ventilation defect. Ascites passes into the pleural space through defects in the diaphragm and leads to pleural effusions. Conservative management includes diuretic therapy and salt restriction. Thoracentesis and pleural catheters may be indicated in refractory patients.[26] Hepatic hydrothorax is reversible after LT.

The pulmonary vascular endothelium is a vital organ that impacts vasoregulation, the fluidity, antithrombosis, laminar blood flow, permeability, and growth of the surrounding smooth muscle. Portal hypertension exposes the pulmonary vascular endothelium to inflammatory cytokines and stress forces owing to high laminar flow. This leads to endothelial dysfunction with either a predominantly vasodilatory pulmonary circulation (HPS) or a restrictive, vasoconstrictive circulation resulting in POPH (**Fig. 2**).

HPS is characterized by a triad of a decreased oxygen saturation in the presence of advanced liver disease and intrapulmonary vascular dilatation. It is present in 5% to 30% of patients evaluated for LT. Pulmonary arteriovenous shunts and capillary vasodilation caused by portal hypertension lead to a reduced capillary transit time and diminished oxygen diffusion.[27–29] The end result is that many of the red cells are not fully saturated with oxygen.

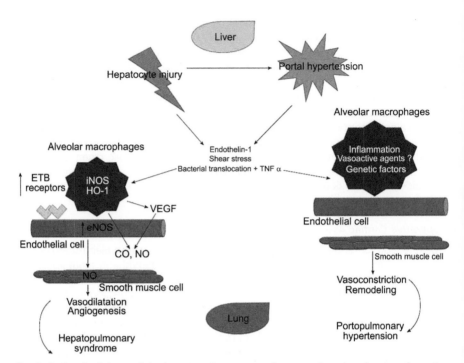

Fig. 2. Pathophysiology of the hepatopulmonary syndrome and portopulmonary hypertension. [a] Worsening cirrhosis or sepsis lead to a further reduction in Systemic Vascual Resistance (SVR), whereas a rapid increase in SVR is seen after liver transplant. CO, carbon monoxide; eNOS, endothelial nitric oxide synthase; ETB, endothelin type B; HO-1, heme oxygenase 1; iNOS, inducible nitric oxide synthase; NO, nitric oxide; TNF-α, tumor necrosis factor alpha; VEGF, vascular endothelial growth factor. (*Adapted from* Surani SR, Mendez Y, Anjum H, et al. Pulmonary complications of hepatic diseases. World J Gastroenterol 2016;22(26):6010; with permission.)

Pulse oximetry can be used to screen for HPS. Oxygen saturations (SpO2) of less than 96% require further evaluation. Diagnosis is confirmed by transthoracic echocardiography showing a delayed right-to-left shunt using agitated saline. After administration of agitated saline into the venous system, contrast microbubbles appear in the left heart after a delay of 3 to 6 heart beats; with intracardiac shunts, contrast microbubbles are seen moving from the right to left heart immediately. The decrease in oxygen content is defined by an increased alveolar–arterial oxygen gradient of equal to or greater than 15 mm Hg while breathing room air in the sitting position.[29]

Clinical signs in patients with HPS are digital clubbing, cyanosis, and platypnea (dyspnea that is worse upon moving from supine to upright position). This form of dyspnea is unique to HPS. Patients diagnosed with HPS have a 2-fold increased risk of mortality compared with cirrhotic patients without HPS. They are granted MELD exception points for higher waitlist priority. There is currently no medical treatment for HPS.

In severely hypoxic patients, extracorporeal membrane oxygenation can facilitate successful LT.[30] After transplantation, resolution of HPS can be expected within 1 to 2 years.[31]

POPH results when the pulmonary vascular endothelium is exposed to inflammatory cytokines, including endothelin-1. This leads to vasoconstriction, proliferation of endothelium and smooth muscle, and platelet aggregation. Eventually fibrosis results. This obstruction to flow leads to pulmonary hypertension and right heart failure. The severity of POPH is graded based on right heart catheterization data (**Table 2**).

Adequate right ventricular (RV) function is essential for survival during LT. Even mild RV dysfunction can cause the new liver graft to become congested and fail. Severe RV dysfunction can lead to intraoperative death.[32] The use of venous–arterial extracorporeal membrane oxygenation improves survival in this patient group. Both POPH and HPS may exist together; however, POPH may not reverse after LT.[33]

All LT candidates must be screened for POPH. The prevalence is about 5%.[34] An RV systolic pressure of greater than 50 mm Hg and/or significant RV hypertrophy or dysfunction is an indication for right heart catheterization to characterize the pulmonary hemodynamics. True POPH must be differentiated from pulmonary hypertension generated from high cardiac output, volume overload, or venous hypertension (**Fig. 3**).

Without treatment, POPH is associated with a 1-year survival of 35% to 46%.[35,36] The medical treatment for POPH is improving. There are 3 therapeutic classes available: prostacyclin analogues, phosphodiesterase inhibitors, and endothelin receptor antagonists. Mild POPH presents with normal perioperative risk for LT. Moderate POPH is associated with increased perioperative mortality, and severe POPH is considered a contraindication to LT. Patients with severe POPH can undergo LT only if their pulmonary arterial pressures can be lowered using medical therapy and if RV function is adequate.

Patients diagnosed with POPH in the operating room immediately before LT should have an assessment of RV function by TEE. If there is evidence of RV dysfunction, LT must be deferred. Patients with a mean pulmonary artery pressure of less than 35 mm Hg and a PVR of less than 240 dyn.sec.cm^{-5} can safely undergo LT. Reperfusion is the most critical period during LT. Cardiac output can significantly increase with reperfusion, causing an acute increase in the mean pulmonary artery pressure, which can lead to RV failure. The following interventions have salvaged some transplants: inhaled nitric oxide, intravenous or inhaled prostacyclins, milrinone, and extracorporeal membrane oxygenation.[37]

THE RENAL SYSTEM

Hepatorenal syndrome (HRS) is a functional renal impairment in patients with advanced liver disease or severe fulminant liver injury. It is characterized by increased renal vasoconstriction, a reduced glomerular filtration rate, subsequent increase in creatinine, and impaired sodium and water excretion.

Portal hypertension leads to profound systemic and splanchnic vasodilatation and intravascular volume depletion. This increases renal vasoconstriction via both the renin–angiotensin–aldosterone pathway and sympathetic nervous system activation. Renal vasoconstriction leads to significant hypoperfusion of the kidney.[38] HRS is

Table 2 Classification of portopulmonary hypertension			
	Mean Pulmonary Artery Pressure (mm Hg)	Pulmonary Vascular Resistance (dyn.sec.cm^{-5})	Pulmonary Capillary Wedge Pressure (mm Hg)
Normal	<25	—	—
Mild	25–35	>240	<15
Moderate	35–45		
Severe	>45		

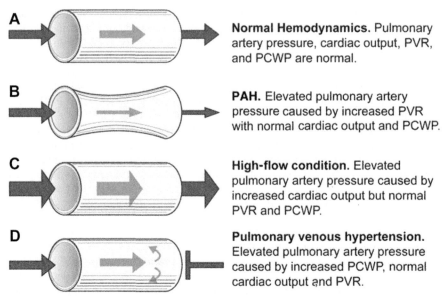

A Normal Hemodynamics. Pulmonary artery pressure, cardiac output, PVR, and PCWP are normal.

B PAH. Elevated pulmonary artery pressure caused by increased PVR with normal cardiac output and PCWP.

C High-flow condition. Elevated pulmonary artery pressure caused by increased cardiac output but normal PVR and PCWP.

D Pulmonary venous hypertension. Elevated pulmonary artery pressure caused by increased PCWP, normal cardiac output and PVR.

Fig. 3. (A–D) Etiologies of pulmonary hypertension in the liver transplant candidate. Only (B) is true portopulmonary hypertension. PAH, pulmonary arterial hypertension; PCWP, pulmonary capillary wedge pressure; PVR, pulmonary vascular resistance. (From Safdar Z, Bartolome S, Sussman N. Portopulmonary hypertension: an update. Liver Transpl 2012;18(8):883; with permission.)

classified as type 1, with rapid deterioration in renal function, and type 2 with a more gradual deterioration in renal function. Type 1 HRS has a 2-week mortality of about 80% whereas in type 2 HRS, kidney function declines more slowly and survival rates without LT are around 6 months. The diagnosis is based on the absence of primary kidney disease, proteinuria, or systemic hypovolemia causing renal hypoperfusion. There is normal urinary sediment, low urinary sodium (<10 mEq/L), uremia, and oliguria. Unfortunately, serum creatinine is a poor marker for renal dysfunction in HRS because these patients are usually cachectic with poor muscle mass. HRS type 1 can be treated with albumin in combination with the vasoconstrictor terlipressin.[38] Other vasoconstrictors used are vasopressin, the alpha-adrenergic receptor agonist midodrine, and norepinephrine. Renal replacement therapy may be used to stabilize the HRS patients before LT. HRS is reversible with LT. Prolonged endothelial damage can lead to irreversible tubular necrosis. A combined liver–kidney transplant should then be considered (**Fig. 4**).

THE COAGULATION SYSTEM

Liver disease has a complex effect on coagulation. It is widely understood to increase risk of bleeding: hepatic synthesis of procoagulant factors such as the vitamin K–dependent coagulation factors II, VII, IX, and X are reduced, and thrombocytopenia is common. However, the liver also produces the anticoagulant factors protein C, protein S, and antithrombin III, which are reduced in liver disease. Coagulation factor VIII, which is synthesized in the endothelium, is increased in patients with liver disease. Despite low platelet counts, platelet adhesion and aggregation might be normal, because of increased endothelial production of von Willebrand factor.[39–41] Thus,

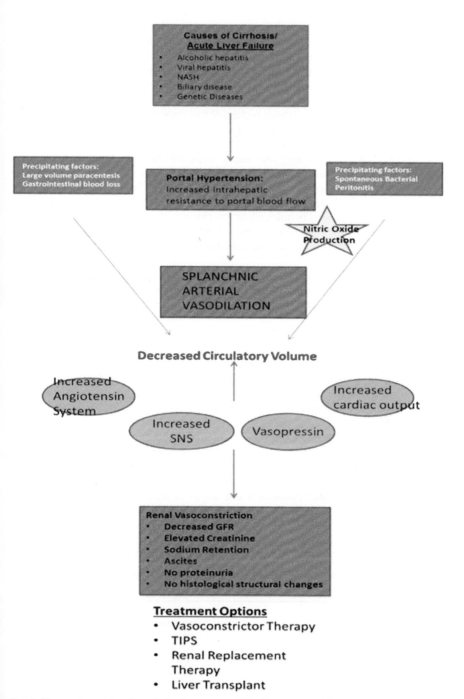

Fig. 4. The basic mechanism of the hepatorenal syndrome. GFR, glomerular filtration rate; NASH, nonalcoholic steatohepatitis; SNS, sympathetic nervous system; TIPS, transjugular intrahepatic portosystemic shunt. (*From* Shah N, Silva RG, Kowalski A, et al. Hepatorenal syndrome. Dis Mon 2016;62(10):367; with permission.)

coagulation dysfunction in liver disease can better be described as a fragile balance between low levels of both procoagulation and anticoagulation factors.[40] During LT, both bleeding as well as thromboembolic complications may occur (**Table 3**). Adequate coagulation requires sufficient amounts of thrombin. Thrombin then triggers the formation of a strong clot made of fibrinogen and platelets that can withstand fibrinolysis. The INR, although often used to assess the risk of bleeding in patients with liver disease, provides only a partial picture of the state of coagulation.[2]

Point-of-care global viscoelastic coagulation tests such as thromboelastography (Haemonetics Corporation, Braintree, MA) and thromboelastometry (TEM International GmbH, Munich, Germany) can help to evaluate clot formation in whole blood. Thromboelastography/thromboelastometry can determine the quality of clot formation (generation of thrombin), clot strength (the effect of fibrinogen and platelets), and fibrinolysis.[42–44] The degree of coagulopathy varies widely with the underlying liver disease. Patients with hepatocellular carcinoma often have normal coagulation profiles. Despite a prolonged INR, some patients show a hypercoagulable profile in thromboelastography. This could likely indicate an increased risk for thromboembolic complications.[45]

In addition, bleeding in patients with liver disease is not always owing to coagulopathy. Other common causes include portal hypertension and varices, endothelial dysfunction, renal failure, and disseminated intravascular coagulation.[46]

ANESTHESIA MANAGEMENT

Except for elective living donor liver transplants, the majority of liver transplants are performed as emergency cases. Many recipients have multiorgan dysfunction at the time of transplantation.

Basic intraoperative monitoring includes central venous and intraarterial pressure monitoring. In patients with suspected cardiac dysfunction or POPH, pulmonary artery catheter placement and/or TEE may be indicated. Echocardiography is a powerful tool to assess major hemodynamic changes and guide inotropic therapy. It also can detect major complications early such as intracardiac thromboembolism or air embolism.[47]

The use of thromboelastography for coagulation monitoring and ultrasound guidance for vascular catheter placement are center specific. Rapid infusion devices and red cell salvage systems are used in some centers. The availability of a rapid

Table 3 Hemostatic system alterations that contribute to bleeding or hemostasis	
Changes That Impair Hemostasis	**Changes That Promote Hemostasis**
Thrombocytopenia	Elevated levels of von Willebrand factor
Platelet function defects	Decreased levels of ADAMTS-13
Enhanced production of nitric oxide and prostacyclin	Elevated levels of factor VIII
Low levels of factors II, V, VII, IX, X, and XI	Decreased levels of protein C, protein S, antithrombin, α2-macroglobulin, and heparin cofactor II
Vitamin K deficiency	Low levels of plasminogen
Dysfibrinogenemia	
Low levels of α2-antiplasmin, factor XIII, and thrombin-activatable fibrinolysis inhibitor	
Elevated tissue plasminogen activator levels	

From Lisman T, Caldwell SH, Burroughs AK, et al. Hemostasis and thrombosis in patients with liver disease: the ups and downs. J Hepatol 2010;53(2):363; with permission.

response laboratory service with rapid turnaround times and blood bank services are essential.[48]

Electrolyte derangements should be monitored closely. With the new MELD-Sodium scoring system, more patients with hyponatramia are likely to be transplanted. If serum sodium is increased too rapidly, central pontine myelinolysis can occur.

The operation is divided into 3 phases: preanhepatic, anhepatic, and the neohepatic phases. During the preanhepatic phase, the native liver is dissected and then removed. Blood loss during this phase can be considerable. Compression or occlusion of major blood vessels can cause further hemodynamic compromise. This phase ends in the clamping of the inferior vena cava, portal vein and hepatic artery, and removal of the liver.

There are 3 basic surgical techniques for liver transplant:

A. Total occlusion of the vena cava and the portal vein ("full clamp," **Fig. 5**): This results in a severe reduction in venous return to the heart during the anhepatic phase. The presence of portal varices and other new vessels in patients with longstanding cirrhosis can ameliorate this effect. Care must be taken not to overcompensate with significant volume expansion, because this volume will return to the circulation upon unclamping. The resulting hypervolemia can lead to venous congestion and poor function of the new liver.

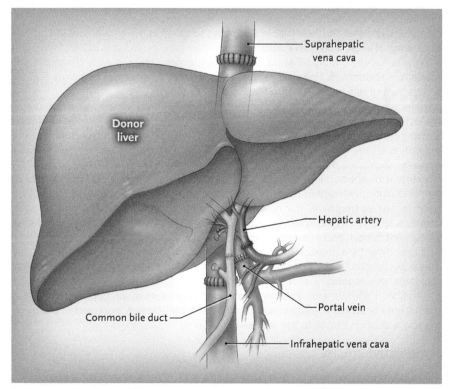

Fig. 5. Liver transplant with replacement of the vena cava ("full clamp"). (*From* Dienstag JL, Cosimi AB. Liver transplantation — a vision realized. N Engl J Med 2012;367(16):1484; with permission.)

B. "Piggy-back" technique: The inferior vena cava is only partially occluded with a side-biting clamp. The portal vein is still fully clamped throughout the anhepatic phase. With partial return of blood from the inferior vena cava to the heart, hemodynamics are usually more stable than with a full clamp.

C. Venovenous bypass: Venous blood from the inferior vena cava and femoral vein is returned into the internal jugular vein using extracorporeal venovenous cannulas and a centrifugal pump. Care must be taken to avoid air emboli, thromboembolism and hypothermia. In theory, this approach might be renoprotective and cause less cardiac strain. But clinical trials proving this advantage are currently lacking. The use of this practice seems to be decreasing.[49]

During the anhepatic phase, the new liver is anastomosed into place and reperfused. As the vena cava is unclamped, adequate return of venous blood volume to the heart is restored. Blood pressure and cardiac output improve. The portal vein is then opened, causing the cold, acidotic, hyperkalemic blood from below the clamp and from the liver graft itself to circulate directly into the right heart. This can cause a significant decrease in blood pressure, bradycardia, other arrhythmias, and occasionally cardiac arrest. Severe hypotension upon unclamping is called reperfusion syndrome and can be ameliorated by administration of calcium chloride, bicarbonate, epinephrine, and vasopressin.[50] The time taken to sew the new graft in place is the warm ischemia time. Warm ischemia is very damaging to the graft, and thus limiting warm ischemia time is critical to graft function.

The neohepatic phase consists of the hepatic artery and bile duct anastomoses, often with a concomitant cholecystectomy. During this time, the anesthesiologist is looking for signs that the new liver is beginning to function—improvement in acidosis and clearing of lactic acid, and improved hemostasis and production of bile. Hemostasis requires excellent surgical skills, temperature control and the early diagnosis and treatment of fibrinolysis. Failure to do so leads to breakdown of existing clots and the development of diffuse bleeding.

Maintenance of a low central venous pressure may reduce venous bleeding during hepatectomy.[51,52] For patients with severe portal hypertension, octreotide infusion may be indicated to reduce the portal venous pressure.[53] Vasopressors commonly used during LT are norepinephrine, vasopressin, and epinephrine.[54] Ionized calcium frequently decreases and needs to be replaced.

Treatment of abnormal laboratory values such as low platelet counts, low fibrinogen, and high prothrombin times is only required if there is clinical bleeding. These laboratory values frequently normalize as the new graft functions and platelets return to the circulation from the spleen. In case of bleeding, patients are treated with factor replacement, blood, and platelets. Approaches to resuscitation and treatment of high blood loss differ by institution.

Renal dysfunction, with poor urine output and rising creatinine, may occur during transplantation, especially after a full caval clamp, long anhepatic time, or prolonged hypotension. Patients with volume overload, hyperkalemia, or hyponatremia may benefit from continuous venovenous hemodialysis that can be instituted in the operating room or upon arrival to the intensive care unit.

POSTOPERATIVE COURSE

Early extubation is feasible in select patients after LT.[55] The new graft must show good function by beginning clearance of acidosis and falling lactate levels. Monitoring of neuromuscular blockade is essential before extubation. Patients must also be cooperative, and pain must be controlled adequately. They must meet usual standard extubation criteria. In some institutions, extubated patients with good liver function can bypass the intensive care unit and are sent to the postoperative recovery unit and then to a regular surgical floor or step-down unit.

Occasionally, the abdominal distension owing to an especially large organ or tissue swelling might prevent primary closure of the surgical wound. These patients are at risk for abdominal tamponade. Abdominal closure can be delayed for several days after transplantation to prevent abdominal compartment syndrome.

Measures must be taken to avoid central line-associated infections. Invasive lines should be removed as soon as appropriate. Function of the new graft must be monitored closely, looking especially for signs of infection, bleeding, and acute rejection. Some patients with bleeding or graft dysfunction may require emergent return to the operating room. Patients may have a difficult postoperative course with significant multiorgan dysfunction, and these patients require expert intensive care.

REFERENCES

1. Abbasoglu O, Levy MF, Testa G, et al. Does intraoperative hepatic artery flow predict arterial complications after liver transplantation? Transplantation 1998;66: 598–601.
2. Volk ML, Biggins SW, Huang MA, et al. Decision making in Liver Transplant Selection Committees A Multicenter Study. Ann Intern Med 2011;155:503–8.
3. Suraweera D, Sundaram V, Saab S. Evaluation and management of hepatic encephalopathy: current status and future directions. Gut Liver 2016;10:509–19.
4. Vilstrup H, Amodio P, Bajaj J, et al. Hepatic encephalopathy in chronic liver disease: 2014 Practice Guideline by the American Association for the Study Of Liver Diseases and the European Association for the Study of the Liver. Hepatology 2014;60:715–35.
5. Vaquero J, Fontana RJ, Larson AM, et al. Complications and use of intracranial pressure monitoring in patients with acute liver failure and severe encephalopathy. Liver Transpl 2005;11:1581–9.
6. Shami V. Recombinant activated factor VII for coagulopathy in fulminant hepatic failure compared with conventional therapy. Liver Transpl 2003;9:138–43.
7. Rabinowich L, Wendon J, Bernal W, et al. Clinical management of acute liver failure: results of an international multi-center survey. World J Gastroenterol 2016;22: 7595–603.
8. Wiese S, Hove JD, Bendtsen F, et al. Cirrhotic cardiomyopathy: pathogenesis and clinical relevance. Nat Rev Gastroenterol Hepatol 2013;11:177–86.
9. Ruíz-del-Árbol L, Serradilla R. Cirrhotic cardiomyopathy. World J Gastroenterol 2015;21:11502–21.
10. Lee SS. Cardiac abnormalities in liver cirrhosis. West J Med 1989;151:530–5.
11. Zardi EM, Zardi DM, Chin D, et al. Cirrhotic cardiomyopathy in the pre- and post-liver transplantation phase. J Cardiol 2016;67:125–30.
12. Zardi EM, Abbate A, Zardi DM, et al. Cirrhotic cardiomyopathy. J Am Coll Cardiol 2010;56:539–49.
13. Karagiannakis DS, Vlachogiannakos J, Anastasiadis G, et al. Diastolic cardiac dysfunction is a predictor of dismal prognosis in patients with liver cirrhosis. Hepatol Int 2014;8:588–94.
14. Ruíz-del-Árbol L, Achécar L, Serradilla R, et al. Diastolic dysfunction is a predictor of poor outcomes in patients with cirrhosis, portal hypertension, and a normal creatinine. Hepatology 2013;58:1732–41.

15. Sonny A, Ibrahim A, Schuster A, et al. Impact and persistence of cirrhotic cardiomyopathy after liver transplantation. Clin Transplant 2016;30:986–93.

16. Carvalheiro F, Rodrigues C, Adrego T, et al. Diastolic dysfunction in liver cirrhosis: prognostic predictor in liver transplantation? Transplant Proc 2016;48:128–31.

17. Torregrosa M, Aguadé S, Dos L, et al. Cardiac alterations in cirrhosis: reversibility after liver transplantation. J Hepatol 2005;42:68–74.

18. Lee BC, Li F, Hanje AJ, et al. Effectively screening for coronary artery disease in patients undergoing orthotopic liver transplant evaluation. J Transpl 2016;2016: 7187206.

19. Carey WD, Dumot JA, Pimentel RR, et al. The prevalence of coronary artery disease in liver transplant candidates over age 50. Transplantation 1995;59(6):859.

20. VanWagner LB, Serper M, Kang R, et al. Factors associated with major adverse cardiovascular events after liver transplantation among a national sample. Am J Transplant 2016;16:2684–94.

21. Wray C, Scovotti JC, Tobis J, et al. Liver transplantation outcome in patients with angiographically proven coronary artery disease: a multi-institutional study. Am J Transplant 2013;13:184–91.

22. Hage FG, Bravo PE, Zoghbi GJ, et al. Hypertrophic obstructive cardiomyopathy in liver transplant patients. Cardiol J 2008;15:74–9.

23. Robertson A. Intraoperative management of liver transplantation in patients with hypertrophic cardiomyopathy: a review. Transplant Proc 2010;42:1721–3.

24. Barbara DW, Rehfeldt KH, Heimbach JK, et al. The perioperative management of patients undergoing combined heart-liver transplantation. Transplantation 2015; 99:139–44.

25. Martin P, DiMartini A, Feng S, et al. Evaluation for liver transplantation in adults: 2013 practice guideline by the American Association for the Study of Liver Diseases and the American Society of Transplantation. Hepatology 2014;59: 1144–65.

26. Porcel JM. Management of refractory hepatic hydrothorax. Curr Opin Pulm Med 2014;20:352–7.

27. Castaing Y, Manier G. Hemodynamic disturbances and VA/Q matching in hypoxemic cirrhotic patients. Chest 1989;96:1064–9.

28. Cosarderelioglu C, Cosar AM, Gurakar M, et al. Hepatopulmonary syndrome and liver transplantation: a recent review of the literature. J Clin Transl Hepatol 2016;4: 47–53.

29. Rodriguez-Roisin R, Krowka M, Herve P, et al. Pulmonary-hepatic vascular disorders (PHD). Eur Respir J 2004;24:861–80.

30. Gupta S, Castel H, Rao RV, et al. Improved survival after liver transplantation in patients with hepatopulmonary syndrome. Am J Transplant 2010;10:354–63.

31. Collisson EA, Nourmand H, Fraiman MH, et al. Retrospective analysis of the results of liver transplantation for adults with severe hepatopulmonary syndrome. Liver Transpl 2002;8:925–31.

32. Ramsay M. Portopulmonary hypertension and right heart failure in patients with cirrhosis. Curr Opin Anaesthesiol 2010;23:145–50.

33. Kaspar MD, Ramsay MA, Shuey CB, et al. Severe pulmonary hypertension and amelioration of hepatopulmonary syndrome after liver transplantation. Liver Transpl Surg 1998;4:177–9.

34. Krowka MJ, Swanson KL, Frantz RP, et al. Portopulmonary hypertension: results from a 10-year screening algorithm. Hepatology 2006;44:1502–10.

35. Robalino BD, Moodie DS. Association between primary pulmonary-hypertension and portal-hypertension - analysis of its pathophysiology and clinical, laboratory and hemodynamic manifestations. J Am Coll Cardiol 1991;17:492–8.

36. Swanson KL, Wiesner RH, Nyberg SL. Survival in portopulmonary hypertension: Mayo Clinic experience categorized by treatment subgroups. Am J Transplant 2008;8:2445–53.

37. Krowka MJ, Fallon MB, Kawut SM, et al. International liver transplant society practice guidelines: diagnosis and management of hepatopulmonary syndrome and portopulmonary hypertension. Transplantation 2016;100:1440–52.

38. Nadim MK, Kellum JA, Davenport A. Hepatorenal syndrome: the 8th International Consensus Conference of the Acute Dialysis Quality Initiative (ADQI) Group. Crit Care 2012;16:R23.

39. Schaden E, Saner FH, Goerlinger K. Coagulation pattern in critical liver dysfunction. Curr Opin Crit Care 2013;19:142–8.

40. Tripodi A, Mannucci PM. The coagulopathy of chronic liver disease. N Engl J Med 2011;365:147–56.

41. Lisman T, Porte RJ. Rebalanced hemostasis in patients with liver disease: evidence and clinical consequences. Blood 2010;116:878–85.

42. Hartmann M, Szalai C, Saner FH. Hemostasis in liver transplantation: pathophysiology, monitoring, and treatment. World J Gastroenterol 2016;22:1541–50.

43. Clevenger B, Mallett SV. Transfusion and coagulation management in liver transplantation. World J Gastroenterol 2014;20:6146–58.

44. Mallett S. Clinical Utility of Viscoelastic Tests of Coagulation (TEG/ROTEM) in patients with liver disease and during liver transplantation. Semin Thromb Hemost 2015;41:527–37.

45. Krzanicki D, Sugavanam A, Mallett S. Intraoperative hypercoagulability during liver transplantation as demonstrated by thromboelastography. Liver Transpl 2013;19:852–61.

46. Tripodi A. The coagulopathy of chronic liver disease: is there a causal relationship with bleeding? No. Eur J Intern Med 2010;21:65–9.

47. Robertson AC, Eagle SS. Transesophageal echocardiography during orthotopic liver transplantation: maximizing information without the distraction. J Cardiothorac Vasc Anesth 2014;28:141–54.

48. Schumann R, Mandell MS, Mercaldo N, et al. Anesthesia for liver transplantation in United States academic centers: intraoperative practice. J Clin Anesth 2013; 25:542–50.

49. Gurusamy KS, Koti R, Pamecha V, et al. Veno-venous bypass versus none for liver transplantation. Cochrane Database Syst Rev 2011;(3):CD007712.

50. Paugam Burtz C, Kavafyan J, Merckx P, et al. Postreperfusion syndrome during liver transplantation for cirrhosis: outcome and predictors. Liver Transpl 2009; 15:522–9.

51. Jones RM, Moulton CE, Hardy KJ. Central venous pressure and its effect on blood loss during liver resection. Br J Surg 1998;85:1058–60.

52. Massicotte L, Lénis S, Thibeault L, et al. Effect of low central venous pressure and phlebotomy on blood product transfusion requirements during liver transplantations. Liver Transpl 2006;12:117–23.

53. Byram SW, Gupta RA, Ander M, et al. Effects of continuous octreotide infusion on intraoperative transfusion requirements during orthotopic liver transplantation. Transplant Proc 2015;47:2712–4.

54. Wagener G, Kovalevskaya G, Minhaz M, et al. Vasopressin deficiency and vaso-dilatory state in end-stage liver disease. J Cardiothorac Vasc Anesth 2011;25: 665–70.

55. Aniskevich S, Pai S-L. Fast track anesthesia for liver transplantation: review of the current practice. World J Hepatol 2015;7:2303–8.

Anesthesia for Intestinal Transplantation

Christine Nguyen-Buckley, MD[a],*, Melissa Wong, MD[b]

KEYWORDS

- Intestinal transplant • Intestinal failure • Multivisceral transplant • Anesthesia

KEY POINTS

- Intestinal transplant is an established treatment for patients with irreversible intestinal failure.
- Intestinal failure leads to systemic manifestations requiring multidisciplinary evaluation at a transplant center.
- Intestinal transplantation is a complex operation with potential for hemodynamic and metabolic instability.
- Patient outcomes for intestinal transplant are improving.

Intestinal transplantation merits attention from the transplant anesthesiologist owing to the complexity of the operation and the unique medical comorbidities associated with intestinal failure. Intestinal transplantation is relatively uncommon compared with other types of solid organ transplants; 2796 were completed in the United States from 1988 to 2016. There were 138 intestinal transplants overall in 2016, down from a peak of 198 in 2007.[1] In 2015, nearly equal numbers of intestinal transplantation patients in the United States received combined liver–intestine grafts versus intestine alone, and more than 40% of intestinal transplantation recipients were younger than18 years of age.[2]

INTESTINAL FAILURE AND PARENTERAL NUTRITION DEPENDENCY

Patients who cannot meet their protein and caloric needs, obtain essential micronutrients, and maintain electrolyte and fluid balance by their oral intake have intestinal failure. Intestinal failure may result from a number of conditions that affect gut function, but are typically classified as anatomic/surgical (short bowel syndrome),

Disclosures: None.
[a] Department of Anesthesiology, David Geffen School of Medicine, University of California at Los Angeles, 757 Westwood Plaza, Suite 3304, Los Angeles, CA 90095, USA; [b] Division of Liver and Pancreas Transplantation, Department of Surgery, David Geffen School of Medicine, University of California at Los Angeles, 757 Westwood Plaza, Los Angeles, CA 90095, USA
* Corresponding author.
E-mail address: Cnguyenbuckley@mednet.ucla.edu

Anesthesiology Clin 35 (2017) 509–521
http://dx.doi.org/10.1016/j.anclin.2017.04.007
1932-2275/17/© 2017 Elsevier Inc. All rights reserved.

functional/motility, or mucosal disorders. In infants, the most common etiologies are gastroschisis, volvulus, and necrotizing enterocolitis; in adults, intestinal failure most often arises after an extensive resection for acute mesenteric ischemia, Crohn's disease, or trauma[3,4] (**Table 1**). Although the threshold intestinal length necessary for nutritional autonomy varies, less than 200 cm of small bowel in an adult, or less than 20 cm in a child, raises the concern of intestinal failure.[5] The syndrome of intestinal failure encompasses large-volume enteral outputs from stoma, fistula, or diarrhea/steatorrhea; electrolyte disturbances (hypokalemia, hypomagnesemia); chronic dehydration leading to renal insufficiency; D-lactic acidosis; gastric hyperacidity and hypergastrinemia; vitamin D deficiency with osteoporosis; micronutrient deficiencies (especially thiamine, vitamin B_{12}, zinc) and toxicities (manganese, copper); cholestasis; hepatic steatosis; and nephrolithiasis.[5]

Rehabilitation after the onset of intestinal failure begins with autoadaptation, both physiologic and behavioral. Adaptive changes include delayed gastric emptying, intestinal dilation and hypomotility, and increased absorptive surface area.[5] Dietary modifications to enhance nutrient absorption include increasing oral intake, choosing low-fat foods with complex carbohydrates, and avoiding caffeine. Medications that slow transit (eg, codeine, loperamide, diphenoxylate/atropine) allow more time for absorption. Teduglutide, a glucagon-like peptide-2 analogue, increases intestinal villi height and crypt depth by 50%, and fluid and macronutrient absorption.[5] Nonetheless, many patients require long-term supplementation with parenteral nutrition (PN) or intravenous fluids and electrolytes. In adults, need for PN beyond 2 years, typically in the setting of 60 to 80 cm of small intestine without an ileocecal valve, constitutes PN dependence; in children, thresholds for PN dependency are less than 30 cm of small intestine and 36 to 48 months on PN.[4–6]

The advent of PN transformed intestinal failure from a catastrophe with nearly uniform mortality, into a chronic condition with a 5-year survival of 75%.[5] Key to this sea change was the commercialization of PN, whereby patients can self-administer infusions at home. But the cost of PN dependency remains high: US$150,000 of

Table 1 Etiologies of intestinal failure	
Infants and Children	**Adults**
• Gastroschisis	• Acute mesenteric ischemia
• Volvulus	○ Arterial thromboembolism
• Necrotizing enterocolitis	○ Venous thrombosis
• Intestinal atresia	○ Nonocclusive mesenteric ischemia
• Pseudo-obstruction	• Crohn's disease
• Hirschsprung disease	• Trauma
• Microvillous inclusion disease	• Desmoid tumor
• Tufting enteropathy	• Carcinoid tumor
	• Pseudoobstruction
	• Volvulus
	• Gardner's syndrome
	• Radiation enteritis
	• Adhesive obstruction or internal hernia not amenable to lysis

Adapted from Bathla L, Langnas A. Intestinal and multivisceral transplantation. In: Busuttil RW, Klintmalm G, editors. Transplantation of the liver. 3rd edition. Philadelphia: Elsevier; 2015. p. 818-34; and Rege A, Sudan D. Intestinal transplantation. Best Pract Res Clin Gastroenterol 2016;30(2):320; with permission.

reimbursed charges per patient-year, with additional out-of-pocket costs.[5] Indwelling central venous access leads to loss of vascular access sites over time and central line-associated blood stream infections, with an incidence ranging from 0.16 to 1.09 per catheter-year, leading to up to 70% of all hospitalizations among patients on home PN.[6,7] Catheter-related sepsis accounts for 70% of PN-related deaths.[6] Quality of life studies show lower scores among intestinal failure patients compared with the general population and even with patients with inflammatory bowel disease.[5,6]

Intestinal failure-associated liver disease (IFALD) is diagnosed by persistently elevated liver function tests greater than 1.5 times normal in a patient on chronic PN without any other identifiable cause. Histologically, pediatric patients demonstrate bile duct proliferation and cholestasis, whereas adults show steatotic changes. Over time, both demonstrate periportal inflammation, fibrosis, and ultimately cirrhosis. Almost 50% of pediatric patients and 30% of adults demonstrate evidence of IFALD after 4 to 12 weeks of total PN (TPN).[3] Some liver recovery may be achieved by cycling PN, minimizing lipids, and favoring formulations with antiinflammatory omega-3 fatty acids.[5,7] Nevertheless, 5% to 15% of chronic PN patients develop liver failure, with pediatric patients being at highest risk.[5,6]

INDICATIONS FOR INTESTINAL TRANSPLANTATION

Intestinal transplantation is indicated in patients who develop complications of PN dependence: recurrent central line-associated blood stream infections, limited central venous access, and IFALD[4] (**Table 2**). These patients have a 1-year mortality rate as high as 70%.[10] Patients who fail intravenous support, manifesting recurrent, severe dehydration episodes, also warrant intestinal transplantation. Other indications for intestinal transplantation have emerged, including unresectable mesenteric tumors and liver cirrhosis with extensive portomesenteric venous thrombosis (PMVT), precluding liver transplantation alone[8] (see **Table 2**). Profound comorbid conditions without potential for improvement by transplantation are considered contraindications, such as active malignancy or uncontrolled infection that would not be removed during transplantation, or severe immunologic deficiency (see **Table 2**).

Table 2	
Intestinal transplant indications and contraindications	
Indications	**Contraindications**

• Complications of parenteral nutrition
  ○ Recurrent central line-associated blood stream infections
  ○ Limited central venous access
  ○ Intestinal failure-associated liver disease
  ○ Recurrent dehydration despite parenteral nutrition and intravenous fluids
• Unresectable tumors in close proximity to mesenteric vessels (desmoid, gastrointestinal stromal tumors, and carcinoid tumors)
• Liver cirrhosis with extensive portomesenteric venous thrombosis
• Frozen abdomen
	• Metastatic disease or malignancy not at site of transplant
	• Uncontrolled infection
	• Severe immunologic deficiency

Data from Refs.[4,8,9]

PREOPERATIVE EVALUATION AND LISTING

Intestinal transplantation candidates require a comprehensive, multidisciplinary evaluation at a transplant center.[11] This evaluation should include representatives from transplant surgery, anesthesiology, gastroenterology/hepatology, cardiology, pulmonology, psychiatry, nutrition, and social work. Factors specific to intestinal transplantation candidates are discussed elsewhere in this article.

Cardiovascular evaluation assesses risk factors for perioperative major adverse cardiac events.[12,13] An electrocardiogram and transthoracic echocardiogram is sufficient for young patients with no or few risk factors. Older patients or those with cardiovascular risk factors should undergo nuclear stress testing followed by coronary angiography in patients with reversible ischemia.[12–15] Patients with echocardiographic evidence of elevated pulmonary artery pressures should undergo right heart catheterization for definitive diagnosis of pulmonary hypertension. The diagnosis of significant pulmonary hypertension warrants consultation with cardiology and pulmonary specialists for potential treatment with preoperative pulmonary arterial vasodilators.[15,16] Pulmonary function testing, chest imaging, and determination of functional capacity are necessary to characterize the severity of preexisting pulmonary disease.

Baseline quantitative coagulation function (prothrombin time/International Normalized Ratio, partial thromboplastin time, fibrinogen, and platelets) should be assessed; qualitative function may be evaluated using viscoelastic testing. In a single-center study of intestinal transplantation patients, preoperative thromboelastogram demonstrated reduced reaction times (time to formation of fibrin strands) and increases in alpha angle (speed of clot formation influenced by platelets and fibrinogen).[13] If a thrombophilia is found during workup, the patient should be considered for therapeutic anticoagulation to prevent clot propagation, which jeopardizes remaining bowel, and new thrombus formation with risk of future thromboembolic events.[8] Anticoagulation is usually deferred until after transplantation, particularly in intestinal failure patients with concomitant liver failure and coagulopathy. Workup of a thromboembolic event should also include echocardiography to rule out a patent foramen ovale, which should be addressed preoperatively if found, because it can be an ongoing source of embolism.[12]

Most intestinal transplantation candidates have undergone multiple prior abdominal surgeries before referral to an intestinal transplantation center. Operative notes from the original resection(s) and pathology reports documenting the length of intestine removed and significant histopathologic findings should be obtained. Contrast studies of any remaining intestine should be performed to define remaining length and anatomic or functional abnormalities. Endoscopy with biopsies rules out inflammatory bowel disease, aganglionosis, and mucosal abnormalities. Nutritional status should be optimized, because postoperative liver graft failure is associated with preoperative growth failure.[17]

Because of the incidence of IFALD with PN dependence, evaluation of liver dysfunction determines whether the patient should be listed for intestine alone, or liver-inclusive intestinal transplantation. Any personal or family history of liver dysfunction may signify an increased susceptibility to irreversible liver injury, and should prompt further investigation. Laboratory assessment begins with liver function tests, serum chemistry, viral hepatitis panel, and autoimmune antibodies. Upper endoscopy assesses for evidence of portal hypertension, such as esophageal or gastric varices, or portal hypertensive gastropathy. A liver biopsy may be necessary to evaluate the severity of fibrosis and rule out underlying liver pathology, which would make recovery from IFALD unlikely.

Most patients who come to intestinal transplantation have limited central venous access. Risk factors associated with central venous obstruction include hypercoagulable states and a preoperative inferior vena cava (IVC) filter.[18] Magnetic resonance venogram is more reliable and sensitive than ultrasound imaging in determining the patency of central veins.[4,12] If the innominate, superior vena cava, or IVC are thrombosed and venous drainage is by collaterals, the access may be inadequate for the high-velocity flow needed during the transplant operation (dialysis, pulmonary artery catheter monitoring, or venovenous bypass). Chronic central venous occlusions may be traversed by interventional radiology to reestablish vascular access; albeit high risk, sharp needle recanalization and radiofrequency wire recanalization have been successfully used to maintain transplant candidacy.[19,20]

The number of patients listed for intestinal transplantation nearly doubled from 2000 to 2009, and nearly one-half are younger than 5 years old.[3] The median time to transplantation for pediatric patients (age <18 years) decreased from 5.8 to 2.6 months during that period.[3] Waitlist mortality is predicted by age less than 1 year, multiple abdominal surgeries, liver biopsy showing bridging fibrosis, serum bilirubin greater than 3 mg/dL, and thrombocytopenia.[4] These factors are primarily related to the onset of liver failure, which is consistent with a 2007 Markov analysis predicting better life expectancy and quality-adjusted life years by early listing for isolated intestinal transplantation before the onset of IFALD.[21] Waitlisted patients should be reassessed every 3 months at minimum for changes that may affect their candidacy, particularly worsening liver function and diminishing vascular access. Close outpatient follow-up is important to minimize catheter-associated complications. Patients coming from home for intestinal transplantation have better graft and patient survival than those who are hospitalized at the time of transplantation.[9,22] In addition, psychiatric disorders and chronic pain syndromes are common in intestinal transplantation patients; appropriate consultations should be obtained.[23,24]

TYPES OF INTESTINAL ALLOGRAFTS

Although nomenclature varies, there are 4 anatomic deceased donor allografts, defined by intestine, liver, and stomach.[9,25] The pancreas is included for technical reasons, because removing it increases the risk of portal vein thrombosis owing to twisting. Despite early unfounded concerns of bacterial translocation, sepsis, and increased rejection, the right colon is now included in 30% of intestinal allografts.[9] Indeed, patients receiving a colon-inclusive allograft demonstrated a 5% higher rate of PN independence, likely owing to enhanced fluid absorption and uptake of free fatty acids.[9,11]

Isolated Intestine Allografts

This is the most commonly performed type of intestinal transplantation worldwide, comprising 46.6% of all small bowel-containing allografts.[9] It is suitable for patients with preserved liver function and no evidence of portal hypertension or diffuse PMVT.[22] Inflow to the graft superior mesenteric artery is brought from the recipient's infrarenal aorta; outflow is through the portal vein to the recipient's infrarenal IVC. Interposition grafts (from the donor's external iliac artery and vein) are sometimes necessary to avoid kinking of this anastomosis.

Liver–Intestine Allografts

The second most common intestinal transplantation (26.6%), the liver–intestine allograft, benefits patients who have developed irreversible liver damage.[9] Although these recipients have higher pretransplant waitlist mortality, and lower short-term patient and graft survival after transplantation, they demonstrate better long-term patient and graft survival attributable to the liver's protective effect against acute rejection.[9]

Multivisceral and Modified Multivisceral Allografts

A classic multivisceral allograft includes stomach, pancreatoduodenal complex, liver, intestine, and sometimes colon; a modified multivisceral allograft excludes the liver. These types are indicated for patients with complex abdominal pathologies who require foregut evisceration at the time of transplantation.[22] Multivisceral and modified multivisceral transplants comprise 21.3% and 5.5% of worldwide intestinal transplantations, respectively.[9]

Living Donor Intestine Allografts

Only 2 intestinal transplants using living donors were reported in the United States in 2015.[2,12] Advantages of living donor intestinal transplantation include decreased cold ischemia time, better HLA matching, and time for pretreatment of sensitized recipients with plasmapheresis and intravenous immunogolbulin.[12]

INDUCTION IMMUNOSUPPRESSION

According to the Intestinal Transplant Registry, 72% of patients received induction immunosuppression with either an interleukin-2 receptor antagonist (IL2RA) such as basiliximab, or a T-cell–depleting agent such as antilymphocyte globulin or alemtuzumab.[9] A corticosteroid is often given before reperfusion. Antilymphocyte globulin or alemtuzumab are preferred for higher immunologic risk patients, such as those who are presensitized or receiving an allograft without a liver.[26] Induction with these agents has been associated with improved short-term survival and reduced rates and severity of acute rejection episodes.[3,27]

CONDUCT OF INTESTINAL TRANSPLANTATION

Most intestinal transplantation recipients have a hostile abdomen from multiple prior surgeries, requiring extensive adhesiolysis to mobilize the viscera. If the patient has concomitant liver failure, this initial period may be particularly bloody. If a liver-inclusive graft is planned, the operation proceeds to mobilization of the native liver, and the caval and portal dissections. When extensive PMVT is present, adequate portal flow can sometimes be reestablished by thromboendovenectomy.[8] If successful, the patient can proceed with a liver transplant alone, and the pancreas reallocated to a backup recipient.[8]

The amount of native foregut removed is individualized to the recipient; a typical enterectomy removes the proximal jejunum to the transverse or descending colon. The stomach is transected either midbody or close to the gastroesophageal junction. If the liver is not being transplanted, the hilar structures are divided to preserve as much native length as possible. If the stomach, duodenum, pancreas, and spleen are retained, mesenteric drainage is maintained by creating a portocaval shunt.

Once adhesiolysis, mobilization, and enterectomy are complete, a brief period of hemostasis and resuscitation prepares the patient for implantation. A supraceliac aortic conduit is prepared to provide inflow to the allograft; this necessitates temporary aortic cross-clamping at the diaphragmatic crura.

If a bicaval hepatectomy is planned, test clamping the suprahepatic IVC is performed to assess the patient's hemodynamics and make a final decision regarding the use of venovenous bypass for the anhepatic phase. If this test precipitates instability, the IVC is unclamped and the patient volume loaded. When the patient's hemodynamics can tolerate it, the IVC is clamped and the hepatectomy completed.

For an isolated intestinal transplantation, arterial inflow from the aortic conduit is anastomosed to the graft superior mesenteric artery; the outflow may be the recipient's portal vein or SMV. For a multivisceral allograft, the liver's suprahepatic and infrahepatic caval anastomoses are sewn first, similar to a liver transplant. Then the allograft's descending thoracic aorta is anastomosed to the prepared supraceliac aortic conduit. Once the anastomoses are complete, the graft is reperfused.

Upon reperfusion, the primary surgical goal becomes hemostasis, but the patient is often cold, coagulopathic, acidotic, hypotensive, and has electrolyte abnormalities. Some patients benefit from a damage control approach wherein a longer period of resuscitation follows reperfusion, particularly as liver function recovers and bowel edema decreases; after adequate hemostasis, the patient is packed, temporarily closed, and transferred to the intensive care unit.[28]

Enteric continuity is reestablished with a jejunojejunostomy or a Roux-en-Y gastrogastrostomy proximally, and an ileocolostomy with proximal diverting loop ileostomy or end ileostomy distally. A gastrojejunal tube for proximal decompression and distal feeding is placed.

Abdominal closure after intestinal transplantation often presents challenges. The fascia cannot be closed under tension owing to the risk of vascular compression to the allograft. Patients often have abdominal wall hernias and loss of domain from prior surgeries. Stomas, enteral tubes, and the surgical incision limit flap mobilization for skin coverage.[3,29] Edema of the abdominal wall and bowels from intraoperative resuscitation make closure more difficult. Various methods of staged abdominal closure have been reported, using meshes or Silastic sheets, negative pressure dressings, delayed skin grafting, or pretransplant placement of subcutaneous tissue expanders.[30–32] Finally, transplantation of abdominal wall fascia, procured from the same intestinal allograft donor, offers low immunogenicity and durable abdominal closure.[3,29]

ANESTHETIC MANAGEMENT

Most intestinal transplantation patients have delayed gastric emptying; therefore, a rapid sequence induction should be performed.[13,15,24] Additional airway equipment should be considered if a difficult airway is anticipated.[15] In addition to peripheral access, a large-bore introducer placed in a supradiaphragmatic central vein is necessary for fluid resuscitation and vasopressor administration, because intestinal transplantation may be complicated by significant blood loss and hemodynamic instability. Both peripheral and central access may be challenging in intestinal transplantation patients. If difficult central access is anticipated based on imaging, preoperative fluoroscopically guided line placement may be indicated. Intraoperative surgical placement of central lines may be undertaken in selected cases, including direct IVC access.[15] A Teflon glidewire may be considered when advancing a standard central line guidewire proves difficult.[24]

In addition to standard monitors, a radial arterial line is recommended for beat-to-beat monitoring of arterial blood pressure, measurement of systolic pressure variation for volume assessment, and serial assessments of arterial blood gasses, hemoglobin, and electrolytes. Pulmonary artery catheterization is not compulsory for intestinal transplantation; however, it is useful for determining thermodilution cardiac output, assessing systemic vascular resistance and pulmonary vascular resistance, and measuring blood temperature.[13,33] Transesophageal echocardiogram allows rapid assessment of left and right ventricular function, left ventricular end-diastolic volume, valvular function, and visualization of intracardiac thrombi.[12,13] A nasogastric tube is placed for gastric decompression.[24]

After induction, a standard approach to anesthesia maintenance includes a volatile agent, an opioid, and a neuromuscular blocking agent.[13] Patients with a history of chronic pain may benefit from a subanesthetic ketamine infusion continued postoperatively, in addition to other nonopioid analgesics.[34] Consultation with a pain management expert may be helpful during the postoperative period in patients with a history of complex pain medication regimens.

Maintenance of normothermia is imperative during intestinal transplantation, thus avoiding coagulopathy and cardiac instability secondary to hypothermia. Active warming measures, including upper and lower body forced air warmers, a fluid warmer, and a circuit humidifier, should be considered.[15,33]

TPN formulations may contain potassium and are discontinued intraoperatively. Blood glucose should be monitored regularly in all patients with recent TPN administration; supplemental dextrose may be necessary to avoid hypoglycemia after TPN discontinuation. The anesthesia team typically administers a broad-spectrum antibiotic and antifungal for infection prophylaxis, and intraoperative immunosuppression.[13,24]

Before surgery, an active type and crossmatch should be initiated. Depending on the center and patient, an intraoperative transfusion protocol including multiple units of packed red blood cells and fresh frozen plasma delivered to the operating room before surgery may be considered. Frequent communication with the blood bank is recommended. A rapid transfuser system may be useful in adult patients. Some centers use cell-salvage for replacement of blood losses.[13] Hemorrhage may be severe in patients who have adhesions from previous abdominal surgeries, portal hypertension, or PMVT.[13,35] Hemodynamic instability may be worsened by vasoactive endotoxins released during manipulation of chronically infected abdominal tissues.[13] Crystalloid, albumin, and blood products are given in a balanced and goal-directed fashion with concomitant administration of vasopressor infusions (norepinephrine, vasopressin, and/or epinephrine) aiming to provide hemodynamic stability while avoiding bowel edema.[13,24] For procedures with IVC clamping, a perfusionist should be available for venovenous bypass if the patient does not tolerate IVC clamping.[15]

Serial viscoelastic testing guides transfusion of blood products and correction of coagulopathy, in addition to standard coagulation tests.[13,24,33,36] Coagulopathy is likely multifactorial owing to surgical stress, hemorrhage, hemodilution, immunosuppression, and ischemia–reperfusion injury.[36,37] A hemoglobin level of 7 to 10 g/dL should be maintained to provide adequate oxygen delivery. Excessive transfusion and overcorrection of coagulopathy should be avoided, because hypercoagulability and polycythemia increase the risk of graft vascular thrombosis.[24]

Patients may develop metabolic acidosis during the initial dissection. Large doses of sodium bicarbonate administered for the treatment of metabolic acidosis and massive transfusion may result in significant increases in serum sodium. Serial sodium measurements should be obtained and treated accordingly to avoid the risk of central pontine myelinolysis.[38,39] Patients may also develop hyperkalemia, especially in cases complicated by massive transfusion and at the time of organ reperfusion. Treatment of hyperkalemia includes maintenance of alkalosis as well as administration of calcium, diuretics, insulin, and washed blood products.[13,40,41] Many authors recommend serial potassium measurements and interventions to maintain potassium levels of less than 4 mmol/L before organ reperfusion.[13,24,42] Intraoperative dialysis for the treatment of hyperkalemia and acidosis may be considered, especially in the setting of preoperative renal failure.[43]

Cross-clamping and release of major venous and arterial vessels may contribute to significant hemodynamic instability during intestinal transplantation. Before IVC clamping, administration of fluid boluses and a vasopressor infusion may prevent significant hypotension associated with preload reduction. Rapid afterload reduction may be required with partial or complete aortic cross-clamping. Aortic cross-clamping may also contribute to renal injury; studies have demonstrated a 50% risk of posttransplant renal failure in intestinal transplantation patients.[12,35] Close communication with surgeons and visualization of the surgical field is imperative during the time of clamping and release of major vessels. Release of vascular clamps may be complicated by thromboembolism that can be diagnosed with a transesophageal echocardiogram; low-dose tissue plasminogen activator (0.5-4.0 mg) has been reported to be effective for the treatment of intracardiac thrombus complicated by severe hemodynamic instability.[44]

Reperfusion of the intestinal graft may be associated with acute metabolic and hemodynamic instability. Liver-inclusive intestinal transplantation patients have a higher incidence of hyperkalemia, severe base deficit, and postreperfusion syndrome (PRS) than liver transplant recipients, likely through a synergistic effect of the 2 grafts.[40] Acute acidosis results from release of an organic acid load from the ischemic graft and a concomitant increase in arterial CO_2 from increased graft metabolism.[37] Transient hyperkalemia associated with electrocardiographic changes may occur. Some centers prophylactically administer calcium, sodium bicarbonate, and vasopressor boluses before reperfusion.

PRS has been defined as a decrease in the mean arterial pressure of less than 60 mm Hg or 30% lower than baseline for at least 1 minute within the first 5 minutes after reperfusion.[45] Mechanisms contributing to PRS include an acute increase in capacitance associated with the new mesenteric circulation; massive release of inflammatory cytokines, free radicals, and endotoxins by the allograft bowel; and significant capillary leak and third spacing in the transplanted bowel and abdominal wall.[46] PRS occurs in nearly one-half of intestinal transplantations.[13,33] Hemodynamic changes after reperfusion include a transient increase in cardiac output and ventricular filling pressures and an acute decrease in systemic vascular resistance that remains low for many hours after reperfusion.[33,37] Some patients may develop right heart dysfunction or overt failure after reperfusion, requiring inotropic support and/or inhaled nitric oxide. Severe PRS may be complicated by cardiac arrest; it is reasonable to routinely place defibrillation pads before surgery.[24] More severe and prolonged postreperfusion instability may occur with poor graft quality and prolonged donor cold ischemia time.[33] PRS is associated with an increased incidence of postoperative renal failure and early postoperative mortality.[33]

After reperfusion, the main anesthetic goals are to maintain adequate graft perfusion while avoiding hepatic congestion.[47] Massive intraoperative fluid shifts and ongoing occult blood loss may contribute to intravascular depletion requiring continued fluid resuscitation and prolonged surgical hemostasis.[12] Abdominal closure may be complicated by the development of abdominal compartment syndrome owing to limited abdominal domain; peak airway pressures should be monitored closely.[24] Upon completion of surgery, most patients are transferred intubated to a surgical intensive care unit.

PEDIATRIC MANAGEMENT

Children represent the majority of patients on the intestinal transplantation waiting list, with the most common indication for transplantation being short gut syndrome, followed by gastroschisis, functional bowel impairment, and necrotizing enterocolitis.[12,48] Preoperative evaluation should be focused on systemic manifestations of the patient's primary disease with attention to associated syndromes such as congenital heart disease.[47] Immunizations should be up to date before surgery.[17] Care must be taken to avoid overtransfusion of blood products with the development of hypercoagulability and high blood viscosity, which may contribute to graft vascular thrombosis.[45,47] Maintenance of normothermia may be challenging in small patients with high surface areas.[47] Basic principles of pediatric organ transplantation will be covered in Nicholas Wasson and colleagues' article, "Anesthetic Management of Pediatric Liver and Kidney Transplantation," in this issue.

OUTCOMES AND POSTOPERATIVE COMPLICATIONS

Intestinal transplantation outcomes continue to improve. The 1- and 5-year graft survivals is 71.5% and 45.2%, respectively, for intestine-only patients, and 70.2% and 50.0%, respectively, for liver–intestine recipients.[2] Pediatric intestine-only patients have the highest 1- and 5-year patient survivals (88.1% and 74.6%, respectively), whereas adult liver–intestine recipients have the lowest (68.6% and 35.7%, respectively).[2] In a large, long-term study of nutritional outcomes in pediatric intestinal transplantation patients, median time to starting enteral nutrition was 8 days after transplant, whereas median time to wean off PN was 31 days.[49]

The leading cause of graft failure in intestinal transplantation is rejection, partially owing to the high immunogenicity of the intestinal graft. Predictors of graft survival include use of a liver-inclusive graft, panel reactive antibody less than 20%, absence of donor-specific antibody, negative T-cell crossmatch, and IL2RA induction.[50] Acute rejection may present subclinically and is often caught on serial surveillance endoscopy with biopsy.[33,35,51] The first sign of rejection may be increased stool output or sepsis owing to bacterial translocation.[33,51] Other postoperative complications include hemorrhage, thrombosis, anastomotic leak, renal failure, and graft-versus-host disease.[24]

SUMMARY

Intestinal transplantation is an established treatment for irreversible intestinal failure. Intestinal transplantation candidates present with systemic manifestations of intestinal failure and the sequelae of chronic PN dependency. They have high waitlist mortality, particularly driven by liver failure. Candidates require a detailed, multidisciplinary evaluation at an intestinal transplantation center. Intestinal transplantation is a complex operation with the potential for hemodynamic and metabolic instability, significant fluid shifts, major hemorrhage, and coagulopathy. Pediatric patients with intestinal failure make up a significant proportion of patients transplanted. Outcomes for intestinal transplantation are improving but acute rejection remains the most common major postoperative complication.

ACKNOWLEDGMENTS

The authors thank Christopher Wray, MD, and Douglas G. Farmer, MD, for their critical review of this article.

REFERENCES

1. US Department of Health and Human Services. Organ Procurement and Transplantation Network. National data. Available at: https://optn.transplant.hrsa.gov/data/view-data-reports/national-data/#. Accessed January 7, 2017.

2. Smith JM, Skeans MA, Horslen SP, et al. OPTN/SRTR 2015 annual data report: intestine. Am J Transplant 2017;17(Suppl 1):252–85.

3. Bathla L, Langnas A. Intestinal and multivisceral transplantation. In: Busuttil RW, Klintmalm G, editors. Transplantation of the liver. 3rd edition. Philadelphia: Elsevier; 2014. p. 818–34.

4. Rege A, Sudan D. Intestinal transplantation. Best Pract Res Clin Gastroenterol 2016;30(2):319–35.

5. Carroll RE, Benedetti E, Schowalter JP, et al. Management and complications of short bowel syndrome: an updated review. Curr Gastroenterol Rep 2016;18:40.

6. Hofstetter S, Stern L, Willet J. Key issues in addressing the clinical and humanistic burden of short bowel syndrome in the US. Curr Med Res Opin 2013;29(5): 495–504.

7. Wanten G. Parenteral approaches in malabsorption: home parenteral nutrition. Best Pract Res Clin Gastroenterol 2016;30(2):309–18.

8. Reyes JD. Intestinal transplantation: an unexpected journey. Robert E. Gross Lecture. J Pediatr Surg 2014;49:13–8.

9. Vianna R, Beduschi T. Multivisceral transplantation for diffuse splanchnic venous thrombosis. Curr Opin Organ Transplant 2016;21(2):201–8.

10. Grant D, Abu-Elmagd K, Mazariegos G, et al. Intestinal transplant registry report: global activity and trends. Am J Transplant 2015;15(1):210–9.

11. Ramisch D, Rumbo C, Echevarria C, et al. Long-term outcomes of intestinal and multivisceral transplantation at a single center in Argentina. Transplant Proc 2016; 48(2):457–62.

12. Dalal A. Intestinal transplantation: the anesthesia perspective. Transplant Rev (Orlando) 2016;30(2):100–8.

13. Planinsic RM. Anesthetic management for small bowel transplantation. Anesthesiol Clin North America 2004;22(4):675–85.

14. Lentine KL, Costa SP, Weir MR, et al. Cardiac disease evaluation and management among kidney and liver transplantation candidates: a scientific statement from the American Heart Association and the American College of Cardiology Foundation: endorsed by the American Society of Transplant Surgeons, American Society of Transplantation, and National Kidney Foundation. Circulation 2012;126(5):617–63.

15. Jacque JJ. Anesthetic considerations for multivisceral transplantation. Anesthesiol Clin North America 2004;22(4):741–51.

16. Raval Z, Harinstein ME, Skaro AI, et al. Cardiovascular risk assessment of the liver transplant candidate. J Am Coll Cardiol 2011;58(3):223–31.

17. Emre S, Umman V, Cimsit B, et al. Current concepts in pediatric liver transplantation. Mt Sinai J Med 2012;79(2):199–213.

18. Matsusaki T, Sakai T, Boucek CD, et al. Central venous thrombosis and perioperative vascular access in adult intestinal transplantation. Br J Anaesth 2012; 108(5):776–83.

19. Lang EV, Reyes J, Faintuch S, et al. Central venous recanalization in patients with short gut syndrome: restoration of candidacy for intestinal and multivisceral transplantation. J Vasc Interv Radiol 2005;16:1203–13.

20. Sivananthan G, MacArthur DH, Daly KP, et al. Safety and efficacy of radiofrequency wire recanalization of chronic central venous occlusions. J Vasc Access 2015;16(4):309–14.

21. Lopushinsky SR, Fowler RA, Kulkarni GS, et al. The optimal timing of intestinal transplantation for children with intestinal failure: a Markov analysis. Ann Surg 2007;246:1092–9.

22. Grant D, Abu-Elmagd K, Reyes J, et al. 2003 report of the intestine transplant registry: a new era has dawned. Ann Surg 2005;241(4):607–13.
23. Pither C, Green J, Butler A, et al. Psychiatric disorders in patients undergoing intestinal transplantation. Transplant Proc 2014;46(6):2136–9.
24. Lomax S, Klucniks A, Griffiths J. Anaesthesia for intestinal transplantation. Contin Educ Anaesth Crit Care Pain 2011;11(1):1–4.
25. Abu-Elmagd KM. The small bowel contained allografts: existing and proposed nomenclature. Am J Transplant 2011;11:184–5.
26. Cheng EY, Everly MJ, Kaneku H, et al. Prevalence and clinical impact of donor-specific alloantibody among intestinal transplant recipients. Transplantation 2017;101(4):873–82.
27. Mazariegos GV, Steffick DE, Horslen S, et al. Intestine transplantation in the United States, 1999-2008. Am J Transplant 2010;10(Part 2):1020–34.
28. DiNorcia J, Lee MK, Harlander-Locke MP, et al. Damage control as a strategy to manage postreperfusion hemodynamic instability and coagulopathy in liver transplant. JAMA Surg 2015;150(11):1066–72.
29. Gondolesi G, Fauda M. Technical refinements in small bowel transplantation. Curr Opin Organ Transplant 2008;13:259–65.
30. Sheth J, Sharif K, Lloyd C, et al. Staged abdominal closure after small bowel or multivisceral transplantation. Pediatr Transplant 2012;16:36–40.
31. Carlsen BT, Farmer DG, Busuttil RW, et al. Incidence and management of abdominal wall defects after intestinal and multivisceral transplantation. Plast Reconstr Surg 2007;119(4):1247–55.
32. Watson MJ, Kundu N, Coppa C, et al. Role of tissue expanders in patients with loss of abdominal domain awaiting intestinal transplantation. Transpl Int 2013; 26(12):1184–90.
33. Faenza S, Arpesella G, Bernardi E, et al. Combined liver transplants: main characteristics from the standpoint of anesthesia and support in intensive care. Transplant Proc 2006;38(4):1114–7.
34. Himmelseher S, Durieux ME. Ketamine for perioperative pain management. Anesthesiology 2005;102(1):211–20.
35. Sudan D. The current state of intestine transplantation: indications, techniques, outcomes and challenges. Am J Transplant 2014;14(9):1976–84.
36. Siniscalchi A, Spedicato S, Lauro A, et al. Intraoperative coagulation evaluation of ischemia-reperfusion injury in small bowel transplantation: a way to explore. Transplant Proc 2006;38(3):820–2.
37. Siniscalchi A, Piraccini E, Cucchetti A, et al. Analysis of cardiovascular, acid-base status, electrolyte, and coagulation changes during small bowel transplantation. Transplant Proc 2006;38(4):1148–50.
38. Morard I, Gasche Y, Kneteman M, et al. Identifying risk factors for central pontine and extrapontine myelinolysis after liver transplantation: a case-control study. Neurocrit Care 2014;20(2):287–95.
39. Crivellin C, Cagnin A, Manara R, et al. Risk factors for central pontine and extrapontine myelinolysis after liver transplantation: a single-center study. Transplantation 2015;99(6):1257–64.
40. Song X, Farmer DG, Xia VW. Intraoperative management and postoperative outcome in intestine-inclusive liver transplantation versus liver transplantation. Transplant Proc 2015;47(8):2473–7.
41. Xia VW, Obaidi R, Park C, et al. Insulin therapy in divided doses coupled with blood transfusion versus large bolus doses in patients at high risk for hyperkalemia during liver transplantation. J Cardiothorac Vasc Anesth 2010;24(1):80–3.

42. de Oliveira Clark RM, Neto AB, Bianchi EH, et al. Evaluation of hemodynamic, metabolic, and electrolytic changes after graft reperfusion in a porcine model of intestinal transplantation. Transplant Proc 2010;42(1):87–91.

43. Wray CL, AV, Scovotti JC, et al. An intraoperative algorithm for the management of liver transplant patients receiving preoperative dialysis: a case series. Int Liver Transplant Soc Congress (abstract O-80). 2016.

44. Boone JD, Sherwani SS, Herborn JC, et al. The successful use of low-dose recombinant tissue plasminogen activator for treatment of intracardiac/pulmonary thrombosis during liver transplantation. Anesth Analg 2011;112(2):319–21.

45. Aggarwal S, Kang Y, Freeman JA, et al. Postreperfusion syndrome: cardiovascular collapse following hepatic reperfusion during liver transplantation. Transplant Proc 1987;19(4 Suppl 3):54–5.

46. Siniscalchi A, Cucchetti A, Miklosova Z, et al. Post-reperfusion syndrome during isolated intestinal transplantation: outcome and predictors. Clin Transplant 2012; 26:454–60.

47. Uejima T. Anesthetic management of the pediatric patient undergoing solid organ transplantation. Anesthesiol Clin North America 2004;22(4):809–26.

48. Lao OB, Healey PJ, Perkins JD, et al. Outcomes in children after intestinal transplant. Pediatrics 2010;125(3):e550–8.

49. Venick RS, Wozniak LJ, Colangelo J, et al. Long-term nutrition and predictors of growth and weight gain following pediatric intestinal transplantation. Transplantation 2011;92(9):1058–62.

50. Farmer DG, Venick RS, Colangelo J, et al. Pretransplant predictors of survival after intestinal transplantation: analysis of a single-center experience of more than 100 transplants. Transplantation 2010;90:1574–80.

51. Yeh J, Ngo KD, Wozniak LJ, et al. Endoscopy following pediatric intestinal transplant. J Pediatr Gastroenterol Nutr 2015;61(6):636–40.

Anesthesia and Perioperative Care in Reconstructive Transplantation

Raymond M. Planinsic, MD[a],*, Jay S. Raval, MD[b],
Vijay S. Gorantla, MD, PhD, FRCS[c]

KEYWORDS

- Anesthesia • Perioperative care • Reconstructive transplantation
- Vascularized composite allografts

KEY POINTS

- Anesthetic management in reconstructive transplantation (RT) requires a thorough knowledge of solid organ transplant anesthesia as well as regional anesthesia strategies in microvascular surgery.
- Anesthetic protocols must be customized for individual RT procedures (eg, upper extremity, craniofacial) for proactive prevention of common complications and aggressive intervention during these complex procedures.
- The RT anesthesiologist must prepare for the perioperative effects of induction immunotherapies, immune risks of the large antigenic burden and microbial load, overwhelming ischemia-reperfusion injury, significant electrolyte imbalances, drastic hemodynamic shifts, massive blood loss, and extended anesthesia times among a host of intraoperative and postoperative challenges.
- RT procedures require intensive intraoperative monitoring of hemodynamics and coagulation, large-volume resuscitation requirements (with induced hypotension and intraoperative cell salvage), maintenance of supranormovolemic status before allograft revascularization, timed utilization of pneumatic tourniquets, and aggressive antimicrobial prophylaxis.
- Optimal anesthesiology management in RT involves close partnership and coordination with the surgical team to plan for and address inherent demands, risks, and challenges unique to these procedures.

Disclosure Statement: None.
[a] Department of Anesthesiology, University of Pittsburgh Medical Center, 200 Lothrop Street, Suite C-200, Pittsburgh, PA 15213, USA; [b] Division of Transfusion Medicine, Department of Pathology and Laboratory Medicine, Transfusion Medicine Service, Hematopoietic Progenitor Cell Laboratory, University of North Carolina at Chapel Hill, 101 Manning Drive, Suite C3162, Chapel Hill, NC 27514, USA; [c] Departments of Surgery, Ophthalmology and Bioengineering, US Air Force, Wake Forest Institute for Regenerative Medicine, Wake Forest Baptist Medical Center, Richard H. Dean Biomedical Building, 391 Technology Way, Winston Salem, NC 27101, USA
* Corresponding author.
E-mail addresses: planinsicrm@anes.upmc.edu (R.M.P.); gorantlavs@upmc.edu (V.S.G.)

Anesthesiology Clin 35 (2017) 523–538
http://dx.doi.org/10.1016/j.anclin.2017.04.008
1932-2275/17/© 2017 Elsevier Inc. All rights reserved.
anesthesiology.theclinics.com

RECONSTRUCTIVE TRANSPLANTATION

Reconstructive transplantation (RT) is an emerging domain, including but not limited to extremity, craniofacial, genitourinary, tracheal, or abdominal tissue allografts (**Box 1**). Vascularized composite allografts (VCAs) derived from deceased or living-related donors are now defined by specific criteria (**Box 2**) under Organ Procurement and Transplantation Network (OPTN) policy guidelines.[1] Since most VCA are primarily vascularized, they are deemed as solid organs for donation and transplantation.

Per the latest reports, there are 53 VCA programs approved by the United Network for Organ Sharing (UNOS) and OPTN, located at 24 RT centers in the United States.[2] These programs are distributed across 11 geographic regions spanning 58 organ procurement organizations that facilitate VCA donation and allocation. Most VCA programs are approved for upper extremity, head and neck, or abdominal wall VCA. A few programs are approved for genitourinary transplantation (eg, penile or uterine) and lower extremity transplantation.

ANESTHESIA IN RECONSTRUCTIVE TRANSPLANTATION

RT is a multidisciplinary specialty that integrates the tenets of transplant surgery with those of reconstructive surgery.[2,3] Thus, the anesthetic management of these challenging and complex VCA procedures mandates a thorough understanding of the principles and practice of transplant anesthesia,[4] and regional anesthesia strategies as applicable to microsurgical reconstruction.[5]

Unlike solid organ transplantation (SOT), RT procedures involve significant microsurgical reconstruction. The primary intraoperative goals of regional anesthesia for RT are to maintain global and local hemodynamics and homeostasis, as well as

---

Box 1
Approved list of body parts classifiable as vascularized composite allografts per United Network for Organ Sharing Vascularized Composite Allograft committee designation

Upper limb, including but not limited to any group of body parts from the upper limb or radial forearm flap

Head and neck, including but not limited to face, including underlying skeleton and muscle, scalp, larynx, trachea, thyroid, or parathyroid gland

Abdominal wall, including, but not limited to symphysis pubis and other vascularized pelvic elements

Genitourinary organs, including but not limited to uterus, internal or external male and female genitalia, or urinary bladder

Lower limb, including but not limited to pelvic structures that are attached to the lower limb and transplanted intact, gluteal region, vascularized bone transfers from the lower extremity, anterior lateral thigh flaps, or toe transfers

Adrenal gland

Spleen

Musculoskeletal composite graft segment, including but not limited to latissimus dorsi, spine axis, or any other vascularized muscle, bone, nerve, or skin flap

From Gorantla VS, Plock JA, Davis MR. Reconstructive transplantation: program, patient, protocol, policy, and payer considerations. In: Subramaniam K, Sakai T, editors. Anesthesia and perioperative care for organ transplantation. New York: Springer New York; 2016. p. 554; with permission.

Box 2
Organ Procurement and Transplantation Network and United Network for Organ Sharing criteria for definition of vascularized composite allografts

Primarily vascularized grafts

Contain multiple tissue types

Recovered from a human donor as an anatomic or structural unit

Transplanted into a human recipient as an anatomic or structural unit

For homologous use (the replacement or supplementation of a recipient organ with that performing the same basic function in recipient as in donor)

Minimally manipulated (ie, processing that does not alter the original relevant characteristics of the organ relating to the organ's utility for reconstruction, repair, or replacement)

Not combined with another article, such as a device

Susceptible to ischemia and, therefore, only stored temporarily and not cryopreserved

Susceptible to allograft rejection, generally requiring immunosuppression, which may increase infectious disease risk to the recipient

From Gorantla VS, Plock JA, Davis MR. Reconstructive Transplantation: program, patient, protocol, policy, and payer considerations. In: Subramaniam K, Sakai T, editors. Anesthesia and perioperative care for organ transplantation. New York: Springer New York; 2016. p. 554; with permission.

---

hemostasis in the VCA. Key priorities are minimizing peripheral vasoconstriction (through adequate pain control; attention to vasoactive medications; preserving normothermia; and preventing hyperoxia, hypocapnia, and hypovolemia) and treating hypotension (through hypervolemic or normovolemic hemodilution, rapid and adequate volume replacement, attention to sympathetic blockade, and maintaining systemic vascular resistance). To achieve these goals, a combination of general and regional anesthesia techniques need to be explored for VCA procedures. In particular, the altered perioperative immune response secondary to prolonged surgery, ischemia reperfusion injury (IRI), and use of transplant medications in VCA procedures must guide the choice of anesthetics and techniques.

Similar to SOT, such as liver transplants, VCA, such as bilateral upper extremity transplants and craniofacial transplants, are often protracted procedures that require robust large-volume resuscitation involving fluids and blood products, intensive intraoperative hemodynamic monitoring (ie, metabolic and coagulation parameters), and aggressive intraoperative and postoperative analgesia to enable successful surgical, immunologic, and functional outcomes.

Our team was the first to establish recommendations for protocols and procedures for anesthesia in upper extremity VCA.[6] Although various VCA are unique in procedural, planning, or patient-related aspects, there is significant relevance and overlap for broad principles of anesthesia and perioperative management across these transplants. Herein, the authors share our experience in anesthetic management in RT with specific emphasis on the procedural and protocol-related aspects.

THE PERIOPERATIVE IMMUNE RESPONSE IN RECONSTRUCTIVE TRANSPLANTATION

The perioperative immune response can be affected by multiple factors, including but not limited to the nature and extent of surgery, anesthetic agents and technique, blood products, and perioperative medications.[7]

Surgical trauma affects both innate and acquired immune responses. In particular, revascularization of ischemic tissues results in IRI triggering a complex inflammatory cascade involving upregulation of danger-associated molecular patterns; activation of pattern-recognition receptors, such as toll-like receptors (TLRs); inflammatory cell trafficking; antibody deposition; and activation of the complement and coagulation pathways.[8] TLRs are primarily found on macrophages, mast cells, and dendritic cells, the 3 sentinel cells of the innate immune response.

Inhalational and intravenous (IV) anesthetics have immunosuppressive effects due to their multifaceted inhibitory effects on lymphocyte apoptosis, neutrophil phagocytosis, and natural killer cell function.[9,10] Anesthetics (eg, propofol or sevoflurane) can mitigate the effects of IRI through their immunosuppressive effect.[11] Drugs, such as opioids or steroids, used as adjuncts in transplant anesthetic management may also affect perioperative immune competence in VCA recipients.[12,13] Evidentially, selection of the appropriate anesthetic agents and implementing the optimal techniques is critical to minimizing the risks of postoperative infection and ensuring perioperative success in VCA. In addition to risks for sensitization, perioperative allogenic blood transfusion can have collateral immunosuppressive effects that can have an impact on infectious risk, especially in major VCA procedures requiring massive transfusion.[14]

Peritransplant Immunosuppression

Induction therapies

The overarching goals of induction therapies in SOT or VCA are to minimize the proinflammatory effects of IRI and prevent early acute rejection (AR) by facilitating a donor graft-permissive, peritransplant immunosuppressive window in the recipient.[15] There is no consensus regarding the choice of induction therapy in VCA. Both depleting polyclonal or monoclonal antibodies, as well as nondepleting antibodies, have been used in VCA.[16,17]

Depleting agents

Common depleting agents include polyclonal antibodies, such as antithymocyte globulin (ATG), or monoclonal antibodies, such as alemtuzumab (Campath 1H, Millennium). The most widely used ATG in VCA is thymoglobulin (rabbit ATG, Genzyme, Sanofi). Both thymoglobulin and alemtuzumab have been used off-label in VCA applications.[17,18]

Thymoglobulin results in rapid T-cell depletion in peripheral blood through complement-dependent cell lysis and T-cell apoptosis in lymphoid tissues. Due to its polyclonal nature, thymoglobulin also affects other antigens, molecules, and pathways that mediate lymphocyte trafficking, adhesion, regulation, and hemostasis.[19,20]

Alemtuzumab is a recombinant DNA-derived humanized monoclonal antibody directed at CD52, which is a cell surface antigen present on B and T lymphocytes, most monocytes, macrophages, natural killer cells, and a subpopulation of granulocytes.[21] A proportion of bone marrow cells, including some CD34+ cells, express variable levels of CD52. The proposed mechanism of action is antibody-dependent cellular-mediated lysis following CD52 binding.

In 2009, the Pittsburgh program was the first in the United States to use alemtuzumab induction in upper extremity VCA.[22] Since then, its use has expanded across other VCA programs (eg, abdominal wall and face transplantation).[23–26] Overall, most VCA programs continue to use thymoglobulin as the preferential induction agent.[17,27]

Nondepleting agents

Basiliximab (Simulect, Novartis) and daclizumab (Zinbryta, Biogen) bind to CD25, which is the alpha subunit of the IL-2 receptor and prevents T-cell activation and proliferation for 5 to 8 weeks without causing cell lysis.[28] Basiliximab was used as induction therapy in the nation's first upper extremity transplant performed in Louisville in 1999. This remains the longest surviving VCA in the world at 19 years after surgery.[29]

Immunomodulatory Protocols

The Pittsburgh Protocol using donor bone marrow (DBM) cell infusion, was the world's first successful implementation of an immunomodulatory therapy in clinical RT.[30] The premise of the Pittsburgh Protocol is to use nonmyeloablative depletional conditioning with induction agents (eg, alemtuzumab) to eliminate alloreactive effector cells while preserving regulatory cells and creating a permissive window. Additionally, the non-T-cell–depleted DBM infusion (along with bone marrow stem cells) is aimed to accomplish clonal exhaustion-deletion of effector cells (coincident with the burst of donor antigen) and help in immunomodulation of the hyporesponsive recipient immune system under lower doses of maintenance therapy. Initial and emerging data from 8 hand or forearm transplants performed in a small cohort of 5 subjects at the University of Pittsburgh confirm the feasibility and tolerability of the protocol.[22]

KEY PERIOPERATIVE ANESTHETIC CONSIDERATIONS

The primary challenge of induction is to achieve profound reductions in T cells for preventing (or delaying) AR while minimizing concomitant increased perioperative risks of drug toxicity and opportunistic infections secondary to reduced immune competence.

Alemtuzumab and thymoglobulin have been used as induction agents in VCA for more than a decade. Overall, induction therapy can cause global immunosuppression (myelosuppression associated with leukopenia and thrombocytopenia) with a prolonged immune reconstitution.[31] Full recovery is debatable, especially in older VCA recipients. However, the published data on perioperative opportunistic infections in VCA recipients are limited,[32] as in SOT.[33] Further, efficacy of antimicrobial prophylaxis after such induction therapy in recipients receiving a specific type of VCA is poorly defined.[34]

Notably, craniofacial VCA composed of nasopharyngeal, dental, buccal, gingival, or upper airway tissues may be inherently contaminated with donor flora (bacterial, viral, or fungal). Despite global antimicrobial or antifungal prophylaxis, immunocompromised recipients receiving such grafts face serious infectious risks in the perioperative period. Indeed, multidrug-resistant sepsis has been reported in 2 patients receiving combination craniofacial and upper extremity transplants, leading to amputations of the limbs in 1 case and death in the other.[35] Most such studies are single-center experiences with inconsistent or incomplete data on other factors that may affect the epidemiology of opportunistic infections (eg, after use of depletional antibodies in AR refractory to maintenance therapy).[36,37] Given the small number of VCA patients worldwide, there is a lack of open-label, randomized, multicenter studies comparing safety and efficacy of different therapies.

Depletional induction is often associated with massive release of effector cytokines from lysed T-cells, such as interferon-γ or interleukin-(IL)-10 or IL-6.[38,39] Such a cytokine release syndrome (CRS), correlates with both toxicity and efficacy in patients receiving these induction therapies. CRS can cause high-grade fever (>39°C), chills, and possibly rigors during preoperative or intraoperative induction therapy. Premedication with steroids (bolus methylprednisolone), along with diphenhydramine and acetaminophen, may be helpful to minimize risk of CRS.

In contrast to alemtuzumab and thymoglobulin, basiliximab and daclizumab have a superior safety profile (similar to placebo) and do not cause CRS.[34,40–42] However, rare hypersensitive reactions can occur with these agents, resulting in intraoperative or perioperative hypotension, tachycardia, cardiac failure, bronchospasm, pulmonary edema, and respiratory failure.[43]

The use of nondepleted DBM infusions in immunomodulatory protocols could be associated with a risk of graft-versus-host disease (GVHD). However, there was no evidence of GVHD with the Pittsburgh Protocol albeit lack of T-cell depletion.[44,45] Several studies have also confirmed that both alemtuzumab and thymoglobulin protect against GVHD.[46–50]

It is also important to note other intraoperative and perioperative risks of alemtuzumab relevant to the anesthetic management of VCA recipients:

- Coagulopathy: Coagulopathic complications have been reported with alemtuzumab in SOT[51,52] and documented with the use of this induction agent in upper extremity VCA.[6] Six hours after administration of alemtuzumab, the recipient developed significant coagulopathy manifested by excessive intraoperative bleeding that continued into the perioperative period, necessitating emergency re-exploration 4 hours and 46 minutes after the transplant.
- Pulmonary edema: Alemtuzumab has been linked to intraoperative pulmonary edema that can cause oxygen desaturation during transplant surgery.[53] Rarely, perioperative pulmonary edema[54] and alveolar hemorrhage[55] have been also reported.
- Other reported risks include immune thrombocytopenia[56,57] and infusion-related side effects that may lead to intraoperative hypotension.

ANESTHETIC PROCEDURES AND PROTOCOLS: PEARLS AND PITFALLS

Although a wide range of VCA are now a clinical reality, significant world experience relates to upper extremity and craniofacial transplantation. These procedures are often protracted and involve complex surgical planning and preparation.

The endothelial surface layer provides the primary vascular barrier between the blood and tissues and is also critically involved in inflammation and coagulation pathways. Both IRI and sepsis can cause breakdown of this barrier, leading to increased vascular leakage. Revascularization following VCA procedures can result in drastic blood volume shifts into the intravascular space. Interestingly, both revascularization and hypervolemia due to high-volume fluid resuscitation can result in damage to the endothelial barrier. This, in turn, could lead to third-spacing of fluid into the interstitial tissues of the VCA, causing potentially serious complications such as edema, reduced cardiac output, and drastic hypotension. These could be compounded because VCAs, such as bilateral high upper extremity or lower extremity transplants, bring with them a large muscular compartment and vascular bed (>30% increase in vascular bed in some cases).

Operative times of up to 14 hours have been reported for upper extremity transplants and 28 hours for craniofacial transplants.[58,59] The surgical sequence may be different across upper extremity or craniofacial VCA; however, in all instances, the primary goal is to minimize ischemia time and facilitate expeditious surgery. Temporary vascular shunts have been used by some teams to minimize ischemia time between tendinous, neuromuscular, and skeletal repairs and definitive vascular anastomoses.

Intraoperative bleeding in these prolonged surgical procedures can be on the order of liters per hour, requiring very large volumes of blood or crystalloid infusions. Such challenging intraoperative transfusion requirements necessitate unique blood management. It is imperative that centers preparing to perform these transplants engage their transfusion medicine service for early assessment of massive transfusion needs and to ensure that appropriate blood components are readily available for these recipients.

For upper extremity transplantation, nadir hemoglobins have been reported to be as low 4.9 g/dL along with prolongations of international normalized ratio (INR) up to 7.3, whereas platelet and fibrinogen levels decreased to 33,000/µL and 31 mg/dL, respectively.[6] To offset these losses, multiple blood component transfusions, including up to 45 units of red blood cells (RBCs), 34 units of plasma, 4 units of platelets, and 2 units of cryoprecipitate have been reported in VCA recipients.[6,60] Expectedly, patients who undergo bilateral upper extremity transplantation have markedly increased intraoperative blood component requirements compared with those who undergo unilateral procedures.[59]

Compared with upper extremity VCA, more liberal transfusion thresholds have been reported in craniofacial transplants (hemoglobin <9 g/dL, activated partial thromboplastin time [APTT]/prothrombin time [PT] >1.5 × upper limits of normal, and platelets <50,000/µL).[58] In some cases, up to 66 RBC units, 63 plasma units, 9 platelet units, and 6 cryoprecipitate doses have been transfused.[61,62] These levels of transfusion are compatible with massive resuscitation mandated for trauma settings.[63] The tissue damage compounded by IRI and risks of coagulopathy with hemorrhage complicate VCA procedures. In trauma patients, plasma/platelet/RBC transfusion strategies involving resuscitation ratios of 1:1:1 versus 1:1:2 have shown improvement in early hemostasis and decreased early mortality due to exsanguination.[64–66] However, it is important to recognize that, although evidence for various transfusion ratios has been established for trauma patients, no data currently exist to support the benefits of pre-emptive transfusion for blood losses in VCA. In fact, it has been suggested that nontrauma patients who receive algorithmic massive transfusion protocol-based blood resuscitation may have poorer outcomes.[67]

Dynamic intraoperative and perioperative monitoring of hematologic status during VCA procedures is critical. Laboratory services must be able to process hourly or, more frequently, stat laboratory results. The Pittsburgh anesthesiology protocol for upper extremity VCA[6] recommends monitoring of arterial blood gases (ABGs), sodium, potassium, calcium, glucose, lactate, hemoglobin, and serum osmolality during surgery in all patients. ABGs are documented at baseline and hourly. Additionally, after reperfusion of the transplant, 30-second, 30-minute, and 60-minute ABGs are determined along with these laboratory values. These time points are defined to help assess peak potassium concentrations, as well as other immediate metabolic and physiologic changes associated with reperfusion.

Routine coagulation panels, including PT, APTT, partial thromboplastin time, INR, platelets, and fibrinogen are performed at baseline, 30 minutes before reperfusion, and 30 and 60 minutes after reperfusion. Although informative, these automated and semiautomated assays have turn-around times of up to an hour. This can complicate or delay intraoperative decision-making on the use of plasma or cryoprecipitate transfusions.

A final coagulation panel must be performed at completion of transplantation. Thromboelastography (TEG) at regular intervals is essential: at baseline, 60 minutes after incision, and then hourly until surgical completion. Additional TEGs are evaluated 30 minutes before reperfusion, and 5, 30, and 60 minutes after reperfusion. The 3 TEGs studied 5, 30, and 60 minutes after reperfusion should include natural, amicar, and protamine channels to exclude coagulopathy related to possible fibrinolysis or heparin from the donor graft. For example, in cases of VCA donors with a documented history of heparin-induced thrombocytopenia and thrombosis, special precautions must be taken to replace heparin with bivalirudin in the recipient, along with modifications of deep vein thrombosis prophylaxis.[68] Though a completed TEG takes up to 30 minutes for completion, important information, such as reaction time (R-time) and maximum amplitude (MA) can be obtained much sooner by seeing the progressive readout on TEG monitors in the operating room. Calcium chloride or gluconate is used to correct for decreases in ionized calcium noted on ABG and/or after large-volume blood transfusion. Base deficits greater than 7 or pH less than 7.2 must be corrected with sodium bicarbonate.

Viscoelastic clot-based testing, such as TEG or ROTEM, has the ability to provide more timely information regarding the coagulation status of patients in the operative suite. These assays involve the measurement of resistance to movement of a developing clot against a metallic probe; the shape and amplitude of curves generated from these tests can indicate depletion of coagulation factors and/or platelets and would provide evidence to support plasma and/or cryoprecipitate transfusion. Viscoelastic clot-based testing has been successfully used to complement complete blood count (CBC) to assess the need for platelet transfusion in upper extremity transplantation.[6] CBC provides quantitative data on platelet counts, whereas viscoelastic clot-based testing gives qualitative insights into platelet functionality.

The published experience with transfusion requirements and blood management in upper extremity and craniofacial VCA is scant (**Table 1**). Based on the authors'

Table 1
Reported data on intraoperative blood use in vascularized composite allograft

Program | (Literature Reference)	Procedure	RBC	Plasma	Platelet
Mexico | (Moran-Romero,[78] 2014)	Bilateral UE	45	32	4
Lyon, France | (Clerc,[79] 2015)	Bilateral UE	8	8	1
Pittsburgh, Hopkins | (Lang et al,[6] 2012 | Raval et al,[59] in press)	Right UE	6	2	0
	Bilateral UE	19	4	1
	Bilateral UE	15	9	0
	Right UE	7	5	0
	Bilateral UE	33	34	3
	Bilateral UE	9 (+500 mL ICS)	9	1
Brigham | (Pomahac et al,[76] 2012)	Face	24 (+17 units ICS)	NR	NR
	Face	2	NR	NR
	Face and bilateral UE[a]	20	NR	NR
Paris, France | (Sedaghati-Nia et al,[58] 2013)	Face	28	23	3
	Face	16	16	1
	Face and bilateral UE[b]	66	63	9
	Face	10	10	0
	Face	22	13	1
	Face	15	15	2
	Face	9	2	0

Abbreviations: ICS, intraoperative cell salvage; NR, not reported; UE, upper extremity.
[a] Patient underwent bilateral limb amputation due to vascular insufficiency following septic shock.
[b] Patient underwent unilateral limb amputation and partial facial allograft removal because of vascular insufficiency and multidrug-resistant sepsis.

experience, it would be reasonable to have the blood bank prepare 10 crossmatch-compatible RBC units, 10 plasma units, and 1 platelet unit to be available in the operative suite at the initiation of surgery. This is compatible with massive transfusion protocols at most trauma centers in the United States.[69] The blood bank should keep an additional 10 crossmatch-compatible RBC units, 10 plasma units, and 1 platelet unit ready at all times until completion of surgery. The authors have successfully used the following formula in VCA patients: 1 unit packed RBC (PRBC), 1 unit fresh frozen plasma, and 250 cc normal saline. This ratio achieves a hematocrit of 26% to 28% in the rapid infusion system (RIS) reservoir. The authors recommend transfusion before reperfusion during blood loss.

All cellular blood components should be leukoreduced to decrease the risk of transfusion-associated cytomegalovirus infection (in recipients who are seronegative) and human leukocyte antigen alloimmunization. Additionally, irradiation of all cellular blood components should be considered to decrease the risk of transfusion-associated GVHD, especially in those recipients receiving DBM cell-based therapies (eg, the Pittsburgh Protocol) involving depletional induction regimens. Whenever possible, intraoperative cell salvage should also be used to decrease the need for allogeneic RBC transfusion. The authors recommend that an evidence-based strategy of blood transfusion for predefined laboratory or clinical parameters as outlined by the American Society of Anesthesiologists Task Force on Perioperative Blood Management be implemented for VCA (**Table 2**).[70]

Because most preservation solutions are potassium rich, the sudden electrolyte imbalances caused during reperfusion can lead to cardiac arrest or anesthetic complications. Further, the cold preservation solution can result in hypothermia on revascularization. Hypothermia alters the distribution and decreases the metabolism of most drugs, including anesthetic drugs and muscle relaxants, thus prolonging recovery. Prefilling the allograft with warm (37°C) crystalloids before microsurgical repair and vascular clamp release can prevent catastrophic blood pressure or body temperature drops by inducing a hemodilution effect (compensated in advance with PRBC transfusion), rather than volume depletion. Additional measures, such as airway heating and humidification and cutaneous warming (Bair Hugger) are important

Table 2
American Society of Anesthesiologists Task Force Criteria on Perioperative Blood Management

Red blood cell transfusion trigger of hemoglobin	<7 g/dL
Plasma transfusion trigger of APTT/PT	>1.5 × upper limit of normal
INR	>2.0 (in the absence of heparin) or prespecified viscoelastic clot-based testing thresholds with concomitant microvascular bleeding
Platelet transfusion trigger	<50,000/μL or prespecified viscoelastic clot-based testing thresholds
Cryoprecipitate or fibrinogen concentrate transfusion trigger of fibrinogen	<100 mg/dL or prespecified viscoelastic clot-based testing thresholds.

Modified from American Society of Anesthesiologists Task Force on Perioperative Blood Management. Practice guidelines for perioperative blood management: an updated report by the American Society of Anesthesiologists Task Force on Perioperative Blood Management*. Anesthesiology 2015;122(2):257; with permission.

considerations. The neuromuscular tissue components of the VCA are sensitive to not only the effects of cold ischemia (from cold preservation) but also IRI after revascularization. IRI can cause multipronged physiologic and immunologic effects ranging from hypovolemic shock and hyperkalemia to oxidative stress and innate immune activation with increased risk of acute and chronic rejection. IRI can also worsen hypovolemia, leading to hypoperfusion or ischemia of transplanted limb muscles. This causes reactive vasodilatation following reperfusion and further worsens hypotension. Ex vivo pulsatile machine preservation with normothermic or subnormothermic perfusion (blood, hemoglobin oxygen carriers) in VCA can minimize risk of IRI and associated complications.[71]

Apart from unilateral or bilateral upper extremity transplants,[60,72] or isolated craniofacial transplants, several combination transplants have been reported in the literature. These include combined face and bilateral hand transplants (see **Table 1**)[35,73] and combined upper and lower extremity transplants. Uniformly, quadruple VCA and triple VCA have been associated with very high failure. In the only reported case of quadruple limb transplantation, intraoperative or perioperative blood and blood product transfusion requirements totaled 200 units.[74] Three of 4 of these reported tandem transplant patients died due to operative or perioperative complications that included overwhelming sepsis or shock.[75] One patient survived but had to undergo removal of both upper extremities only to preserve a face transplant (see **Table 1**).[76] Importantly, in combination transplants, there is an acute change in the body mass index that challenges cardiac adaptations (eg, changes in cardiac output) in the perioperative period, leading to tissue hypoperfusion or shock. The intraoperative use of military antishock trousers or pneumatic antishock garments must be considered.[77]

VCA procedures demand a large surgical team, working in staggered rotating shifts to prevent fatigue and slowing. Extensive preoperative mock rehearsals involving surgeons and anesthesia teams can help prepare for the actual surgery.

MISCELLANEOUS RECOMMENDATIONS
Blood Loss

For procedures involving upper extremity and transplantation, continuous bleeding from dissected tissues can be an underappreciated problem. Constant oozing from exposed tissue beds may occur for hours. Such blood loss is difficult to measure because the blood is not readily accessible for suctioning in the surgical field. Insensible blood loss and third spacing fluid loss, make adequate vascular access an essential prerequisite for VCA procedures.

Intravascular and Airway Access

The authors recommend IV (internal jugular) access via a large-bore (cordis or Shiley) catheter. Central venous pressure monitoring is usually accomplished via a single lumen infusion catheter inserted through the introducer. In unilateral upper extremity VCA, an additional 14-gauge IV catheter is recommended in the nontransplanted limb. Bilateral upper extremity VCA, unlike craniofacial transplants may have limited IV access, requiring an additional 7-French double lumen or equivalent central venous internal jugular catheter. Alternately, a 20-gauge radial artery catheter in the nontransplanted limb and an 18-gauge femoral artery catheter for bilateral upper extremity VCA are recommended. Internal jugular access will not be possible, so large-bore IV access must be obtained from the upper extremity and femoral vessels.

Coagulation Monitoring

Monitoring of coagulation with ROTEM or TEG is essential. An RIS, such as the fluid management system, is also indispensable. Transesophageal echocardiography should be available if required.

Pulmonary Protection

Aggressive protection of the airway for prevention of aspiration is critical, especially in craniofacial VCA. In craniofacial VCA procedures, the airway is normally already secured via tracheostomy. Head-end bed elevation, regular clearance of endotracheal tube secretions, and continuous gastric suctioning are recommended.

Sepsis Prevention

Broad spectrum coverage of both recipient-cultured and donor-cultured flora, as well as viral and fungal species, is essential, especially in craniofacial transplants.[36,37] Concomitant reduction in immunosuppression must be considered in the event of perioperative sepsis to prevent further spread. Worsening of sepsis must be prevented by aggressive and timely debridement of frankly necrotic tissue, including removal of devitalized allografts. The induction immunosuppression prevents AR despite immunosuppression withdrawal.

Preventing Regional Vasoconstriction

A fluid warmer must be used for the infusion of cold solutions. An increase in ambient room temperature, use of forced air warmers (Bair Hugger 3M) and extensive surgical draping help maintain body temperature throughout the procedure. Alpha agonists should be avoided because they may affect graft perfusion. Dopamine is instituted when hypotension is not adequately corrected by infusion of IV fluids or blood products, such as vasodilation in response to donor extremity reperfusion. Low-dose dopamine maintains regional blood flow by increasing cardiac contractility through beta-1 agonist effects and sustains renal perfusion via dopaminergic receptors.

Pain Management

The authors recommend ultrasound-guided preoperative placement of supraclavicular brachial plexus nerve blocks unilaterally or bilaterally, depending on the surgical site. Supraclavicular access is a useful route for brachial plexus blockade and securing indwelling catheters. A single bolus of a short-acting local anesthetic is used during catheter placement to confirm function of the block. However, it is not activated for postoperative analgesia and vasodilatation by continuous infusion until completion of the transplant. This approach avoids the potential contribution of upper extremity vasodilation that may, in theory, contribute to brisk bleeding and hypotension during the procedure. After the initial bolus has worn off, an opioid general anesthetic helps patient tolerance of the tourniquet. Postoperative analgesia, provided by regional anesthetics, also helps diminish stress responses secondary to pain, such as pain during early physical therapy.

FUTURE DIRECTIONS

Program experience with anesthetic considerations, concepts, and challenges in RT is evolving as more VCA procedures continue to be performed across the world. A greater degree of collaboration is needed between anesthesiology teams representing various VCA programs for prompt, rational, effective, objective, rigorous, and deliberate evaluation of existing and novel anesthetic options for RT. Only then can anesthesiologists optimize and standardize protocols, as well as facilitate validation of safety, efficacy, and feasibility of protocols across VCA recipients from different demographic, ethnic, and etiopathologic groups. Agreeing on study standards, uniform assessments or data points, and pooling of data or comparison of results among centers (that individually lack necessary sample size or randomization), may indeed be the best means of increasing the quality of evidence for anesthesia protocols in VCA. This could increase generalizability of anesthetic outcomes and allow development of national society guidelines for VCA.

REFERENCES

1. Glazier AK. Regulatory oversight in the United States of vascularized composite allografts. Transpl Int 2016;29(6):682–5.
2. Gorantla VS, Plock JA, Davis MR. Reconstructive transplantation: program, patient, protocol, policy, and payer considerations. In: Anesthesia and perioperative care for organ transplantation. New York: Springer New York; 2016. p. 553–60.
3. Gorantla VS, Plock JA, Davis MR. Reconstructive transplantation: evolution, experience, ethics, and emerging concepts. In: Anesthesia and perioperative care for organ transplantation. New York: Springer New York; 2016. p. 539–52.
4. Planinsic RM. Anesthesia for composite tissue allografts. In: Anesthesia and perioperative care for organ transplantation. New York: Springer New York; 2016. p. 561–3.
5. Hagau N, Longrois D. Anesthesia for free vascularized tissue transfer. Microsurgery 2009;29(2):161–7.
6. Lang RS, Gorantla VS, Esper S, et al. Anesthetic management in upper extremity transplantation: the Pittsburgh experience. Anesth Analg 2012;115(3):678–88.
7. O'Dwyer MJ, Owen HC, Torrance HDT. The perioperative immune response. Curr Opin Crit Care 2015;21(4):336–42.
8. Salo M. Effects of anaesthesia and surgery on the immune response. Acta Anaesthesiol Scand 1992;36(3):201–20.
9. Kurosawa S, Kato M. Anesthetics, immune cells, and immune responses. J Anesth 2008;22(3):263–77.
10. Procopio MA, Rassias AJ, DeLeo JA, et al. The in vivo effects of general and epidural anesthesia on human immune function. Anesth Analg 2001;93(2):460–5.
11. Hsiao H-T, Wu H, Huang P-C, et al. The effect of propofol and sevoflurane on antioxidants and proinflammatory cytokines in a porcine ischemia-reperfusion model. Acta Anaesthesiol Taiwan 2016;54(1):6–10.
12. Welters I. Opioids and immunosuppression. Clinical relevance? Anaesthesist 2003;52(5):442–52 [in German].
13. Anderson SL, Duke-Novakovski T, Singh B. The immune response to anesthesia: part 2 sedatives, opioids, and injectable anesthetic agents. Vet Anaesth Analg 2014;41(6):553–66.
14. Hill GE, Frawley WH, Griffith KE, et al. Allogeneic blood transfusion increases the risk of postoperative bacterial infection: a meta-analysis. J Trauma Acute Care Surg 2003;54(5):908.
15. Charafeddine AH, Kirk AD. Induction immunosuppressive therapy. In: Kirk AD, Knechtle SJ, Larsen CP, et al, editors. Textbook of organ transplantation. Oxford (United Kingdom): John Wiley & Sons, Ltd; 2014. p. 715–31.
16. Petruzzo P, Lanzetta M, Dubernard JM, et al. The International Registry on Hand and Composite Tissue Transplantation. Transplantation 2010;90(12):1590–4.

17. Petruzzo P, Dubernard JM, Lanzetta M. 2527: The International Registry on Hand and Composite Tissue Allotransplantation (IRHCTT). Vascularized Compos Allotransplantation 2016;3(1–2):7.

18. Weissenbacher A, Boesmueller C, Brandacher G, et al. Alemtuzumab in solid organ transplantation and in composite tissue allotransplantation. Immunotherapy 2010;2(6):783–90.

19. Mueller TF. Mechanisms of action of thymoglobulin. Transplantation 2007; 84(Supplement):S5–10.

20. Brayman K. New insights into the mechanisms of action of thymoglobulin. Transplantation 2007;84(Supplement):S3–4.

21. Calne R. The use of alemtuzumab (Campath 1H) in organ transplant recipients. Curr Opin Organ Transpl 2005;10(4):261–4.

22. Schneeberger S, Gorantla VS, Brandacher G, et al. Upper-extremity transplantation using a cell-based protocol to minimize immunosuppression. Ann Surg 2013; 257(2):345–51.

23. Schneeberger S, Ninkovic M, Margreiter R. Hand transplantation: the Innsbruck experience. In: Hewitt CW, Lee WPA, editors. Transplantation of composite tissue allografts. Boston: Springer US; 2008. p. 234–50.

24. Schneeberger S, Landin L, Kaufmann C, et al. Alemtuzumab: key for minimization of maintenance immunosuppression in reconstructive transplantation? Transplant Proc 2009;41(2):499–502.

25. Marvin M, Ravindra K, Buell J, et al. Alemtuzumab induction in hand transplantation: progress towards minimizing immunosuppression in composite tissue allotransplantation (CTA). Transplantation 2008;86(Supplement):749.

26. Selvaggi G, Levi DM, Cipriani R, et al. Abdominal wall transplantation: surgical and immunologic aspects. Transplant Proc 2009;41(2):521–2.

27. Diaz-Siso JR, Bueno EM, Sisk GC, et al. Vascularized composite tissue allotransplantation - state of the art. Clin Transplant 2013;27(3):330–7.

28. Pascual J. Anti-interleukin-2 receptor antibodies: basiliximab and daclizumab. Nephrol Dial Transplant 2001;16(9):1756–60.

29. Jones JW, Gruber SA, Barker JH, et al. Successful hand transplantation — one-year follow-up. N Engl J Med 2009;343(7):468–73.

30. Gorantla VS, Brandacher G, Schneeberger S, et al. Favoring the risk-benefit balance for upper extremity transplantation–the Pittsburgh Protocol. Hand Clin 2011; 27(4):511–20, ix–x.

31. Sageshima J, Ciancio G, Guerra G, et al. Prolonged lymphocyte depletion by single-dose rabbit anti-thymocyte globulin and alemtuzumab in kidney transplantation. Transpl Immunol 2011;25(2–3):104–11.

32. Broyles JM, Alrakan M, Ensor CR, et al. Characterization, prophylaxis, and treatment of infectious complications in craniomaxillofacial and upper extremity allotransplantation: a multicenter perspective. Plast Reconstr Surg 2014;133(4): 543e–51e.

33. Helfrich M, Ison MG. Opportunistic infections complicating solid organ transplantation with alemtuzumab induction. Transpl Infect Dis 2015;17(5):627–36.

34. LaMattina JC, Mezrich JD, Hofmann RM, et al. Alemtuzumab as compared to alternative contemporary induction regimens. Transpl Int 2012;25(5):518–26.

35. Carty MJ, Hivelin M, Dumontier C, et al. Lessons learned from simultaneous face and bilateral hand allotransplantation. Plast Reconstr Surg 2013;132(2):423–32.

36. Hammond SP. Infections in composite tissue allograft recipients. Infect Dis Clin North Am 2013;27(2):379–93.

37. Avery RK. Update on infections in composite tissue allotransplantation. Curr Opin Organ Transpl 2013;18(6):659–64.
38. Wing MG, Moreau T, Greenwood J, et al. Mechanism of first-dose cytokine-release syndrome by CAMPATH 1-H: involvement of CD16 (FcgammaRIII) and CD11a/CD18 (LFA-1) on NK cells. J Clin Invest 1996;98(12):2819–26.
39. Thiyagarajan UM, Ponnuswamy A, Bagul A, et al. Thymoglobulin and its use in renal transplantation: a review. Am J Nephrol 2013;37(6):586–601.
40. Ciancio G, Gaynor JJ, Roth D, et al. Randomized trial of thymoglobulin versus alemtuzumab (with lower dose maintenance immunosuppression) versus daclizumab in living donor renal transplantation. Transplant Proc 2010;42(9):3503–6.
41. Hao WJ, Zong HT, Cui YS, et al. The efficacy and safety of alemtuzumab and daclizumab versus antithymocyte globulin during organ transplantation: a meta-analysis. Transplant Proc 2012;44(10):2955–60.
42. Burdette SD. Infectious Risks Associated with IL-2R Antagonist [Basiliximab (Simulect) and Daclizumab (Zenapax)]. In: Kumar D, Humar A, editors. The AST handbook of transplant infections. Kumar/The AST handbook of transplant infections. Oxford (United Kingdom): Wiley-Blackwell; 2011. p. 135.
43. Sun ZJ, Du X, Su LL, et al. Efficacy and safety of basiliximab versus daclizumab in kidney transplantation: a meta-analysis. Transplant Proc 2015;47(8):2439–45.
44. Gorantla VS, Schneeberger S, Moore LR, et al. Development and validation of a procedure to isolate viable bone marrow cells from the vertebrae of cadaveric organ donors for composite organ grafting. Cytotherapy 2012;14(1):104–13.
45. Donnenberg AD, Gorantla VS, Schneeberger S, et al. Clinical implementation of a procedure to prepare bone marrow cells from cadaveric vertebral bodies. Regen Med 2011;6(6):701–6.
46. Marsh RA, Lane A, Mehta PA, et al. Alemtuzumab levels impact acute GVHD, mixed chimerism, and lymphocyte recovery following alemtuzumab, fludarabine, and melphalan RIC HCT. Blood 2016;127(4):503–12.
47. Marsh RA, Neumeier L, Mehta PA, et al. Peri-Transplant Alemtuzumab Levels IMPACT ACUTE Gvhd, MIXED Chimerism, and Lymphocyte Recovery Following Reduced Intensity Conditioning with Alemtuzumab, Fludarabine, and Melphalan. Biol Blood Marrow Transplant 2016;22(3):S337.
48. Norlin A-C, Remberger M. A comparison of Campath and Thymoglobulin as part of the conditioning before allogeneic hematopoietic stem cell transplantation. Eur J Haematol 2011;86(1):57–66.
49. Storek J. Impact of serotherapy on immune reconstitution and survival outcomes after stem cell transplantations in children: thymoglobulin versus alemtuzumab. Biol Blood Marrow Transplant 2015;21(3):385–6.
50. Hale G, Bright S, Chumbley G, et al. Removal of T cells from bone marrow for transplantation: a monoclonal antilymphocyte antibody that fixes human complement. Blood 1983;62(4):873–82.
51. Ku G, Ting WC, Lim STK, et al. Life-threatening coagulopathy associated with use of Campath (alemtuzumab) in maintenance steroid-free renal transplant given before surgery. Am J Transplant 2008;8(4):884–6.
52. Farid SG, Barwick J, Goldsmith PJ, et al. Alemtuzumab (Campath-1H)-induced coagulopathy in renal transplantation. Transplantation 2009;87(11):1751–2.
53. Grable B, Sakai T. Isolated left-sided pulmonary edema caused by alemtuzumab (Campath) during kidney transplantation. Transpl Int 2010;23(8):851–4.
54. Muthusamy ASR, Vaidya AC, Sinha S, et al. Alemtuzumab induction and steroid-free maintenance immunosuppression in pancreas transplantation. Am J Transplant 2008;8(10):2126–31.

55. Sachdeva A, Matuschak GM. Diffuse alveolar hemorrhage following alemtuzumab. Chest 2008;133(6):1476–8.
56. Cuker A, Coles AJ, Sullivan H, et al. A distinctive form of immune thrombocytopenia in a phase 2 study of alemtuzumab for the treatment of relapsing-remitting multiple sclerosis. Blood 2011;118(24):6299–305.
57. Reda G, Maura F, Gritti G, et al. Low-dose alemtuzumab-associated immune thrombocytopenia in chronic lymphocytic leukemia. Am J Hematol 2012;87(9):936–7.
58. Sedaghati-nia A, Gilton A, Liger C, et al. Anaesthesia and intensive care management of face transplantation. Br J Anaesth 2013;111(4):600–6.
59. Raval JS, Gorantla VS, Shores JT, et al. Blood product utilization in human upper-extremity transplantation: challenges, complications, considerations, and transfusion protocol conception. Transfusion 2017;57(3):606–12.
60. Iglesias M, Leal P, Butrón P, et al. Severe complications after bilateral upper extremity transplantation: a case report. Transplantation 2014;98(3):e16–7.
61. Edrich T, Cywinski JB, Colomina MJ, et al. Perioperative management of face transplantation. Anesth Analg 2012;115(3):668–70.
62. Siemionow M. The miracle of face transplantation after 10 years. Br Med Bull 2016;120(1):5–14.
63. Kozek-Langenecker S. Monitoring of hemostasis in emergency medicine. In: Vincent J, editor. Intensive care medicine. New York: Springer New York; 2007. p. 847–60.
64. Stephens CT, Gumbert S, Holcomb JB. Trauma-associated bleeding: management of massive transfusion. Curr Opin Anaesthesiol 2016;29(2):250–5.
65. Chang R, Holcomb JB. Implementation of massive transfusion protocols in the United States: the relationship between evidence and practice. Anesth Analg 2017;124(1):9–11.
66. Holcomb JB, Fox EE, Wade CE, PROPPR Study Group. Mortality and ratio of blood products used in patients with severe trauma–reply. JAMA 2015;313(20):2078–9.
67. Wijaya R, Cheng HMG, Chong CK. The use of massive transfusion protocol for trauma and non-trauma patients in a civilian setting: what can be done better? Singapore Med J 2016;57(5):238–41.
68. Edrich T, Pomahac B, Lu JT, et al. Perioperative management of partial face transplantation involving a heparin antibody-positive donor. J Clin Anesth 2011;23(4):318–21.
69. Camazine MN, Hemmila MR, Leonard JC, et al. Massive transfusion policies at trauma centers participating in the American College of Surgeons Trauma Quality Improvement Program. J Trauma Acute Care Surg 2015;78:S48–53.
70. American Society of Anesthesiologists Task Force on Perioperative Blood Management. Practice guidelines for perioperative blood management: an updated report by the American Society of Anesthesiologists Task Force on Perioperative Blood Management*. Anesthesiology 2015;122(2):241–75.
71. Gorantla VS, Davis MR. Vascularized composite allograft preservation: ubi sumus? Transplantation 2016;101(3):469–70.
72. Clerc M, Prothet J, Rimmelé T. Perioperative management of a bilateral forearm allograft. Hand Surg Rehabil 2016;35(3):215–9.
73. Shores JT, Lee WPA, Brandacher G. Discussion: lessons learned from simultaneous face and bilateral hand allotransplantation. Plast Reconstr Surg 2013;132(2):433–4.

74. Nasir S, Kilic YA, Karaaltin MV, et al. Lessons learned from the first quadruple extremity transplantation in the world. Ann Plast Surg 2014;73(3):336–40.
75. Swanson EW, Brandacher G, Gordon CR. Discussion of lessons learned from the first quadruple extremity transplantation in the world. Ann Plast Surg 2014;73(3): 343–5.
76. Pomahac B, Pribaz J, Eriksson E, et al. Three patients with full facial transplantation. N Engl J Med 2012;366(8):715–22.
77. Dickinson K, Roberts I. Medical anti-shock trousers (pneumatic anti-shock garments) for circulatory support in patients with trauma. Cochrane Database Syst Rev 2000;(2):CD001856.
78. Iglesias M, Leal P, Butrón P, et al. Severe complications after bilateral upper extremity transplantation: a case report. Transplantation 2014;98(3):e16–7.
79. Clerc M, Prothet J, Rimmelé T. Perioperative management of a bilateral forearm allograft. Hand Surg Rehabil 2016;35(3):215–9.

Anesthetic Considerations in Transplant Recipients for Nontransplant Surgery

Joshua Herborn, MD[a],*, Suraj Parulkar, MD[b]

KEYWORDS

- Solid organ transplantation • Organ transplantation physiology
- Intraoperative monitoring • Anesthesia methods • Perioperative care

KEY POINTS

- With an increasing number of solid organ transplants and improved long-term survival outcomes, more posttransplant patients will be presenting to the operating room for nonspecific surgery.
- A comprehensive preoperative examination and thorough understanding of the posttransplant physiology is essential in protecting graft function in the perioperative period.
- All types of anesthesia, including general and regional techniques, have been used safely in patients after solid organ transplantation.
- Intraoperative monitoring and invasive access should be dictated by patient's medical status and surgical procedure.

ANESTHETIC CONSIDERATIONS IN TRANSPLANT RECIPIENTS FOR NONTRANSPLANT SURGERY

Organ transplantation has changed and saved many lives, but it requires significant resources from the medical community, including prescription medications, follow-up appointments, and diagnostic procedures, some being quite invasive (cardiac catheterization, organ biopsies, etc). As successful as organ transplantation may be, it is not entirely curative and significant hurdles remain for the posttransplant recipient. The pathophysiologic process that caused the primary organ dysfunction may have other deleterious effects on other organ systems.

Disclosure Statement: The authors have no relevant financial or nonfinancial relationships to disclose.
[a] Department of Anesthesiology, Northwestern University Feinberg School of Medicine, Chicago, IL, USA; [b] Department of Anesthesiology, Northwestern University Feinberg School of Medicine, 251 East Huron Street, F5-704, Chicago, IL 60611, USA
* Corresponding author. 1523 N Mohawk, Unit 4, Chicago, IL 60610.
E-mail address: Jherborn@nm.org

The United Network for Organ Sharing (UNOS) reported that 30,974 solid organ transplants were performed in the United States in 2015. From 1988 to 2016, there were more than 403,614 kidney, 147,128 liver, 65,433 heart, and 33,148 lung transplants according to the Organ Procurement and Transplant Network. As the number of solid organ transplants increases and patient survival improves, it will become more common for these patients to present for surgery, even at nontransplant centers. Many recipients will present with medical problems unique to the transplant and important steps are required to keep the transplanted organ functioning.

IMMUNOSUPPRESSION

Immunosuppression is critical in the prevention of an immune-mediated rejection of the transplanted organ and pharmacologic advances are directly responsible for the improvement of graft and patient survival. The regimen of these medications must balance their immunosuppressant effects of preventing organ rejection with deleterious actions of infection, malignancy, bone marrow suppression, and organ-specific side effects. Specific immunosuppressant medications are discussed in Curtis D. Holt's article, "Overview of Immunosuppressive Therapy in Solid Organ Transplantation," in this issue.

PREOPERATIVE EVALUATION

A comprehensive preoperative evaluation is instrumental in preparing the transplanted patient for surgery. A thorough history and physical examination should specifically focus on graft function. Laboratory tests have the potential to provide critical information about the functional status of the allograft, and obtaining results within 3 months of the surgical procedure is advisable in all but the most low risk of surgical procedures. Blood urea nitrogen and creatinine levels, urine albumin, and calculation of the glomerular filtration rate are useful measurements to evaluate renal function in renal transplant recipients or those on significant immunosuppressive therapy. Prothrombin time, serum bilirubin, albumin, and standard liver enzymes should be obtained for liver transplanted patients. The biomarkers cystatin C and troponin T are increased in patients with reduced left ventricular ejection fractions, although brain natriuretic peptide does not display prognostic power.[1] Any significant worsening of laboratory values should prompt an evaluation made by the appropriate members of the posttransplant medical team.

The 2014 American College of Cardiology/American Heart Association Guidelines for Perioperative Cardiovascular Evaluation and Management of Patients Undergoing Noncardiac Surgery[2] recommend patients with greater than 4 metabolic equivalents or functional capacity (walking up 1 flight of stairs without symptoms) proceed to surgery without further testing, irrespective of major cardiac risk factors. For those with a functional capacity of less than 4 metabolic equivalents or whom cannot be evaluated, clinical and surgical risk factors determine cardiac workup. Recipients may have an overall increased risk of atherosclerotic heart disease after transplantation[3] and it should be considered as an additional risk factor. A history of heart failure or impaired cardiac contractility in the setting of procedures that involve fluid shifts should prompt ventricular function evaluation.

The most recent posttransplant medical evaluation should be available when transplant recipients present for surgery. Specifically, overall graft function, changes in immunosuppressive medication, history of rejection episodes requiring steroid or potent immunosuppressive treatment, and relevant objective data (biopsies, cardiac catheterization, gastrointestinal procedures) should be included.

BLOOD PRODUCT ADMINISTRATION

Appropriate blood product management in transplant recipients is critical, because certain aspects of blood product administration are more prevalent or unique to transplant recipients.

Anemia

Posttransplant anemia (PTA) is an important consideration in patients presenting for surgery, having a prevalence rate between 45% and 78% in solid organ transplant recipients.[4–7] Immunosuppressants, especially the antimetabolite agents, can directly have antiproliferative effects on the bone marrow.[4] Certain chronic viral infections, such as cytomegalovirus (CMV) or parvovirus B19, have been associated with PTA. Although no definitive correlation between PTA and graft or patient outcome exists,[5] treatment of PTA before surgery could potentially reduce red cell transfusion and important associated complications, such as HLA allosensitization, transfusion-associated circulatory overload, and transfusion-associated lung injury. A hemoglobin level of 11 g/dL for transplant recipients presenting for surgery is a reasonable goal to minimize transfusions.[6] Treatment options for PTA include nutritional supplementation, adjustment of immunosuppressant medication, and erythrocyte-stimulating agents. Such alteration of immunosuppression either reduces medication dosage or changes to another agent, risking rejection, infection, or malignancy. Few data exist with regard to erythrocyte-stimulating agent in transplant recipients, but erythrocyte-stimulating agent use with increased blood viscosity has been shown to be a strong predictor of cardiovascular disease in the general population.[7] The risks and benefits of each intervention should be made after considering associated medical conditions and circumstances of the surgical procedure.

Blood Bank Considerations

Sensitization to HLA antigens on white blood cells can occur even after solid organ transplantation and can lead to antibody-mediated rejection against the donor organ. Any potential units of packed red blood cells to be transfused should be leukocyte reduced. Leukoreduction can be achieved by the application of appropriate filters in the operating room or at the blood bank. For CMV-seronegative transplant recipients, low-risk CMV packed red blood cells should be available. What process makes packed red blood cell units CMV safe is still up for debate. White blood cells are the most likely vehicle of transmission of CMV in blood products; very little CMV if any is present in the blood outside the leukocyte. Most blood banks consider leukocyte-reduced blood, defined by the Food and Drug Administration as containing fewer than 5 million leukocytes per unit, safe for administration in CMV-negative transplant recipients. The use of CMV-seronegative donors has been used as a method of reducing CMV transmission, but potential disadvantages include difficulty obtaining donor blood in high CMV prevalent areas and the potential false negatives in the antibody screening assays. Comparison of filtered blood with that of seronegative donors showed no difference in the transmission of CMV in bone marrow transplant recipients,[8] and that has led many blood banks to replace CMV-seronegative units to those with leukocyte-filtered blood components.

Platelet units are apheresed at most blood banks in the United States and are considered leukoreduced. Leukocyte filters need to be applied when pooled platelets are used. Both fresh frozen plasma and cryoprecipitate have less than 1 to 5 million white blood cells per unit and are considered CMV safe by most blood centers.[9]

CONSIDERATIONS OF ANESTHETIC MANAGEMENT IN TRANSPLANT PATIENTS

As transplant outcomes and longevity improve, more of these patients are going to present for surgical procedures. All different anesthesia techniques (general, regional, neuraxial) have been used successfully and all have stood the test of time. Successful anesthetic management considers the effects of the organ transplant on the patient's medical condition, accounts for associated comorbidities, and considers aspects of the surgical procedure.

MONITORING

No specific equipment is necessary for the transplant recipient undergoing nontransplant surgery, and monitoring should be dictated by the patient's medical status and the surgical procedure. Immunosuppressive agents, associated comorbidities, and the transplant procedure itself[10] alter the pharmokinetic and pharmodynamic properties of anesthetic agents; processed electroencephalographic modalities may aid in the assessment of the depth of anesthesia. Urinary catheters should only be placed where urine measurement or bladder drainage is necessary owing to concerns about catheter-associated urinary tract infection. Arterial line placement may be indicated for operations involving hemodynamic instability, frequent blood gases, or postoperative mechanical ventilation. The incidence of infection was found to be quite low in the general population (2.4 per 10,000 patients)[11] and the high pressure and flow of the arterial system is thought to be protective against arterial catheter blood stream infection. Radial artery occlusion may occur with prolonged arterial line monitoring in complicated transplant patients, complicating later placement of arterial catheters and necessitating ultrasound guidance. Central venous access or pulmonary artery catheters provide intravenous access and hemodynamic data for guidance in procedures with significant fluid shifts, but carry the risk of central line-associated bloodstream infection. Large-bore peripheral access and noninvasive hemodynamic monitoring, such as arterial waveform pressure analysis or transesophageal echocardiography, may be reasonable alternatives.

Strict sterile technique should be used with the placement of invasive monitors, but the risk of the catastrophic complication of infection needs to be considered. Patients who have undergone solid organ transplantation have substantially increased risk of infectious complications, but the greatest risk of nosocomial health care–associated infections occur in the first 30 days after transplantation. After 6 months, infections tend to be community acquired.[12]

GENERAL ANESTHESIA

All inhalational and intravenous anesthetics have been used safely in transplant recipients. Benzodiazepines are reasonable for choices as premedication, but their effects may be prolonged in the presence of hepatic or renal dysfunction. Propofol and volatile anesthetics have been shown not to cause graft dysfunction in solid organ recipients[13] and are reasonable to use when considering their cardiovascular effects. Despite being metabolized by the liver and excreted by the kidney, there is no need to alter the dose of propofol in patients with hepatic or renal impairment.[14] Etomidate provides cardiovascular stability in those at risk for decompensation during the induction of anesthesia. Single dose administration has been shown to decrease serum concentration of cortisol for at least 24 hours,[15] but this factor has never been shown to clinically relevant. The use of nitrous oxide is controversial in transplant patients, being implicated in bone marrow suppression and immunosuppression by its inhibitory effect on methionine synthetase. However, definitive studies demonstrating clear increased risk of nitrous oxide are lacking.[16] Nitrous oxide may increase pulmonary vascular resistance and worsen preexisting pulmonary hypertension, potentially present in some types of transplant recipients.

Cyclosporine has been described as prolonging muscle relaxants[17]; this effect has not been shown in patients on mycophenolate mofetil and tacrolimus. Succinylcholine facilitates rapid intubating conditions and minimizes the risk of aspiration, a devastating complication in the immunosuppressed patient. There is no contraindication to the use of succinylcholine in solid organ transplant recipients, excluding the standard conditions of hyperkalemia, myopathy, and so on. Concern has been raised about succinylcholine administration in heart transplant patients owing to its complex interaction with the denervated heart, but its use has been well-established in the literature.[18]

NEURAXIAL AND REGIONAL ANESTHESIA

Spinal or epidural anesthesia is reasonable in transplant recipients assuming there are no contraindications per the American Society of Regional Anesthesia guidelines.[19] Although patients on immunosuppressive therapy are at higher risk for developing infectious complications, limited data have not demonstrated this occurrence for regional or neuraxial procedures.[20] Risk/benefit considerations need to be made for the placement of indwelling catheters for the postoperative period. Transplant recipients may develop osteoporosis and vertebral fractures,[21] potentially complicating neuraxial anesthesia administration.

Transplant patients may develop neurologic complications including peripheral neuropathy.[22] Peripheral nerve blockade is not contraindicated in these patients, but reduction of the concentration of local anesthetic and omission of epinephrine should be considered.

SPECIAL CONSIDERATIONS FOR LIVER TRANSPLANT RECIPIENTS

Orthotopic liver transplantation (OLT) recipients may present quite early in their post-transplant course for surgery. Overall, 10% to 15% of OLT recipients return to the operating room for abdominal exploration for hemorrhage and the procedures are not always staffed by a transplant anesthesiologist. Early hepatic artery and portal vein thrombosis can be salvaged by surgical intervention. Later reasons for these patients to require anesthesia include diagnostic imaging, endoscopic gastrointestinal procedures, and further abdominal surgery.

Pharmacologic Implications

The recipient liver recovers the capacity for drug metabolism initially after reperfusion, but interaction between preoperative encephalopathy and long-acting sedatives may prolong emergence from anesthesia. Correction of hypoalbuminemia may take weeks to recover after transplantation, potentially increasing the free fraction of administered anesthetic drugs.

Cardiovascular Changes

OLT recipients have a prevalence of posttransplant hypertension of up to 70%.[23] Reasons for this include reversal of the systemic vasodilatory state, increased sympathetic stimulation of the calcineurin inhibitors,[24] and the mineralocorticoid effects of steroids. posttransplant hypertension has been shown to be a risk factor for cardiac events, such as acute coronary syndrome or congestive heart failure.[25] Recipients have a significant risk of developing cardiovascular disease postoperatively despite having a low incidence of it pretransplant.[26] This change is thought to occur as a result of transplant-induced of metabolic factors.

Patients with advanced liver disease may have impaired cardiac contractile function and/or altered diastolic relaxation known as cirrhotic cardiomyopathy. This disorder may be masked by an increased cardiac output and the appearance of normal cardiac function owing to the systemic vasodilatory state.[27] OLT typically leads to the reversal of the hyperdynamic syndrome[28] and may lead to heart failure in these patients. Severe portopulmonary hypertension used to be considered an absolute contraindication to liver transplantation because the outcome was quite poor.[29] More centers are transplanting these patients with treatment with pulmonary vasodilators and recipients may present for later surgery with some element of pulmonary hypertension and impaired right ventricular function.[30] Hepatopulmonary syndrome may take months to improve after transplantation and patients may still require supplemental oxygen.[31] In patients with a transplant-specific cardiac history, the appropriate workup is indicated, judicious fluid administration should be given for routine procedures, and invasive monitoring should be used when appropriate.

Renal Failure

Acute kidney injury is commonly seen before OLT, mostly hypovolemia-induced prerenal azotemia and hepatorenal syndrome. Most patients recover renal function after OLT. However, transplant recipients have a significant risk of chronic renal failure with a 5-year cumulative incidence of end-stage renal disease of 18% to 22%.[32] Risk factors for posttransplant end-stage renal disease include advanced recipient age, diabetes mellitus, malignancy, greater body mass index, a dialysis 1 week before transplantation, serum creatinine, and liver donor risk index.[33] Strategies to attenuate posttransplant chronic renal disease include minimizing calcineurin inhibitor immunosuppression, control of posttransplant hypertension, and glycemic control in the presence of new-onset diabetes.[34] Intraoperative goals include appropriate dosing of renally metabolized drugs, hemodynamic management to optimize renal blood flow, and optimal blood pressure management in patients at risk for impaired autoregulation.

Metabolic Factors

Patients who have undergone OLT are at risk for metabolic complications, such as hyperlipidemia, diabetes mellitus, and nonalcoholic fatty liver disease. Treatment of hyperlipidemia has been shown to be essential in the management of cardiovascular disease,[35] a significant source of morbidity and mortality in the posttransplant patient. Recipients who develop diabetes have an increased risk of cardiovascular events and graft dysfunction,[36] and it is reasonable to provide a strict glycemic control regimen. Regardless of the mechanism of liver disease, recurrent nonalcoholic fatty liver disease remains a concern for the transplant recipient. Although patients who develop nonalcoholic fatty liver disease do not have reduced long-term survival, there is an increased incidence of cardiovascular disease.[37]

SPECIAL CONSIDERATIONS FOR HEART TRANSPLANT RECIPIENTS

Procedures immediately after orthotopic heart transplantation (OHT), such as mediastinal exploration or removal of assist device hardware, are usually managed by the cardiac anesthesia team. Potential noncardiac surgeries OLT recipients may undergo include intraabdominal procedures, abscess drainage, and vascular procedures.[38]

Physiology of the Transplanted Heart

OHT interrupts the parasympathetic and intrinsic postganglionic sympathetic fiber innervation to the myocardium, causing autonomic denervation. This blockage of afferent nerves to the myocardium impairs the response of the heart to sensory input. The resting heart rate is increased, typically at 90 to 100 beats per minute. During exercise or periods of stress, where increased oxygen delivery is required, circulating catecholamines and the Frank Starling mechanism maintain cardiac output by increasing stroke volume.[39] Although some early reinnervation occurs,[40] there is a significantly blunted increase in the heart rate in response to hypotension or hypovolemia, Some later sympathetic innervation is seen with nerve regrowth, typically occurring at 5 to 6 months after translantation.[41]

Drugs that work on the autonomic nervous system have minimal effects on the transplanted heart. Indirect-acting sympathomimetics like ephedrine tend not to be very effective at treating hypotension and maintaining cardiac output. Ketamine may not display hemodynamic stability in heart transplant patients in extremis. Direct-acting sympathetic agents, like norepinephrine, epinephrine, isoproteronolol, and dopamine, are effective, although the beta-adrenergic inotropic effects are attenuated in early heart transplant recipients.[42] Phosphodiesterases have been shown to increase inotrophy in the transplanted heart. The alpha-adrenergic response of phenylephrine is effective, but the reflex bradycardia is absent. The denervated heart has been found to be responsive to beta-blockers.

Anticholinergics (atropine, glycopyrrolate) and anticholinesterases (neostigmine, edrophonium) all act indirectly and have no effect on the heart rate of the cardiac allograft. Anticholinesterases given for reversal of neuromuscular blockade may cause bradycardia by activation of cholinergic receptors on cardiac ganglionic cells.[43] Case reports exist in the literature describing severe bradycardia/asystole after neostigmine administration in heart transplant recipients,[44] but the safety of neuromuscular reversal has been demonstrated in a large-scale study with no instances of severe bradycardia or cardiac arrest.[45] Sugammedex directly inhibits the neuromuscular blocking agents, is devoid of any direct cholinergic effects, and is a reasonable alternative in heart transplant recipients.[46]

Cardiac Rhythm Disturbances

OHT can lead to significant rhythm disturbances. The suture line between the donor and recipient atria in the OHT biatrial technique[47] blocks transmissions of electrical impulses. OHT bicaval technique preserves the integrity of the right atrium and sinus node by separately connecting the pulmonary vein cuffs and vena cava to the donor heart. Two separate P waves may be present in the electrocardiogram with biatrial technique.

Bradyarrhythmias requiring pacemaker implantation are thought to occur as the result of surgical anastomotic factors, allograft ischemic injury, and chronic rejection. The overall incidence of pacemaker implantation is 7% to 10%.[48] Risk factors for postoperative pacemaker requirement are biatrial surgical technique and advanced donor/recipient age.[48] Guidelines for perioperative management of implantable devices are similar to those for nontransplant patients.[49]

Tricuspid Regurgitation

Tricuspid regurgitation after OHT is a concern owing to an association between right ventricular dysfunction and mortality[50] and has been shown to have an incidence of around 17% beyond 1 year.[51] Tricuspid regurgitation is a concern for liver dysfunction in patients transplanted for congenital causes with long-standing hepatic enlargement. A bicaval technique reduces the incidence of tricuspid regurgitation as compared with a biatrial technique.[51]

Endomyocardial Biopsies

Multiple endomyocardial biopsies are standardly performed after OHT to detect cellular or antibody-mediated rejection, most commonly via the right internal jugular vein. Many authors recommend avoiding central line placement in this location because of concern of difficulty with later biopsies, but a large-scale series studying endomyocardial biopsies described no instances of internal jugular vein stenosis.[52] Superior vena cava stenosis has been has been described in OHT[53] and may be a more of a concern when obtaining central access.

Cardiac Allograft Vasculopathy

Cardiac allograft vasculopathy is a major cause of mortality after OHT, accounting for 1 in 8 of all deaths beyond a year posttransplantation. The incidence is 29% at 5 years[54] and described as an accelerated fibroproliferative disease as a result of immune and nonimmune factors. As a result of afferent denervation, symptoms of myocardial ischemia are usually absent. Noninvasive imaging is not particularly successful at detecting cardiac allograft vasculopathy[55] and it is best screened with yearly cardiac catheterizations. Cardiac allograft vasculopathy may predispose OHT recipients to perioperative myocardial ischemia with the increased myocardial oxygen demands associated with surgery.

ANESTHESIA FOR PATIENTS AFTER LUNG TRANSPLANTATION

As the field of lung transplantation continues to mature and the science of preserving donor lungs continues to expand, the anesthesiologist should expect to see posttransplant patients returning to the operative theater for nonspecific surgery. Perioperative physicians should be aware of the unique challenges in caring for these patients.

Pulmonary Physiology After Lung Transplantation

Although not clinically significant, patients may experience mild airway hyperactivity, especially in response to provocation. Lung transplant patients are known to have an impairment in mucociliary clearance, perhaps owing to ciliary dysfunction, epithelial damage, or a disruption in the relationship between the cilia and the mucus layer.[56] Additionally, the afferent limb of the cough reflex is disrupted during organ retrieval, and as such lung transplant recipients demonstrate a markedly decreased cough reflex. Esophageal dysmotility and gastroesophageal reflux disease have been observed at a higher incidence posttransplant.[57] These physiologic perturbations place these patients at a higher risk of infection, mucous plugging, and aspiration pneumonitis.

In general, pulmonary function testing tends to reflect an improvement spirometry values. Double lung transplant patients experience a near-normalization of pulmonary function tests by 6 months to 1 year with one study noting a 2.14-fold and 3.75-fold improvement in FEV_1 and forced vital capacity, respectively.[58] Patients with obstructive lung disease who undergo single lung transplant demonstrate a 50% to 60% improvement in these pulmonary function test values, whereas those who were transplanted for restrictive lung disease are noted to have mild residual restrictive disease on spirometry.[59,60] The A-a gradient in patients who undergo double lung transplantation tends to normalize, whereas those who undergo single lung transplantation experience only a mild increase from normal. Patients with emphysema who underwent single or double lung transplantation experienced a 150% and 300% improvement in carbon monoxide diffusing capacity, respectively, whereas those with interstitial lung disease who underwent a single lung transplant experienced a 50% increase.[61]

Despite these dramatic improvements, the expected change in exercise performance had a tendency to lag behind the measured parameters suggesting that factors such as deconditioning, poor strength, or other peripheral factors that limit the exercise benefit after transplantation.[62]

Bronchiolitis Obliterans Syndrome

Bronchiolitis obliterans syndrome is a late-stage, immune-mediated lung injury without an identifiable alternate and possibly a reversible cause, which is thought to represent a form of chronic rejection. Histologically, the lung displays evidence of chronic inflammation, fibrosis and obliteration of small airways.[63] The new consensus definition developed in 2002 by the International Society for Heart and Lung Transplantation used the FEV_1 and FEV_{25-75} to grade the severity of the disease.[64] Bronchiolitis obliterans syndrome is rare in the first 6 months after transplantation, but its incidence increases dramatically as survival increases. If suspected, elective surgery should be postponed and the patient should be directed to further evaluation and treatment.

Preoperative Evaluation

The preoperative examination should focus on the presence any new symptoms such as dyspnea, fatigue, fever, cough, exercise intolerance, and supplemental oxygen requirements. For patients with single lung transplants, it is essential to know the underlying disease and status of the native lung. If the patient was exposed to prolonged postoperative intubation, he or she could be at risk for airway stenosis or vocal cord dysfunction. Any new or worsening declines in function or spirometry values should warrant investigation by the patient's transplant center and pulmonologist to exclude episodes of acute rejection, bronchiolitis obliterans syndrome, or infection.

Intraoperative Care

As it stands, there has been no demonstrable difference between various techniques for patients after lung transplantation, although it is empirically proven that these patients can safely undergo anesthesia. Many authors advocate the use of regional anesthesia for these patients, citing benefits such as the avoidance of airway manipulation and concomitant positive pressure ventilation, neuromuscular blockade, decreased postoperative opiate requirement, and improved analgesia, which can decrease respiratory splinting. However, it should be noted that impaired ventilation can occur iatrogenically owing to hemidiaphragmatic paralysis or pneumothorax from upper extremity regional techniques as well as accessory respiratory muscle weakness from neuraxial techniques.

In addition to the standard American Society of Anesthesiologists monitors, the choice of invasive intraoperative monitoring should take into account the patient's preoperative cardiopulmonary status, the nature of surgery, and the potential for fluid shifts and blood loss during the procedure. Owing to incomplete lymphatic drainage from the transplanted lung(s), these patients tend to be sensitive to fluid overload and pulmonary edema.[65,66] As such, the anesthesiologist may benefit from more invasive monitors to approximate left ventricular end-diastolic volume such as pulmonary arterial catheters, transesophageal echocardiography, and peripheral intraarterial continuous cardiac output monitors.

Airway Management and Ventilation

The decision regarding airway management should take into account the duration and nature of the procedure along with patient comorbidities. The use of supraglottic airways can avoid potential disruption of anastomoses or complications owing to the presence of subglottic stenosis. Tracheal intubation is best performed orally using a larger sized endotracheal tube to facilitate passage of suction catheters and/or a fiberoptic bronchoscope. Single or differential lung ventilation can be safely performed using a double lumen tube or single lumen tube with endobronchial blockade. The double lumen tube should be inserted under direct visualization to avoid damaging weakened tracheobronchial structures and should avoid bronchial intubation on the side of the transplanted lung.

Although there are no clearly defined guidelines for the application of positive pressure ventilation to patients with transplanted lungs, much of the practice is derived using data from nontransplant patients and conclusions extrapolated from acute respiratory distress syndrome protocols. In general, parameters are based on recipient characteristics: tidal volume, 6 mL/kg; adjusting Fio_2 versus increasing positive end-expiratory pressure for arterial oxygen desaturation; minimum positive end-expiratory pressure of 5 cm H_2O; median maximum end-expiratory pressure of 11.5 cm H_2O; and a median plateau pressure limit to trigger reduction in tidal volumes of 30 cm H_2O.[67] If 1 lung ventilation is required on a double lung transplant patient, tidal volumes of 5 to 6 mL/kg are suggested, similar to patients with normal lungs.[68]

After single lung transplantation, patients with native emphysematous disease are at risk of volutrauma, pneumothorax secondary to bled rupture, and compression of the transplanted lung owing to dynamic hyperinflation. Those with native restrictive disease may require higher airway pressures for expansion, which can place the transplanted lung at risk of barotrauma and volutrauma. Should ventilation place the allograft at risk of compromise, advanced intensive care ventilators or differential lung ventilation with a double lumen tube and 2 ventilators should be considered.

Every attempt should be taken to facilitate early extubation in this patient population given the established risk of respiratory infection in patients with prolonged tracheal intubation. Extubation criteria should be the same as in patients without lung transplant.

ANESTHESIA FOR PATIENTS AFTER KIDNEY TRANSPLANTATION

Renal transplantation is the most common transplant procedure performed and the number of patients alive with functioning grafts has more than doubled since 2000.[69] These patients tend to have a high incidence of multisystem diseases that persist after transplant such as diabetes mellitus, coronary artery disease, hypertension, hyperlipidemia and congestive heart failure. Additionally, these patients presenting for anesthesia tend to be older than those with other types of organ transplants.[70]

Assessment of graft function is vital when assessing these patients for subsequent surgery. Although practice varies from center to center, recipients are usually followed by a transplant nephrologist for approximately 1 year with routine testing such as serum chemistry and complete blood count, trough immunosuppressant levels, urinalysis, and screening for urine protein. The routine evaluation thereafter includes monitoring serum creatinine levels as well as screening for proteinuria. In general, transplanted patients tend to have an approximated 20% decrease in function,[71] evidenced by a decreased glomerular filtration rate (<60 mL/min/1.73 m^2) and a creatinine level of greater than 1.1 mg/dL. Reasons for this include single kidney transplant and graft–recipient mismatch.[72] Should the patient have an increase in creatinine from baseline, elective surgery should be delayed and consultation with the patient's nephrologist should be sought.

ANESTHESIA FOR PATIENTS AFTER PANCREAS TRANSPLANTATION

Pancreas transplantation as a treatment for diabetes was first described in 1966 and only relatively recently has the yearly number of transplants begun to increase. In 2012, 630 transplants were performed and only 25% were performed in isolation of other transplanted organs.

The preoperative evaluation of these patients should focus on the comorbidities associated with diabetes, which have the potential of causing multiorgan dysfunction. Additionally, laboratory investigation should focus on volume status, metabolic and electrolyte disturbances, and glucose levels.

One population that merits special mention is the subset of patients whose pancreatic transplant drains exocrine secretions to the bladder. This configuration has the potential for urinary bicarbonate loss and the development of metabolic acidosis and resultant dehydration. Should this occur, exogenous bicarbonate replacement and interval arterial blood gas measurements may be indicated. If the initial surgical technique included exocrine drainage of the pancreas into the patient's intestine, the bicarbonate is reabsorbed and this complication is avoided.

SUMMARY

As surgical outcomes continue to improve and the availability of donor organs increases, anesthesiologists will see an increasing number of transplanted patients presenting for nonspecific surgery. Knowledge of posttransplant physiology, comorbidities and implications of the immunosuppressive regimen is essential in caring for these complex patients in the perioperative setting.

REFERENCES

1. Franeková J, Hošková L, Sečník P, et al. The role of timely measurement of galectin-3, NT-proBNP, cystatin C and hsTnT in predicting prognosis and heart function after heart transplantation. Clin Chem Lab Med 2016;54(2):339–44.
2. Fleisher LA, Fleischmann KE, Auerbach AD, et al. 2014 ACC/AHA guideline on perioperative cardiovascular evaluation and management of patients undergoing noncardiac surgery: a report of the American College of Cardiology/American Heart Association Task Force on practice guidelines. J Am Coll Cardiol 2014; 64(22):e77–137.
3. Pisano G, Fracanzani AL, Caccamo L, et al. Cardiovascular risk after orthotopic liver transplantation, a review of the literature and preliminary results of a prospective study. World J Gastroenterol 2016;22(40):8869–82.
4. Kuypers DR, de Jonge H, Naesens M. Current target ranges of mycophenolic acid exposure and drug-related adverse events: a 5-year, open-label, prospective, clinical follow-up study in renal allograft recipients. Clin Ther 2008;30(4): 673–83.
5. Blosser CD, Bloom RD. Posttransplant anemia in solid organ recipients. Transplant Rev 2010;24(2):89–98.

6. Małyszko J, Watschinger B, Przybyłowski P, et al. Anemia in solid organ transplantation. Ann Transplant 2012;17(2):86–100.
7. Jeong SK, Cho YI, Duey M, et al. Cardiovascular risks of anemia correction with erythrocyte stimulating agents: should blood viscosity be monitored for risk assessment? Cardiovasc Drugs Ther 2010;24(2):151–60.
8. Bowden RA, Slichter SJ, Sayers M, et al. A comparison of filtered leukocyte-reduced and cytomegalovirus (CMV) seronegative blood products for the prevention of transfusion-associated CMV infection after marrow transplant. Blood 1995;86(9):3598–603.
9. Heddle NM, Boeckh M, Grossman B, et al. AABB committee report: reducing transfusion-transmitted cytomegalovirus infections. Transfusion 2016;56(6 Pt 2): 1581–7.
10. Pai SL, Aniskevich S, Rodrigues ES, et al. Analgesic considerations for liver transplantation patients. Curr Clin Pharmacol 2015;10(1):54–65.
11. Nuttall G, Burckhardt J, Hadley A, et al. Surgical and patient risk factors for severe arterial line complications in adults. Anesthesiology 2016;124(3):590–7.
12. Fishman JA. Infection in solid-organ transplant recipients. N Engl J Med 2007; 357(25):2601–14.
13. Gajate martín L, González C, Ruiz torres I, et al. Effects of the hypnotic agent on primary graft dysfunction after liver transplantation. Transplant Proc 2016;48(10): 3307–11.
14. White P, Romero G. Nonopioid intravenous anesthesia. In: Barash PG, Cullen BF, Stoelting RK, editors. Clinical anesthesiology. 5th edition. Philadelphia: Lippincott Williams & Wilkins; 2006. p. 334–52.
15. De jong FH, Mallios C, Jansen C, et al. Etomidate suppresses adrenocortical function by inhibition of 11 beta-hydroxylation. J Clin Endocrinol Metab 1984; 59(6):1143–7.
16. Schallner N, Goebel U. The perioperative use of nitrous oxide: renaissance of an old gas or funeral of an ancient relict? Curr Opin Anaesthesiol 2013;26(3):354–60.
17. Sidi A, Kaplan RF, Davis RF. Prolonged neuromuscular blockade and ventilatory failure after renal transplantation and cyclosporine. Can J Anaesth 1990;37(5): 543–8.
18. Cheng DC, Ong DD. Anaesthesia for non-cardiac surgery in heart-transplanted patients. Can J Anaesth 1993;40(10):981–6.
19. Horlocker TT, Wedel DJ, Rowlingson JC, et al. Regional anesthesia in the patient receiving antithrombotic or thrombolytic therapy: American Society of Regional Anesthesia and Pain Medicine evidence-based guidelines (third edition). Reg Anesth Pain Med 2010;35(1):64–101.
20. Gronwald C, Vowinkel T, Hahnenkamp K. Regional anesthetic procedures in immunosuppressed patients: risk of infection. Curr Opin Anaesthesiol 2011;24(6): 698–704.
21. Stein E, Ebeling P, Shane E. Post-transplantation osteoporosis. Endocrinol Metab Clin North Am 2007;36(4):937–63.
22. Zivković SA. Neurologic aspects of multiple organ transplantation. Handb Clin Neurol 2014;121:1305–17.
23. Watt KD, Pedersen RA, Kremers WK, et al. Evolution of causes and risk factors for mortality post-liver transplant: results of the NIDDK long-term follow-up study. Am J Transplant 2010;10(6):1420–7.
24. Zbroch E, Małyszko J, Myśliwiec M, et al. Hypertension in solid organ transplant recipients. Ann Transplant 2012;17(1):100–7.

25. Albeldawi M, Aggarwal A, Madhwal S, et al. Cumulative risk of cardiovascular events after orthotopic liver transplantation. Liver Transpl 2012;18(3):370–5.
26. Fussner LA, Heimbach JK, Fan C, et al. Cardiovascular disease after liver transplantation: when, what, and who is at risk. Liver Transpl 2015;21(7):889–96.
27. Zardi EM, Zardi DM, Chin D, et al. Cirrhotic cardiomyopathy in the pre- and post-liver transplantation phase. J Cardiol 2016;67(2):125–30.
28. Gadano A, Hadengue A, Widmann JJ, et al. Hemodynamics after orthotopic liver transplantation: study of associated factors and long-term effects. Hepatology 1995;22(2):458–65.
29. Krowka MJ. Portopulmonary hypertension and the issue of survival. Liver Transpl 2005;11(9):1026–7.
30. Khaderi S, Khan R, Safdar Z, et al. Long-term follow-up of portopulmonary hypertension patients after liver transplantation. Liver Transpl 2014;20(6):724–7.
31. Eriksson LS, Söderman C, Ericzon BG, et al. Normalization of ventilation/perfusion relationships after liver transplantation in patients with decompensated cirrhosis: evidence for a hepatopulmonary syndrome. Hepatology 1990;12(6):1350–7.
32. Kida Y. Chronic renal failure after transplantation of a nonrenal organ. N Engl J Med 2003;349(26):2563–5.
33. Israni AK, Xiong H, Liu J, et al. Predicting end-stage renal disease after liver transplant. Am J Transplant 2013;13(7):1782–92.
34. Moon JI, Barbeito R, Faradji RN, et al. Negative impact of new-onset diabetes mellitus on patient and graft survival after liver transplantation: long-term follow up. Transplantation 2006;82(12):1625–8.
35. Baigent C, Blackwell L, Emberson J, et al. Efficacy and safety of more intensive lowering of LDL cholesterol: a meta-analysis of data from 170,000 participants in 26 randomised trials. Lancet 2010;376(9753):1670–81.
36. Bodziak KA, Hricik DE. New-onset diabetes mellitus after solid organ transplantation. Transpl Int 2009;22(5):519–30.
37. Dureja P, Mellinger J, Agni R, et al. NAFLD recurrence in liver transplant recipients. Transplantation 2011;91(6):684–9.
38. Bhatia DS, Bowen JC, Money SR, et al. The incidence, morbidity, and mortality of surgical procedures after orthotopic heart transplantation. Ann Surg 1997;225(6):686–93.
39. Kavanagh T, Yacoub MH, Mertens DJ, et al. Cardiorespiratory responses to exercise training after orthotopic cardiac transplantation. Circulation 1988;77(1):162–71.
40. Bengel FM, Ueberfuhr P, Hesse T, et al. Clinical determinants of ventricular sympathetic reinnervation after orthotopic heart transplantation. Circulation 2002;106(7):831–5.
41. Doering LV, Dracup K, Moser DK, et al. Evidence of time-dependent autonomic reinnervation after heart transplantation. Nurs Res 1999;48(6):308–16.
42. Koglin J, Gross T, Uberfuhr P, et al. Time-dependent decrease of presynaptic inotropic supersensitivity: physiological evidence of sympathetic reinnervation after heart transplantation. J Heart Lung Transplant 1997;16(6):621–8.
43. Backman SB, Fox GS, Ralley FE. Pharmacological properties of the denervated heart. Can J Anaesth 1997;44(8):900–1.
44. Cachemaille M, Olofsson M, Livio F, et al. Recurrent asystole after neostigmine in a heart transplant recipient with end-stage renal disease. J Cardiothorac Vasc Anesth 2017;31(2):653–6.

45. Barbara DW, Christensen JM, Mauermann WJ, et al. The safety of neuromuscular blockade reversal in patients with cardiac transplantation. Transplantation 2016; 100(12):2723–8.

46. Tezcan B, Şaylan A, Bölükbaşı D, et al. Use of sugammadex in a heart transplant recipient: review of the unique physiology of the transplanted heart. J Cardiothorac Vasc Anesth 2016;30(2):462–5.

47. Lower RR, Shumway NE. Studies on orthotopic homotransplantation of the canine heart. Surg Forum 1960;11:18–9.

48. Cantillon DJ, Tarakji KG, Hu T, et al. Long-term outcomes and clinical predictors for pacemaker-requiring bradyarrhythmias after cardiac transplantation: analysis of the UNOS/OPTN cardiac transplant database. Heart Rhythm 2010;7(11): 1567–71.

49. Crossley GH, Poole JE, Rozner MA, et al. The Heart Rhythm Society (HRS)/American Society of Anesthesiologists (ASA) Expert Consensus Statement on the perioperative management of patients with implantable defibrillators, pacemakers and arrhythmia monitors: facilities and patient management this document was developed as a joint project with the American Society of Anesthesiologists (ASA), and in collaboration with the American Heart Association (AHA), and the Society of Thoracic Surgeons (STS). Heart Rhythm 2011;8(7):1114–54.

50. Anderson CA, Shernan SK, Leacche M, et al. Severity of intraoperative tricuspid regurgitation predicts poor late survival following cardiac transplantation. Ann Thorac Surg 2004;78(5):1635–42.

51. Aziz T, Burgess M, Khafagy R, et al. Bicaval and standard techniques in orthotopic heart transplantation: medium-term experience in cardiac performance and survival. J Thorac Cardiovasc Surg 1999;118(1):115–22.

52. Awad M, Ruzza A, Soliman C, et al. Endomyocardial biopsy technique for orthotopic heart transplantation and cardiac stem-cell harvesting. Transplant Proc 2014;46(10):3580–4.

53. Blanche C, Tsai TP, Czer LS, et al. Superior vena cava stenosis after orthotopic heart transplantation: complication of an alternative surgical technique. Cardiovasc Surg 1995;3(5):549–52.

54. Lund LH, Edwards LB, Kucheryavaya AY, et al. The registry of the international society for heart and lung transplantation: thirty-second official adult heart transplantation report–2015; focus theme: early graft failure. J Heart Lung Transplant 2015;34(10):1244–54.

55. Sade LE, Eroğlu S, Yüce D, et al. Follow-up of heart transplant recipients with serial echocardiographic coronary flow reserve and dobutamine stress echocardiography to detect cardiac allograft vasculopathy. J Am Soc Echocardiogr 2014; 27(5):531–9.

56. Herve P, Silbert D, Cerrina J, et al. Impairment of bronchial mucociliary clearance in long-term survivors of heart/lung and double-lung transplantation. The Paris-Sud Lung Transplant Group. Chest 1993;103(1):59–63.

57. Wood RK. Esophageal dysmotility, gastro-esophageal reflux disease, and lung transplantation: what is the evidence? Curr Gastroenterol Rep 2015;17(12):48.

58. Pêgo-fernandes PM, Abrão FC, Fernandes FL, et al. Spirometric assessment of lung transplant patients: one year follow-up. Clinics (Sao Paulo) 2009;64(6): 519–25.

59. Pochettino A, Kotloff RM, Rosengard BR, et al. Bilateral versus single lung transplantation for chronic obstructive pulmonary disease: intermediate-term results. Ann Thorac Surg 2000;70(6):1813–8.

60. Chacon RA, Corris PA, Dark JH, et al. Comparison of the functional results of single lung transplantation for pulmonary fibrosis and chronic airway obstruction. Thorax 1998;53(1):43–9.
61. Miyoshi S, Mochizuki Y, Nagai S, et al. Physiologic aspects in human lung transplantation. Ann Thorac Cardiovasc Surg 2005;11(2):73–9.
62. Bartels MN, Armstrong HF, Gerardo RE, et al. Evaluation of pulmonary function and exercise performance by cardiopulmonary exercise testing before and after lung transplantation. Chest 2011;140(6):1604–11.
63. Aguilar PR, Michelson AP, Isakow W. Obliterative bronchiolitis. Transplantation 2016;100(2):272–83.
64. Estenne M, Maurer JR, Boehler A, et al. Bronchiolitis obliterans syndrome 2001: an update of the diagnostic criteria. J Heart Lung Transplant 2002;21(3):297–310.
65. Ruggiero R, Muz J, Fietsam R Jr, et al. Reestablishment of lymphatic drainage after canine lung transplantation. J Thorac Cardiovasc Surg 1993;106:167–71.
66. Baker J, Yost CS, Niemann CU. Organ transplantation. In: Miller RD, editor. Miller's anesthesia. 6th edition. Philadelphia: Elsevier; 2005. p. 2271.
67. Beer A, Reed RM, Bölükbas S, et al. Mechanical ventilation after lung transplantation. An international survey of practices and preferences. Ann Am Thorac Soc 2014;11(4):546–53.
68. Montes FR, Pardo DF, Charrís H, et al. Comparison of two protective lung ventilatory regimes on oxygenation during one-lung ventilation: a randomized controlled trial. J Cardiothorac Surg 2010;5:99–104.
69. Hart A, Smith JM, Skeans MA, et al. OPTN/SRTR 2015 annual data report: kidney. Am J Transplant 2017;17(Issue Supplement S1):21–116.
70. Liu LL, Wiener-Kronish JP. Perioperative anesthesia issues in the elderly. Crit Care Clin 2003;19:641–56.
71. Tran S. Anesthetic considerations for patients post-organ transplantation. Semin Anesth Periop Med Pain 2003;22(2):119–24.
72. Chandraker A, Yeung M. Overview of care of the adult kidney transplant recipient. In: Post TW, editor. UpToDate. Waltham (MA): UpToDate. Accessed January 4, 2017.

Moving?

Make sure your subscription moves with you!

To notify us of your new address, find your **Clinics Account Number** (located on your mailing label above your name), and contact customer service at:

Email: journalscustomerservice-usa@elsevier.com

800-654-2452 (subscribers in the U.S. & Canada)
314-447-8871 (subscribers outside of the U.S. & Canada)

Fax number: 314-447-8029

Elsevier Health Sciences Division
Subscription Customer Service
3251 Riverport Lane
Maryland Heights, MO 63043

*To ensure uninterrupted delivery of your subscription, please notify us at least 4 weeks in advance of move.

Printed and bound by CPI Group (UK) Ltd, Croydon, CR0 4YY

08/05/2025

01864703-0009